AF574829

WOMAN

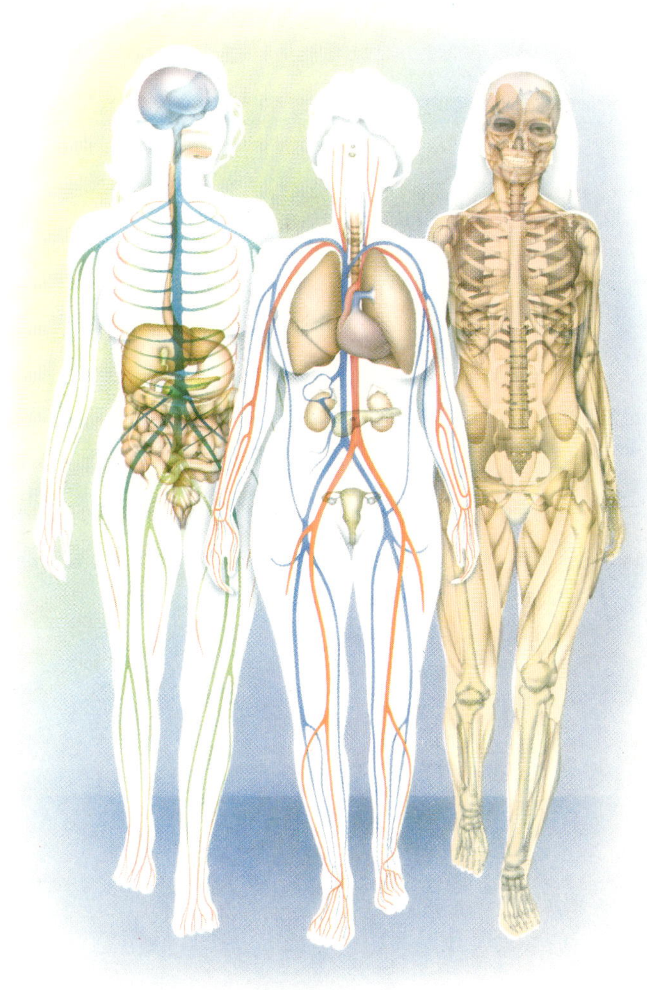

WOMAN

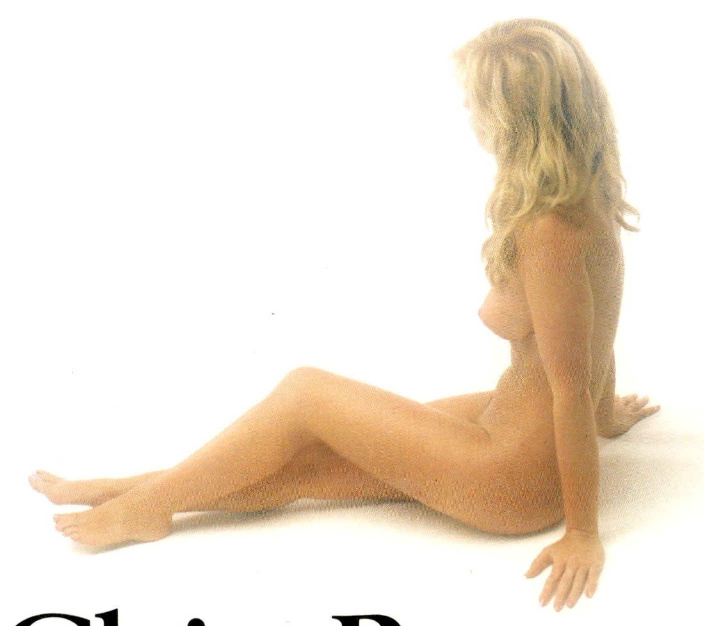

Claire Rayner

Airbrush illustrations by Bill Botten

HAMLYN

For Amanda, the most
important woman in my life

Published 1986 by Hamlyn Publishing
a division of The Hamlyn Publishing Group Limited
Bridge House, London Road,
Twickenham, Middlesex, England

Published simultaneously in Australia
by Pitman Publishing

ISBN 0 600 50285 6

Woman was edited and designed by
Thames Head Limited, Avening, Tetbury, Gloucestershire, Great Britain.

Editorial and Marketing director
Martin Marix Evans

Design and Production director
David Playne

Art editor
Tony De Saulles

Medical consultant
Peter Diggory FRCS, FRCOG

Editor
Alison Goldingham

Pencil illustrations
Jacquie Govier

Designers
Nick Allen Heather Church

Photography
Steve Teague

Typeset in ITC Berkeley on Scantext by Thames Head Limited and
processed by Topic Typesetting Limited, Great Britain

Printed and bound by
Royal Smeets Offset bv Weert, The Netherlands

Reproduction by Albany Graphics Limited, Great Britain

CONTENTS

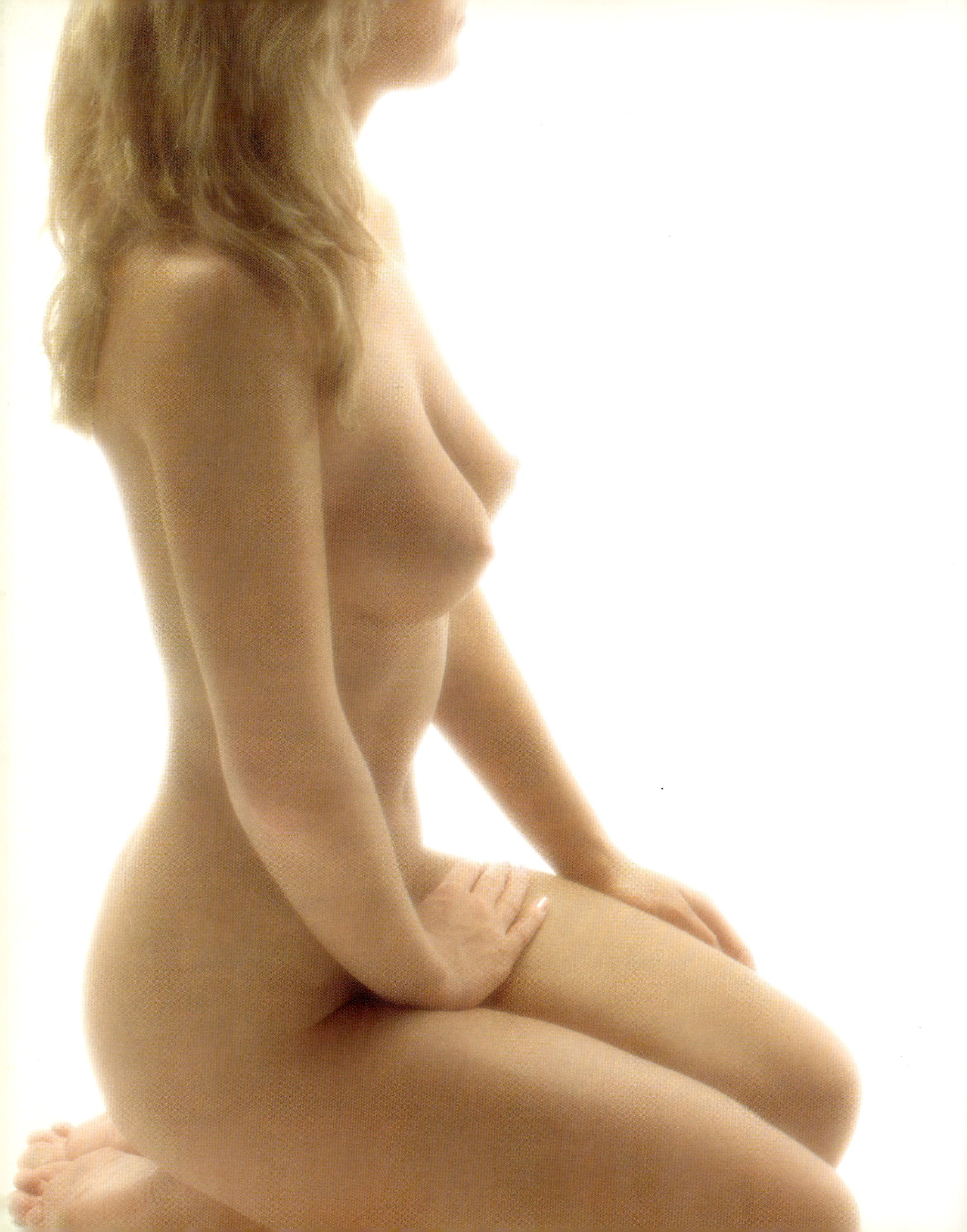

1

WOMAN'S BODY

Small children don't show much in the way of sexual differences. Boys and girls are so much alike that if you look at a naked pair from the back, you'd be hard put to it to tell which is which. Both have rounded buttocks. Both have dimpled hands, arms and knees. Both have smooth skins and soft hair. Even if they turn round so that you can see them from the front the ambiguity persists, if they're wearing pants; the same little pot bellies and pinkish nipples, the same putty noses and round faces. Only the display of the surface sex organs can provide an accurate gender label.

But within a very few years this ambiguity disappears. Even allowing for the vast range of body types there are, most of us develop recognizably masculine or feminine appearances of face and body once we pass puberty. However eagerly young people may adopt so-called unisex fashions in clothes and hair styling, it's fairly easy in the vast majority of cases to label people accurately according to gender. The hard muscularity of the male body differs from the softer roundness of the female; the hair distribution on face, belly and chest is generally obvious on the male, absent in the female; the narrower bony hips of the male contrast markedly with the swelling wideness of the female.

But all these adult differences are based on that original childhood similarity. We as women are far more like our men than we are different from them. That means that no woman can fully understand the aspects of herself that make her a woman until she understands the aspects of herself that make her simply a person. So, before considering what makes a small girl become a woman, we need to look at the body structure she shares with small boys. And as good a way as any of looking at it is to start from the surface and go inside the body, system by system.

The skin

It's the biggest organ in the human body, and just about the most flexible in every sense of the word.

It is a bulwark that keeps unwanted water, germs of all kinds and many noxious substances out of the body while at the same time allowing excess material from the inside of the body to escape. (People who eat a lot of highly aromatic material actually get rid of some of it in their sweat; it isn't only your breath that smells if you eat a highly seasoned curry.)

It can stretch, twist, enlarge to accommodate growth and shrink back to accept

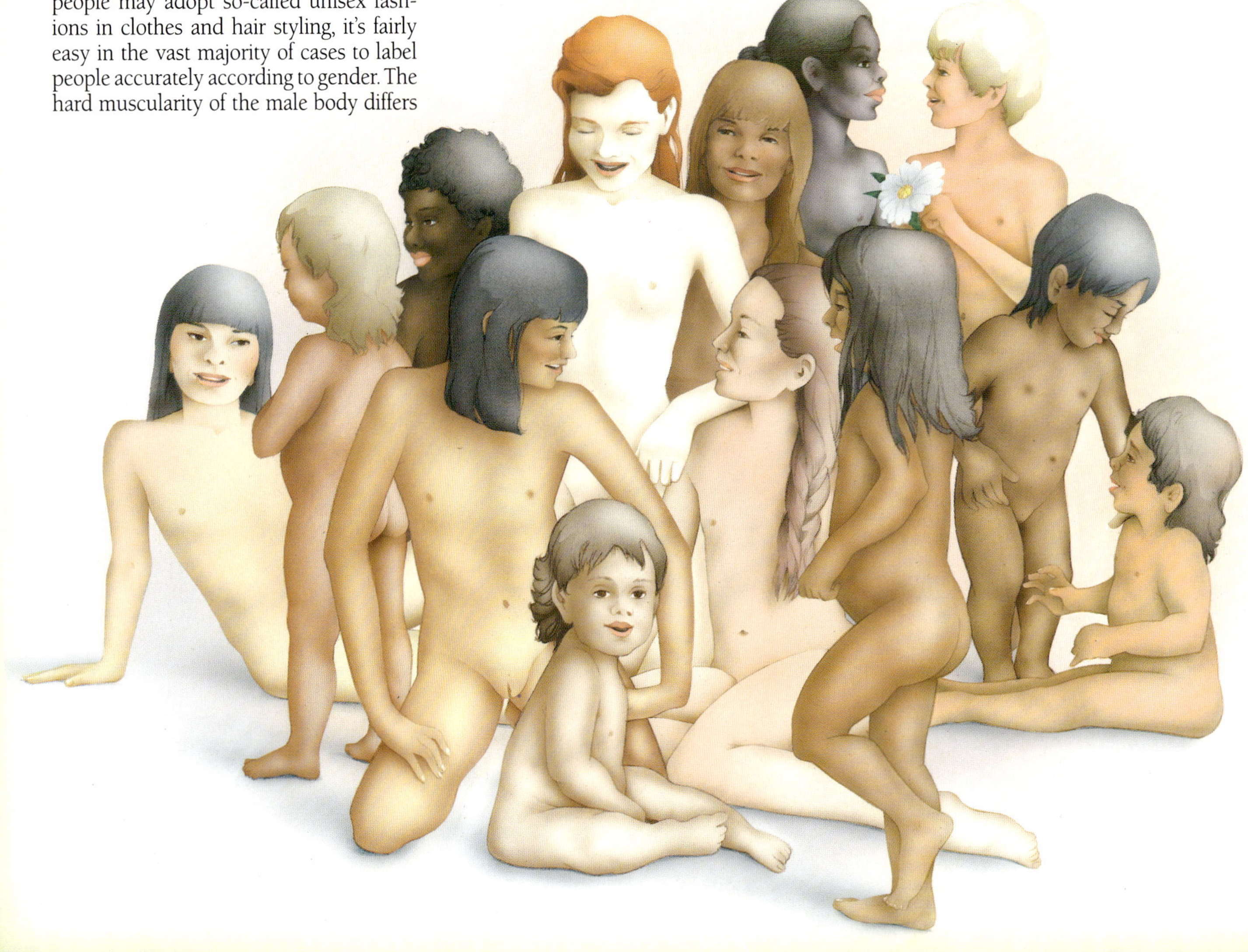

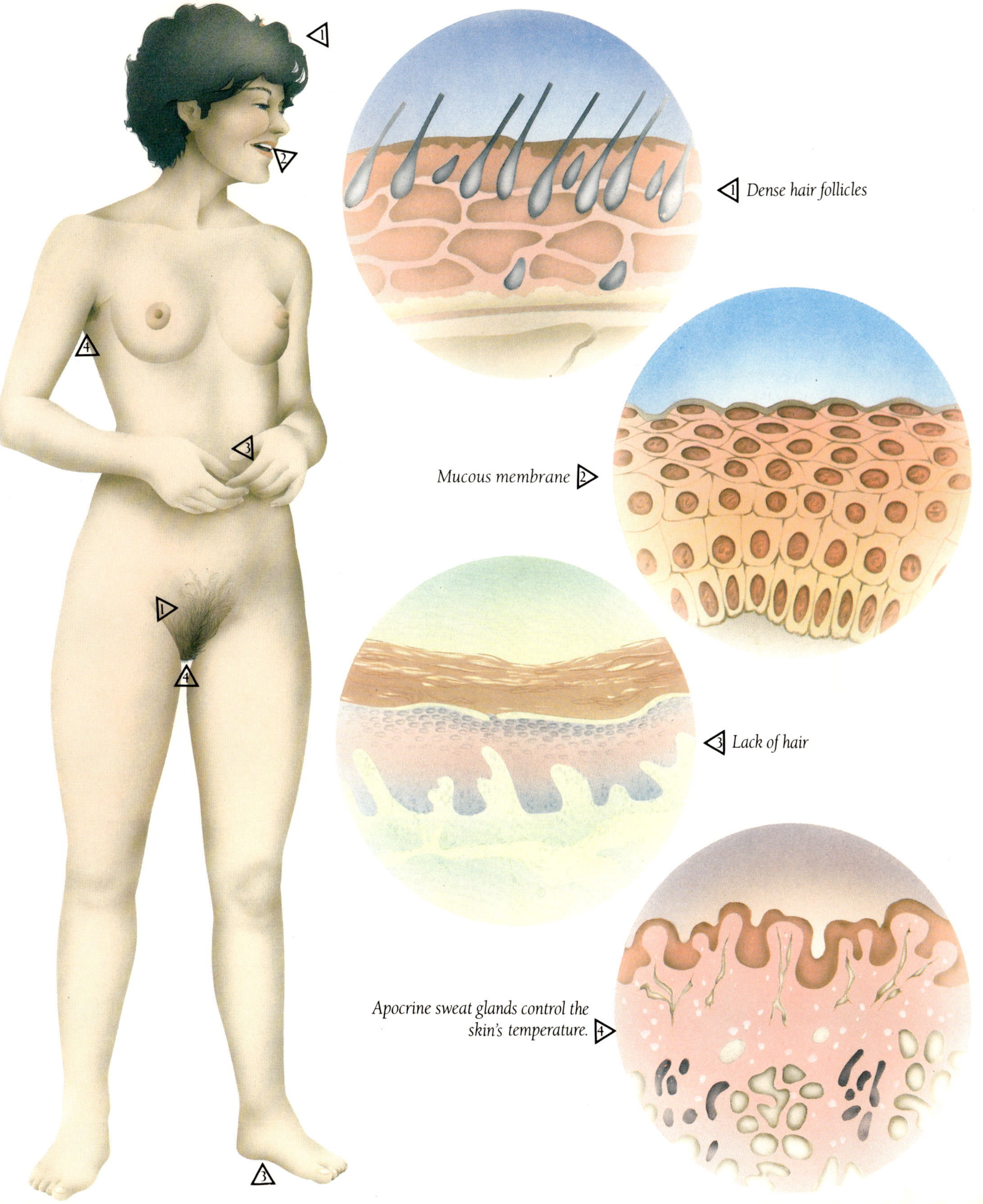
1
2
4
3
1
4
3
1 Dense hair follicles
Mucous membrane 2
3 Lack of hair
Apocrine sweat glands control the skin's temperature. 4

reduction in the size of underlying structures, without unduly injuring itself. It is truly elastic.

It has its own self-protective mechanisms, producing germ-killing substances as well as its own lubrication oil, and can thicken and darken to protect itself from the sun's damaging rays. (And, incidentally, when it does that it also manufactures Vitamin D, also called calciferol — which is essential to the wellbeing of the whole body, in that it works with calcium to produce healthy bones; lack of Vitamin D is the cause of the disease rickets.)

It is self-renewing and self-repairing. All through life, the skin is producing new lower layers which push up and away the surface layers, so that they are shed steadily. This self-sacrificing surface, the epidermis, is actually made of dead cells which have deliberately destroyed themselves by filling up with a horny substance called keratin (hair and nails are made of the same material — they are in fact modified skin).

If the living lower layer — the dermis — is injured it can join together and grow across the rift and become as sound and as active as ever, and often without any mark to show for the damage. And if marks — scars — do appear, they eventually fade, in most cases, to become almost invisible (although there is a form, called a keloid scar, in which there is prominent overgrowth of tissue — but they are really relatively rare).

It is essential to the whole body's heat control mechanisms. When you're too hot, the skin radiates extra heat away, as well as creating a cooling system via the sweat; a lot of sweat is produced in hot conditions, and as it evaporates it cools the surface. In cold conditions, the skin conserves heat by shutting down on heat sources; blood vessels in the skin constrict, so sending warm blood to deeper structures to retain the heat there. That is why when you're hot you go red, and when you're cold you go pale (all of which is particularly relevant at the beginning of a woman's reproductive life — menarche — and at the end of it — menopause — as will be seen later). It helps regulate blood pressure, again by means of constricting or relaxing its blood vessels.

Skin types

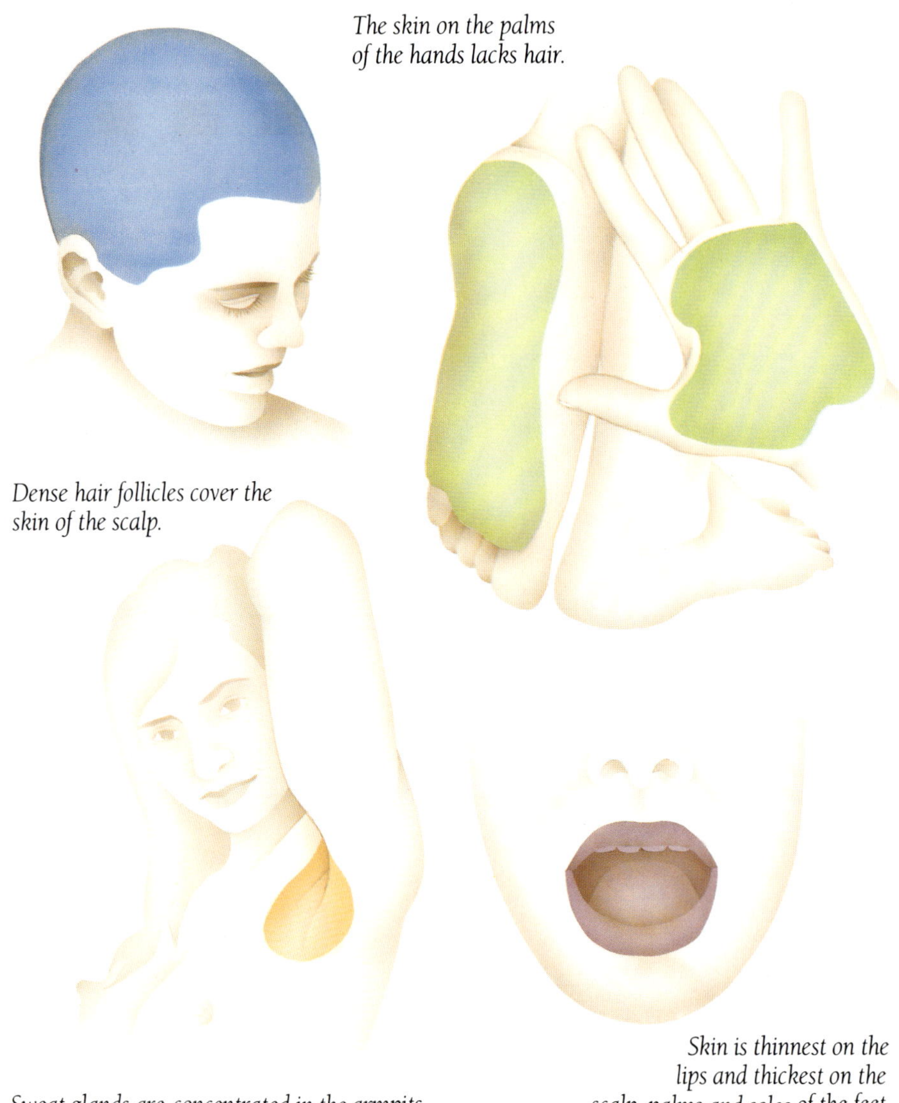

The skin on the palms of the hands lacks hair.

Dense hair follicles cover the skin of the scalp.

Sweat glands are concentrated in the armpits.

Skin is thinnest on the lips and thickest on the scalp, palms and soles of the feet.

It is the essential organ of touch; without it we would be unable to identify a vast range of messages from the outside world.

It is a vital part of our communication system, including and perhaps especially sexual communication. Without skin we could never be truly intimate with another human being. There is an apt old French proverb which says that 'Love is the contact of two skins'.

And finally, each and every one of us has a skin of unique design. On the surface many human skins appear to match — all black skins, all pink ones, all olive and all sallow ones may seem the same, but the pattern of ridges, whorls and loops that can be seen when you look closely at an area of skin (try your fingertips) is unique. Even identical twins have different patterns, though they are very similar; which is why fingerprinting is so essential a part of criminal investigation.

Skin is rather thinner in the child than in the adult but no less versatile, and like other body structures it undergoes a considerable degree of change as adulthood approaches — as we'll see later.

The body's structure

Bones give the human body its basic structure and its rigidity; muscles give it shape and movement. Both together they give the body its strength.

Bones

It is said there are about 206 individual bones making up the individual human scaffolding. About, because there is a surprising amount of variation, with some people having an extra bone in their spines, and some having extra ribs.

The size range is considerable; the femur (the thigh bone), is a great heavy bone, and the ossicles, of which there are three in each inner ear, are tiny. Some are long and rounded — the femur, the humerus (the upper arm) — while others are flat — the scapula (shoulder blade) and the ilium (the spread of the pelvis which creates the hip).

The long bones are hollow, to give them added strength; as any engineer knows, solid structures are far more liable to shatter under strain than those with hollow centres. But the hollows aren't only to confer strength; they also contain the bone marrow, which has the essential job of making blood. In infancy, blood cells are made in all bones, but by the time adulthood is reached, blood factories are confined mainly to the skull, the spine, the ribs, the femurs and the sternum (breastbone). Other body structures make blood cells (the liver, the spleen, the small glands called lymph nodes) but the bones are of prime importance.

In children there is provision for bones to grow. Each bone has a special area where the tissue is like a thick stiffish jelly — called cartilage — from which bone cells develop to lengthen and strengthen the bones. These areas are called epiphyses and the last of them disappears — signalling the completion of bony growth and therefore the attainment of adult height — usually in the late teens or early twenties. It happens rather earlier in girls than in boys.

The size of individual bones, and therefore individual people, is governed partly by inheritance (tall parents generally have tall children) and by environmental pressures. People who eat a lot and so carry extra weight tend to have stronger bones, which thicken to the size they need to be to carry their burdens. People who live in areas where air pressure is low (high on mountains, say) will have lighter bones than those in areas like deep valleys where the pressure is greater. Astronauts living in weightless conditions tend to lose bone mass for this reason. (There are other reasons for loss of bone mass, especially in women, see page 126, Section nine, on Woman in maturity.)

Rigid as the bony scaffolding can be, yet it has provision for movement. Joints between each bone allow an incredible range of movement; from simple bending to the sort of contortions that fairground performers show. Children are generally better at using the full range of actions allowed by their joints than are adults who tend to be more cautious, but that isn't because their joints aren't capable of movement; it is generally because their minds are not — they lack the confidence of the young and so far unalarmed.

There is a wonderful assortment of joints; sliding ones and rotating ones and hinged ones and pivoting ones and many more. Each is beautifully designed for its job, each is self-protecting, with cushions of cartilage to prevent bone surfaces from rasping against each other, each produces its own liquid lubrication, and each will operate in concert with others to allow the full range of activity.

Cut-away section of a long bone

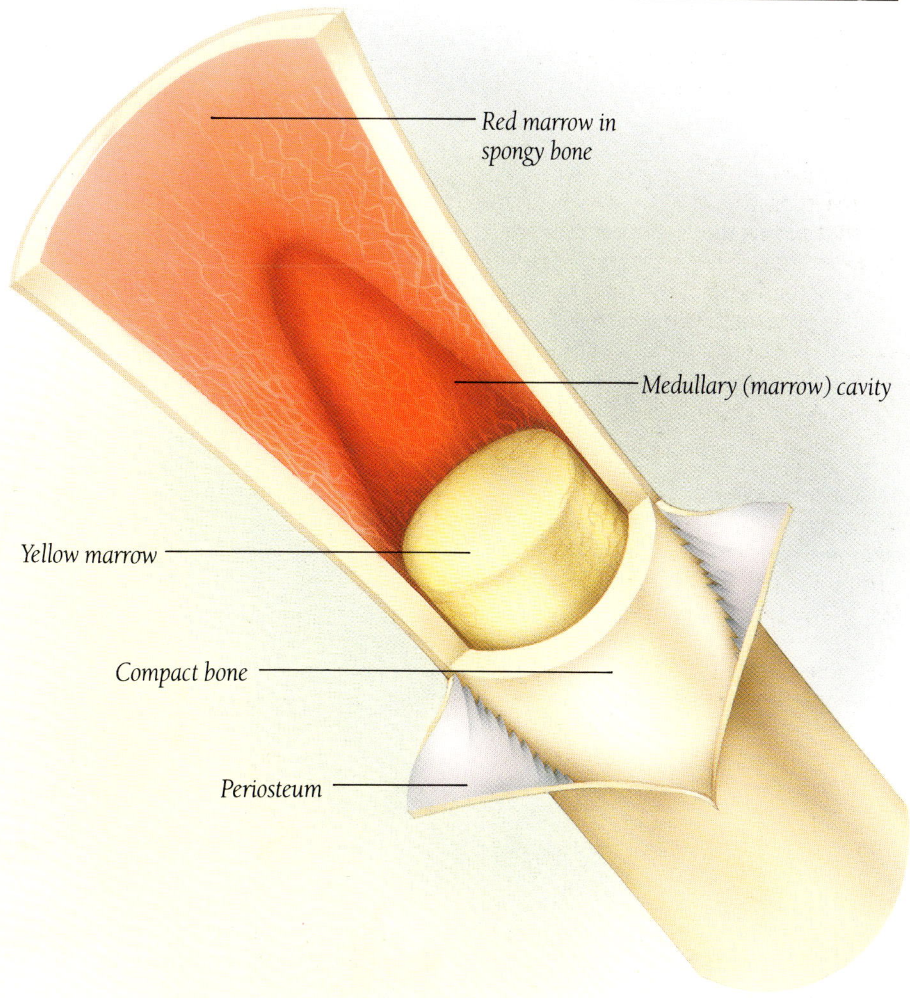

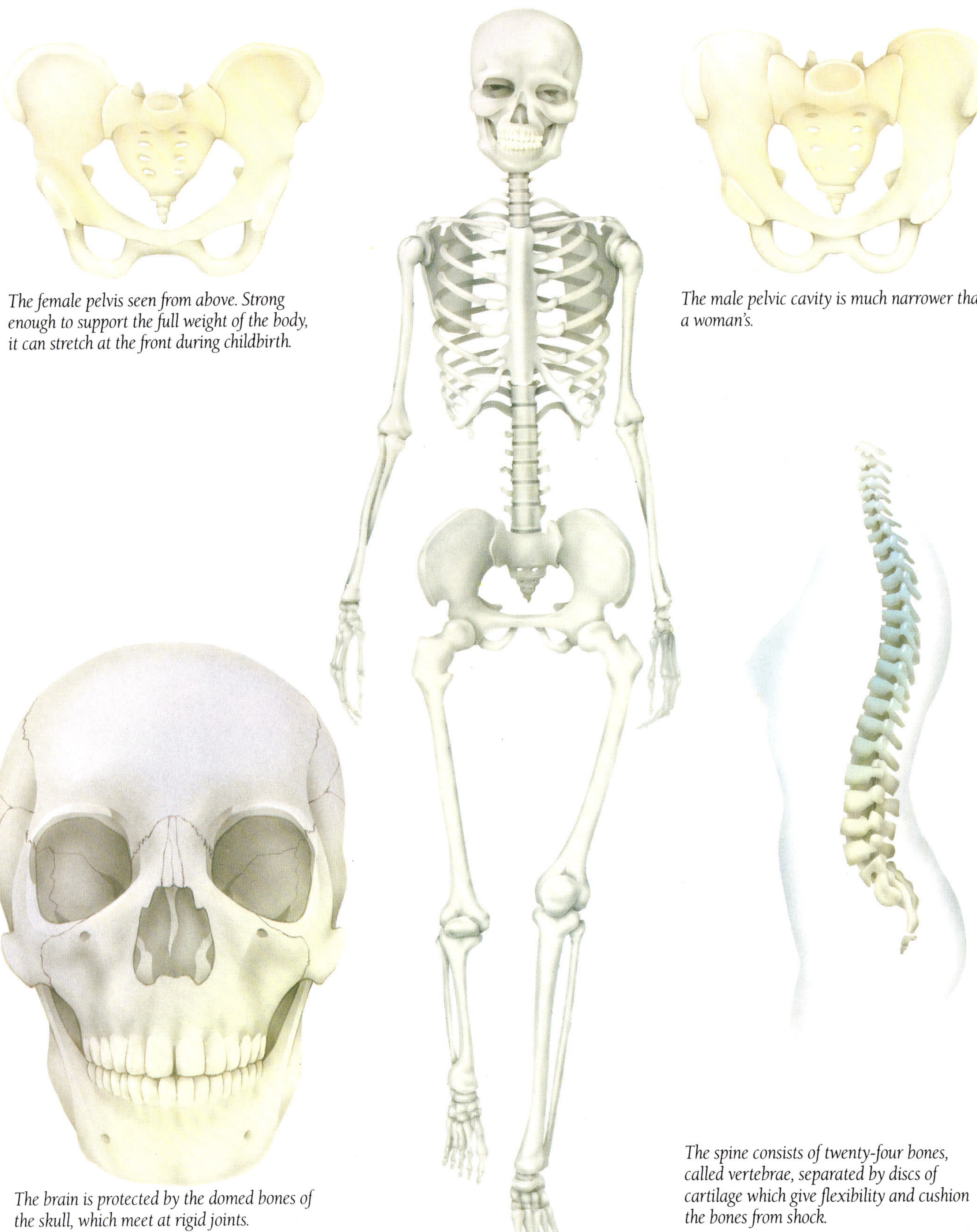

The female pelvis seen from above. Strong enough to support the full weight of the body, it can stretch at the front during childbirth.

The male pelvic cavity is much narrower than a woman's.

The brain is protected by the domed bones of the skull, which meet at rigid joints.

The spine consists of twenty-four bones, called vertebrae, separated by discs of cartilage which give flexibility and cushion the bones from shock.

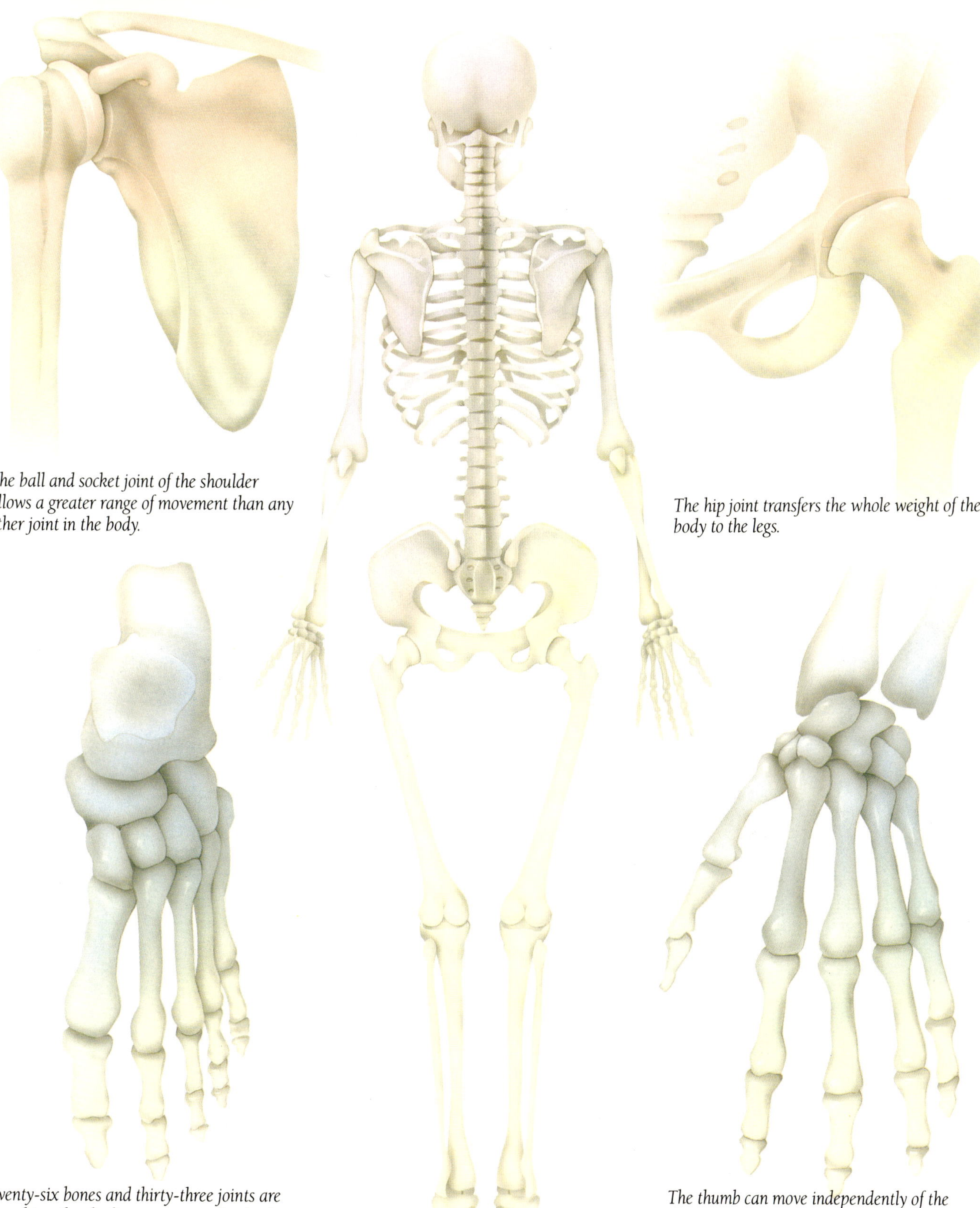

The ball and socket joint of the shoulder allows a greater range of movement than any other joint in the body.

The hip joint transfers the whole weight of the body to the legs.

Twenty-six bones and thirty-three joints are bound together by ligaments to make the foot remarkably flexible.

The thumb can move independently of the fingers to achieve precise grip and manipulation.

Muscles

But the bones can't use their joints without muscles: it is they which actually give us our ability to move. Each one — and we have more than 650 — is made of bunches of fibres, which have the remarkable ability to contract, thus storing up energy, and then to relax, thus releasing the energy in the form of work.

Some of the cells in the fibres are up to twelve inches long. Some go lengthwise, and can therefore shorten, some go round, and can therefore tighten. All burn up sugar and oxygen and other substances in order to do their work, and all create by-products of their activity — heat as well as movement, and waste materials as well as usable substances (when overworked muscles go into cramp it is the accumulation of wastes that causes some of the pain).

There are three types of muscle. The ones you know best are the skeletal muscles — those which are under conscious control. When you lift your leg you do so of your own choice; you could choose to leave it still. That is why these muscles are labelled 'voluntary'. When they are viewed with the naked eye they have a striped appearance — so they are called striped muscles.

We also have involuntary muscles which do their work with no reference to us — to the conscious mind, that is. These muscles are part of the blood vessels, of the gut, of the urinary tract and many other places in the body. Often working with the heart's action, they move blood along the circulation system, send food along the gut and waste materials out of it, and keep the products of the kidneys moving through into the bladder and then out of it. These muscles are smooth, and are therefore described as unstriped.

In some areas there is a mixture of voluntary and involuntary muscle action. For example, the gut sends its contents spanking along, whatever your mind says, but when they reach the rectum — the last few inches — and demand to be excreted your mind insists that they cannot do that unless you're in a suitable place. So, voluntary muscular activity overrides the involuntary, and the contents of the rectum are deliberately contained until it's convenient for the controlling muscles to yield to the clamour of the self-controlling ones. If the two types of muscle have to resist each other's actions for too long because the suitable place can't be reached, the resulting bellyache and discomfort can be considerable, to put it mildly.

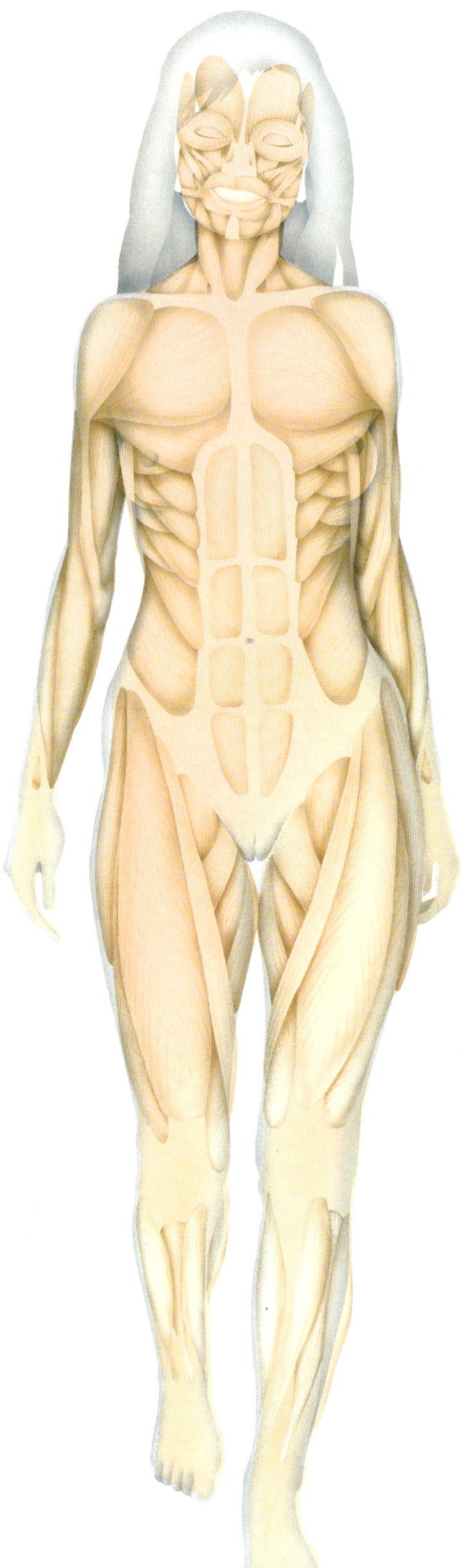

Voluntary muscles are under our conscious control and are striped.

The involuntary muscles

Involuntary muscles are unstriped and can perform their work automatically.

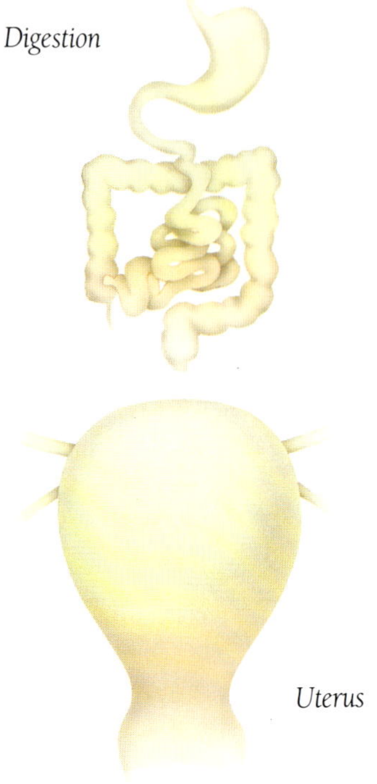

The third kind of muscle is that which makes up the heart. It looks like voluntary muscle in that it has stripes, but behaves like involuntary muscle (which everwhere else in the body has no stripes) in that it keeps on its regular action without reference to our conscious minds. This is just as well, since it has to keep on pumping day and night for seventy to eighty years or more, especially for women who tend to live longer than men. In order to function, muscles need fuel — food and water and oxygen. This they get from the blood.

Bladder

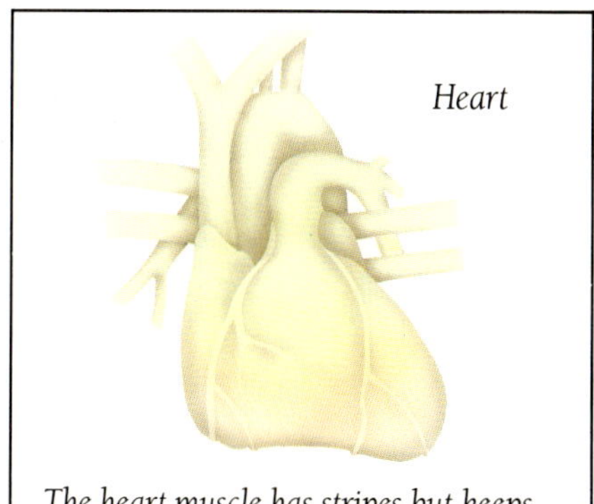

The heart muscle has stripes but keeps up its regular pumping without our active control.

The tracking of a muscle

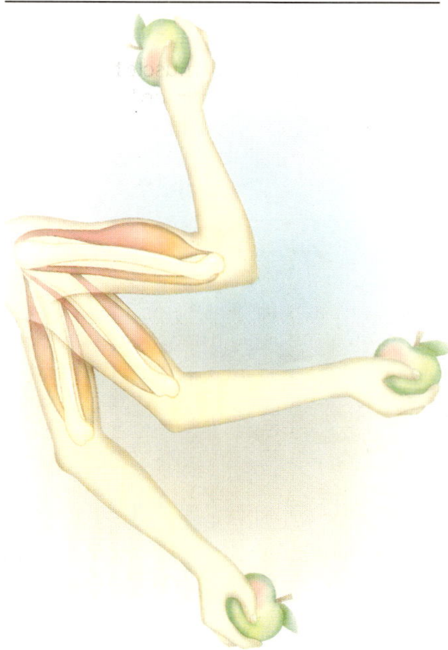

Muscles contracting and relaxing to give smooth, controlled movement.

Heart and lungs

Rich, red and robust, blood is pumped around the system by the heart and is a remarkable body organ in its own right. At birth, a baby has about half a pint, but by adulthood a woman, depending on her size, will have six or seven pints, except when she is pregnant, when she has an extra pint or two to cope with the extra work her body has to do. Men have nine to ten pints of blood, again depending on size.

Blood is made up of liquid and solid parts and it is the essential traffic of the human body. It carries food and oxygen as well as waste products and carbon dioxide. Its water content, like its sugars, salts and subtle chemical cargoes maintain the whole human engine. It is constantly changing, constantly being renewed. The value of blood has given a vivid imagery to human affairs; blood is thicker than water; I'd give my heart's blood for you; my blood ran cold; blood brothers; blood money; bad blood; blood bath; blue blooded; hot blooded; full blooded — and so on.

The basis of blood is plasma, a straw coloured slightly sticky sweetish liquid which is a solution of sugars, salts and proteins. Its constituents vary greatly, depending on its owner's nutrition level, general health, and state of mind (anxious people have different levels of certain hormones in their blood, of which more later). Plasma also carries a number of other essential substances. (The Rhesus factor, which comes into prominence in pregnancy is discussed in Section six.) Plasma forms about fifty-five per cent of the whole blood (and ninety per cent of plasma is water), the rest being cells.

Basically, there are three kinds of cells. Red cells, which look like double-sided frisbees, or, if you prefer the image, doughnuts with the hole covered over, carry oxygen. They are simply envelopes full of haemoglobin, which is made of iron and which has the ability to combine with oxygen and carbon dioxide. The red cells carry oxygen from the lungs around the body and return its waste product — carbon dioxide — back to the lungs to be disposed of. Each cubic millimetre of blood contains about five million red cells. Each one lives for

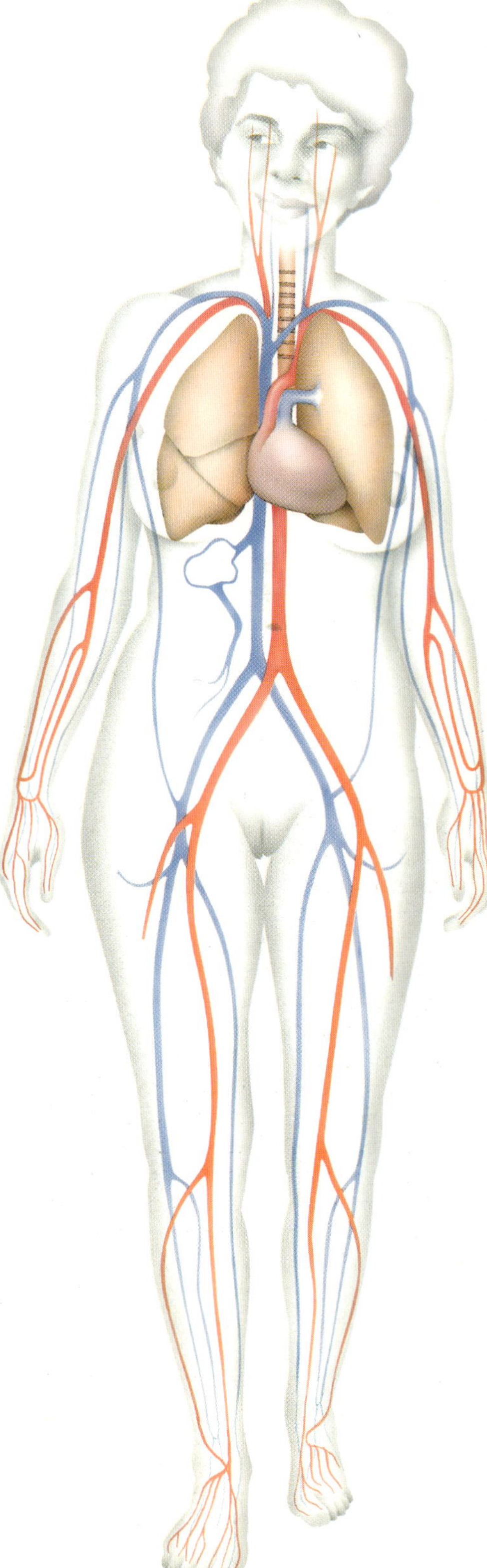

The heart pumps the blood along a system of intricate pathways.

The constituents of blood

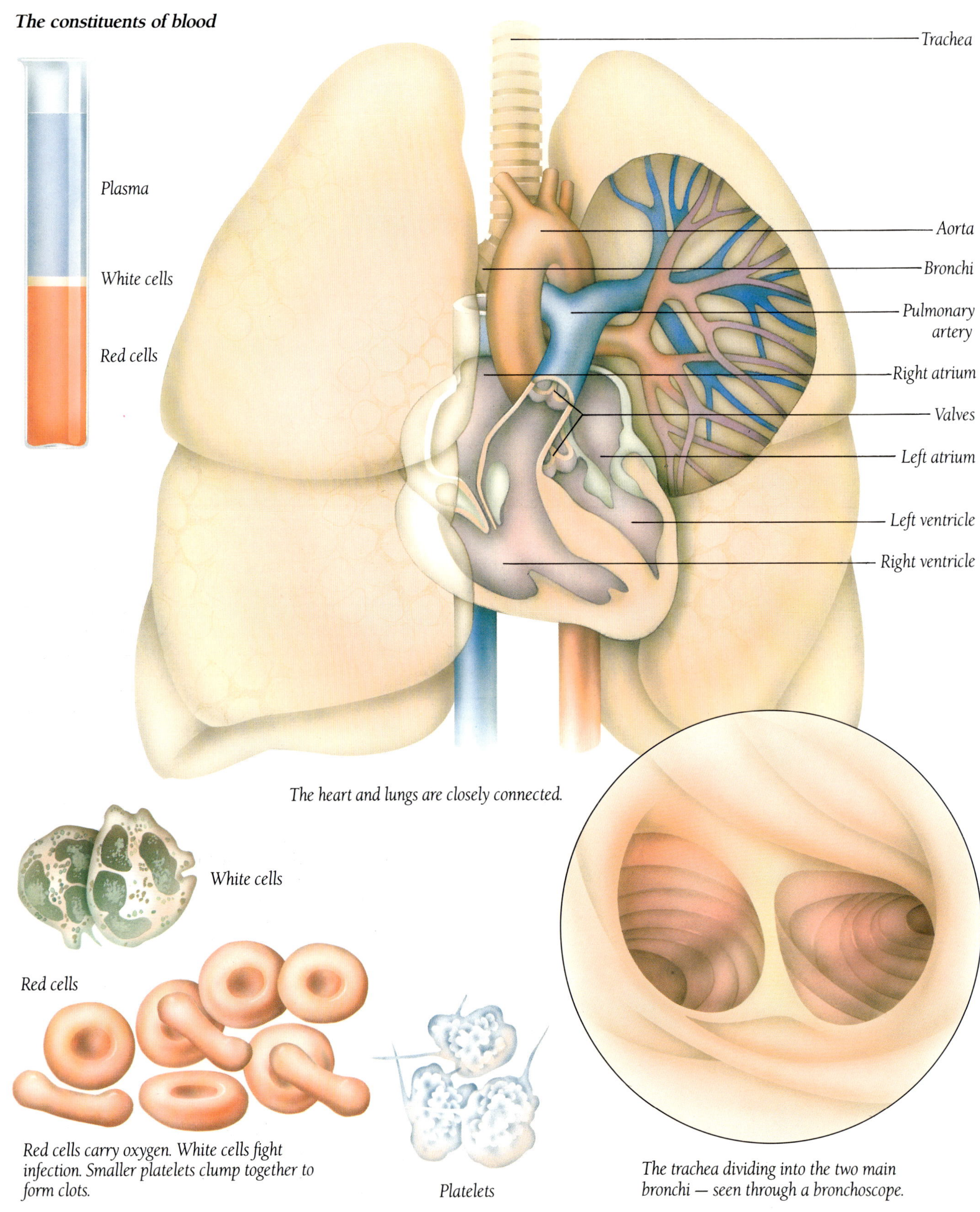

The heart and lungs are closely connected.

Red cells carry oxygen. White cells fight infection. Smaller platelets clump together to form clots.

The trachea dividing into the two main bronchi — seen through a bronchoscope.

around 120 days and about two million of them are destroyed and replaced every second, the bones being the place of manufacture. (The pigments released by the breakdown of worn out red blood cells colour the waste material in the gut. They also form part of the deodorant system used to deal with gut waste. A human body is an exceedingly economical creation; Nature wastes nothing.)

White cells come in five different forms, and in comparatively small numbers (between 4,000 and 10,000 in one cubic millimetre of blood), and mainly have the function of fighting infection. They swallow invading germs whole. They also act as scavengers; if you get a splinter in your finger and can't pull it out it is a particular type of white cell which literally eats it up.

Finally, there are platelets, cells much smaller than reds or whites (there are about 250,000 in one cubic millimetre of blood) and their job is to clump together to form clots. These are the plugs needed to close off a blood vessel if it is broached and so prevent loss of the precious fluid. (There are times when clots are unwanted because they form inside unbroken blood vessels, a matter to be returned to later.)

Blood is carried via a transport network that is both stunningly simple — it is just a series of pathways — and amazingly complex — the vessels pleat and interleave with each other without ever becoming tangled. Every cell in the human body — and there are countless millions of them — has to be served its own balanced diet of food, oxygen and chemicals and each must have its useful products delivered to other cells as well as having its wastes cleaned away. So a blood vessel has to reach each cell — and a blood vessel does.

From the heart, the central pump of the system, great arteries send freshly oxygenated, and therefore brightly red, blood surging along in pulses powered by the heart's beat. Each artery forks and then again and again, and so spreads its branches to smaller and smaller ones, finally to become arterioles and then capillaries, threadlike vessels so narrow that only one blood cell at a time can squeeze along the central channel.

The kidneys

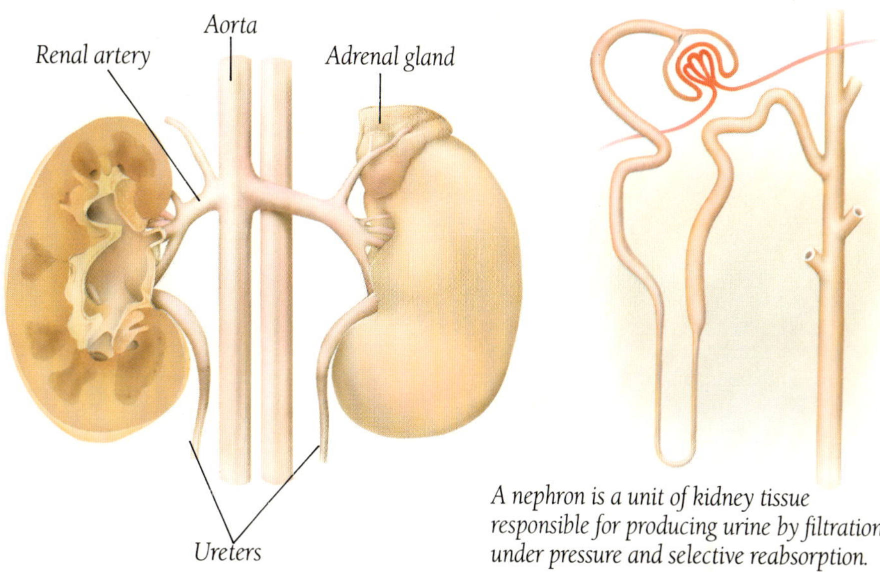

A nephron is a unit of kidney tissue responsible for producing urine by filtration under pressure and selective reabsorption.

As the blood pulses along the system towards the capillaries (and the pulsing can be felt at a very remote distance from the central pump) some of the plasma oozes out through the blood vessel walls to carry cargo to waiting cells and collect waste products. It then enters an adjacent system of vessels, the lymphatic, which carries the cell-less blood (plasma) back into the circulation by pouring it into particularly important veins deep in the neck (near the jugular vein of which everyone has heard. 'Going for the jugular' is seen as a very violent action. Now you know why).

Capillaries don't carry only arterial — oxygen rich — blood. When they reach the distant structures at the end of their journey from the heart they meet other capillaries, which take the now oxygen-depleted blood cells, already beginning to fill up with carbon dioxide instead. The capillaries carry them, in their plasma, to larger vessels, first venules — tiny veins — and then larger and larger ones, until two massive veins, called the inferior and superior *venae cavae,* carry it to the heart. The circular journey is complete — or seems so. In fact it is not.

Before the blood can usefully be sent back on its circular tour, it must rid itself of its burden of carbon dioxide and wastes, and collect more oxygen; so there is a double circuit, via the lungs. And here the language of anatomy has to break a rule. Generally, arteries carry only blood rich in oxygen, and veins carry blood depleted in oxygen. But when blood goes to the lungs, (rather bluish in colour because it is so low in the vital gas) it is carried in the pulmonary arteries, and when it returns, bright red and fizzing with fresh oxygen, it is carried in the pulmonary veins. This isn't as confusing as it sounds, for these vessels have another anatomical definition. Veins enter the heart, arteries leave it.

Whatever the labels used, the basic system is there to be marvelled at; a constantly self-renewing, constantly balanced, constantly working transport method that keeps itself in order and performs all its essential functions without any conscious involvement of the central intelligence that inhabits the body. It is able to cope with an amazing set of demands, from finding the extra energy needed to fuel a short burst of running like that needed to catch a bus, to providing the extra needs of a growing infant in the uterus. Even this short and simple account of the way heart, lungs and blood function is enough to make a person gasp and stretch their eyes with amazement. To have such an incredibly efficient inner system is indeed remarkable, but if you study the design in greater detail its workings are even more startling.

Digestion

'It's a very strange thing, as strange as can be, whatever Miss T eats turns into Miss T,' is a children's rhyme which, like many other such, explains an often disregarded basic truth in a very memorable manner. Food does provide more than energy to fuel the human machine; it *is* the human machine. The food a women eats when she is pregnant creates her child; the food that child eats as she grows creates the woman.

The systems that convert food into active people are as beautiful and as complex as all the other body systems, and interact with them with great elegance. The centre of them is the alimentary canal, which travels from mouth to anus and in the adult is about nine metres (thirty feet) long. More mind boggling statistics: in the average lifetime the canal deals with about 10,000 kg (23,000 pounds) of solid food and 42,000 litres (90,000 pints) of fluid; the surface – digesting – area of the gut in an adult is about 240 square metres (350 square yards); it takes twelve to fifteen hours for food to complete the journey from mouth to rectum – depending on circumstances; some studies have shown that swallowed dye appears at the rectum twenty-four hours later and may go on being disposed of for several days. The stomach produces, without damaging itself, usually, hydrochloric acid strong enough to dissolve iron.

Food starts being digested in the mouth; the salivary glands in the cheek and beneath the tongue produce enzymes which begin to break the basic constituents of food into fragments which the system can handle. Enzymes are specific; there are different ones to deal with different sorts of foods – fats, proteins, carbohydrates. When the food is swallowed it travels to the stomach which continues the digestive process, but which actually performs a storage role more than anything else (and by the way, the controlling mechanisms that ensure that swallowed food goes into the right hole – the gullet – instead of into the adjacent windpipe – the trachea – are another set of beautifully organized reactions). The juices the stomach produces – that fearsome hydrochloric acid included – break down the food into a mush, but don't completely change it; it continues to

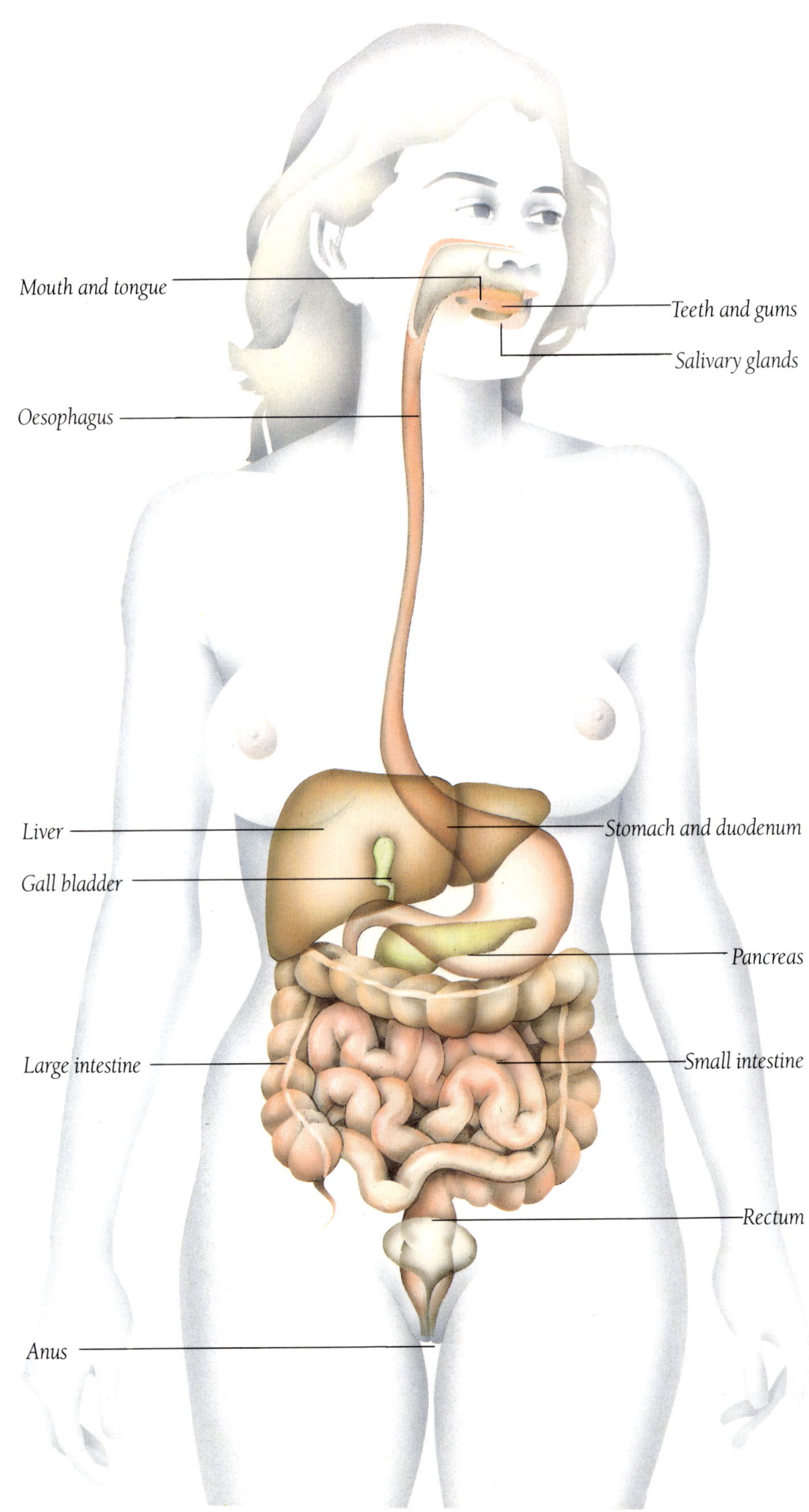

be recognizable food (as anyone who has ever thrown up knows perfectly well). Some of the food's constituents may begin to enter the bloodstream, via the stomach walls, but very little. Some simple sugars may be able to do so, and certain drugs (such as aspirin) but that is all.

The mixture is squirted into the main organ of digestion — the small intestine — by waves of contraction of the smooth muscle layers of the stomach's walls, each wave happening about three times a minute. Since the adult stomach has the capacity of about one and half litres ($2\frac{1}{2}$ pints), it takes some time to empty into the gut. Two to four hours is the average time needed to pass an average breakfast onwards, which is why you're ready for lunch at noon after your cereal and toast at eight. An empty stomach signals 'hunger' to the brain, and as it continues its regular squirting actions create the hunger pangs with which we are so familiar (some of us more than others).

The sounds of the stomach churning and squirting can easily be heard, if you put your ear to the belly; it tends to be noisier when the stomach is empty. Anxious people may find that they can hear it much more than relaxed ones. This is because the smooth muscle of the stomach, like all smooth muscle, is very responsive to the effects of stress.

Once in the small intestine, the real work of digestion can be done. As the food mixture, now a liquid called chyme, enters the first section of the gut (it's called the duodenum, the Latin for twelve being *duodecion*, and the section measuring twelve finger widths — about ten inches) special hormones are triggered into production.

One hormone has the task of calling in bile from an adjacent storage organ, the gall bladder, which lies tucked neatly under the liver, where the bile is made; bile's job is to split fats in foods and produce an emulsion.

Another hormone calls up juices from an organ on the left-hand side, called the pancreas (in a butcher's shop it's called sweetbreads — a delicacy to some) and that has the job of calming down the fierce acidity left in the food by the stomach. When the chyme is more alkaline, the various enzymes can get on with their job, which is splitting foods of various kinds into absorbable substances.

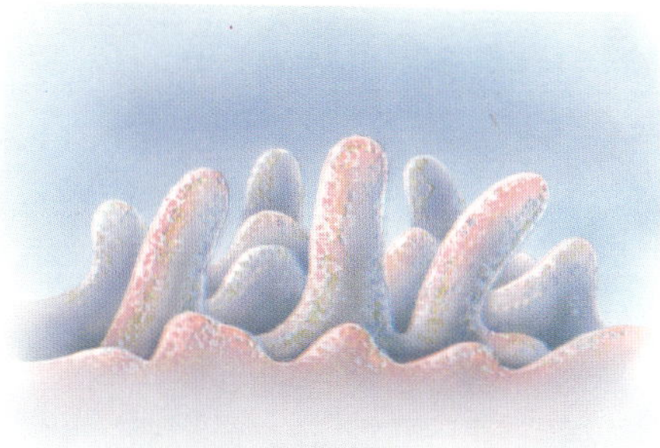

Food is absorbed through tiny finger-like projections called villi, which line the small intestine.

The mixture, in which the enzymes and juices are busily at work, now travels along the small intestine at a rate of about two and a half centimetres (an inch) a minute. The rate slows down as the journey progresses, and while it goes on tiny finger-like projections in the small intestines (called villi) which are rich in minute capillaries, allow the nutriments in the food to pass through into the bloodstream. Each villus contains smooth muscle so it can lengthen and shorten, and that means the nutrients are actually pumped out into the blood.

And now the circulation system gets involved in the work of the digestive system. The blood vessels from the small gut drain their food-rich contents into the portal vein, which goes to the liver. This vast organ, it is the biggest gland in the body, weighing about one and a half kilograms (3-4 pounds) in the adult and occupying two fifths of the belly space in the infant, which is why babies have such round little bellies, has a bewildering range of tasks. It is like a chemical factory in which over five hundred different jobs are done to render food useful to the cells, and to render poisons harmless.

In the course of a lifetime we swallow a good deal that is not designed to be healthful for humans and it is the liver which must deal with this. Alcohol is a case in point; agreeable though it seems, it is a poison and the liver knows it. Taking the sting out of a bottle of wine can put a great strain on a sick or tired liver, which is why people with inflammation of it (hepatitis) have to go on the wagon.

Blood from the liver is rich in safe nutrients ready to be used by the cells, and under stress a large volume is pumped out. While we sleep, around a quarter of our total blood volume is in the liver; sudden waking can make the oxygen send out a couple of pints; exercise — or the threat of it — also makes the liver's circulation more brisk, as it sends essential fuel to the cells which will use it. It takes a little while for the nutrients to reach all the cells, which explains why there is often an energy lag early in exercise. A swimmer, for example, finds the first length or two of the pool hard work, but after that she 'gets her second wind' and loses her fatigue. That is because fuel is now reaching the cells steadily.

Fat is one form of food which does not travel to the liver from the small intestine. It is collected by special little vessels in the villi and shipped to the lymphatic system. Then, when the lymph is poured into the bloodstream — at the jugular, you'll remember — the fat content is immediately available to the blood for sending to distant body cells.

This isn't the end of the alimentary canal's story. When the swallowed food reaches the end of the small intestine anything not digested — and foods heavy in fibre are not — is passed on to the large intestine, the colon. It's pretty watery stuff when it arrives there and during its slow progression round the belly — up the right-hand side, across the top, down the left-hand side to the rectum — the water is slowly absorbed, leaving behind the familiar faeces (a word that comes from the Latin for 'dregs') which though much drier still consists of up to eighty per cent water. Up to a third of the dry matter consists of the dead bodies of bacteria (a dispiriting thought!) and the rest contains some of the secretions and debris of the gut itself (it makes mucus to help the faeces slip along easily) and a very small amount of food residue. People living on highly refined modern foods, low in fibre, may have hardly any food leftovers at all, yet still they'll have to empty their bowels. Even starving people do — remember all those dead bacteria.

At the point where the small intestine meets the big one, there is a blind pouch, called the caecum, from which a small structure hangs. It's called the vermiform appendix (that is, worm-shaped attachment) and in primitive man probably had a digestion job to do: It acted as a place where cellulose (fibre) was broken down and absorbed. It no longer does this job, and is little more than a tiresome leftover that can get infected and may need removing.

While all this alimentary activity is going on in the gut, there is a parallel clearing-out system — the urinary.

Blood is sent to the kidneys, and there it is filtered for all noxious substances, and also balanced for water content. If the body cells have too much water in them, the kidneys will make extra urine; if they are shrunken because there is too little, the kidneys will conserve fluid by making less urine. So, sometimes urine is sparse and dark, with lots of dissolved wastes in it (the chemicals left over from the cells' burning of foods — such as urea) and sometimes copious and pale. It has a characteristic smell, which may be masked by substances swallowed (if you eat asparagus you are aware of the fact when you pee a short time later — it smells faintly metallic) but it never smells of ammonia when it it fresh. That only happens after it is passed and exposed to the air, which seizes on the urea and converts it to, among other things, ammonia.

The kidneys use the dump-and-pick cleaning method. First they remove everything dissolved in the blood that passes through them, and then they put back into the blood what is needed — sugars, salts, chemicals, hormones. If there is too much for the blood's needs it stays in the urine; which is why people with diabetes, for example, excrete sugar. The kidneys work to keep the blood sugar at the right level by removing excesses.

The kidneys work very hard; one and a quarter litres ($2\frac{1}{4}$ pints) of blood pass through them every minute, which means that all the blood in the body goes through a great many times in twenty-four hours, and ninety-nine per cent of what is extracted from the blood is filtered right back in again. Only one per cent is turned into urine, making around one and a half litres (2-3 pints) a day. When a woman is pregnant, her kidneys have a particularly hard job to do. (See Section six.)

The bladder, where urine is stored until it is convenient to dump it, is rather like the rectum in that it — and its outlet — contain both voluntary and involuntary muscle fibres. You can close the outlet by an effort of will (mind you, not for long if the bladder is very full) and the muscular effort can be very uncomfortable if at the same time the bladder's smooth muscle is trying to contract to push out its contents. As will be seen later, this action of the bladder can cause problems to a woman in later life if the voluntary muscles which close the bladder mouth become weakened.

Metabolism

Most people are particularly interested in what they eat and drink and what they get rid of and how the whole process affects their bodies. It is a subject of unending fascination and very sensibly so. Understanding the way food and fluid is handled is an important part of understanding how it is used.

The process of food usage, together with oxygen and water usage, is called metabolism. It is an unbelievably complicated affair, and full understanding of it demands a deep knowledge of biochemistry, biophysics and any number of other highly academic disciplines. This is not surprising, when you consider the remarkable fact

The food chain

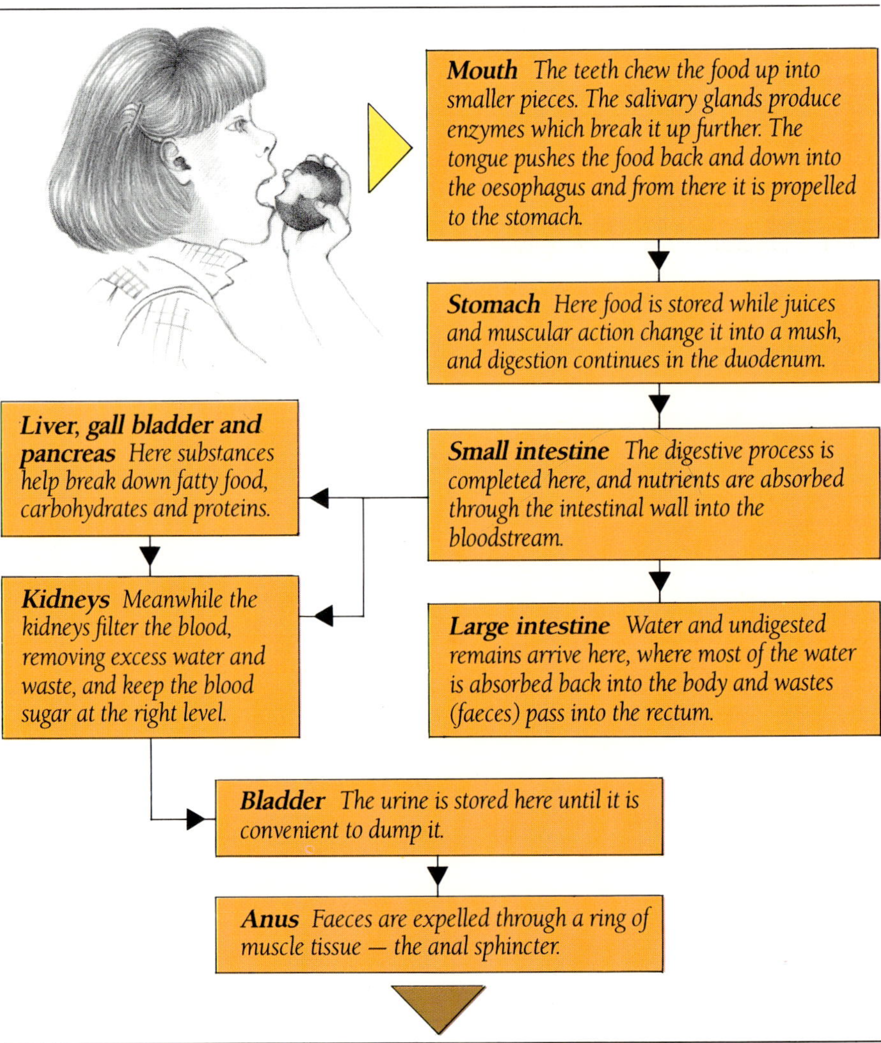

that most people maintain a fairly steady body weight once they reach adult life, while eating very varying amounts of food. It's estimated that we eat about fifty tonnes (tons) of food between birth and death — luckily we don't end up weighing that.

At the time of writing, the world — or certainly the Western part of it — seems obsessed with body weight; a singularly stupid woman of some power (she was a duchess) said in the thirties that no woman 'could be too rich or too thin'. She was wrong on moral grounds with the first statement and on health grounds with the second, but unfortunately, her philosophy seems to have spread widely.

There are millions of women who are constantly trying to control their body weight, and keep it down to an artificially low level, instead of trusting their own inherent metabolic systems to maintain them at the level they are designed by nature to be.

More awareness of what good food is and how best to enjoy it is what they need rather than obsessive calorie counting and painful self starvation that damages them not only physically but psychologically.

But it is important to remember that a woman's eating patterns are based on her diet as a child, so, making sure small girls eat well is an essential part of good mothering. The food charts, on pages 144 and 145 will therefore be as useful for children as for adults, but there is no need to become too anxious about what is eaten and what is not; quite severe psychological illnesses can result when girls get too concerned about food (see page 145).

And it isn't necessary to worry about it; the human frame is a remarkably resourceful creation. It can — and in the less rich parts of the world often does — manage to survive and operate on diets that are both bizarre and sadly depleted. The body has a quite extraordinary ability to make the most use of what is available. As long as the mind that inhabits the body does not interfere too much in its systems and does not deliberately push against the body's natural inclinations and demands, it can be perfectly trusted to do exactly what it was designed to do.

Brain and nerves

The brain has been compared to the computer centre of a vast organization, and when you consider how many body cells there are to be kept in harmonious balance with each other and the way the brain and its attending nerves manage to keep the whole lot running smoothly it's a fair enough analogy. But unlike a computer, the human brain is not just an electrical/electronic machine, even though it does use electric impulses to send its messages within itself, and through its attached nerves. It is also a chemical machine using very complex transmitter substances to link up the body cells into a busy yet efficient whole.

The brain, the centre of the system, is a pinkish grey structure of several different parts. It has a surface made larger by having a great number of folds in it — so that it looks rather like a walnut-shaped blancmange — and sits neatly inside the skull where it is safe from most sorts of buffeting. It has only one very small part of itself in direct contact with the outside world — the eyes. All other information that reaches it, therefore, apart from light, has to be taken in via other structures — nerves.

They are a network of branching filaments that reach out from the brain, and its long 'tail' the spinal cord (also pretty well protected inside the bony arches of the spinal bones) to every part of the body: ears and fingertips, nose and tongue and toes and legs; different parts have different amounts of nerve supply. The tongue and lips for example are richly endowed, and so provide a great deal in the way of information

Synapse

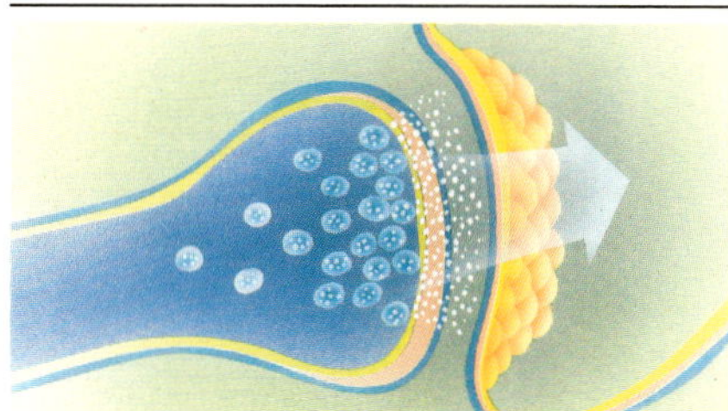

Nerve cells are called neurons. To pass from one neuron to the next, the nerve impulse has to cross their junction — called the synapse.

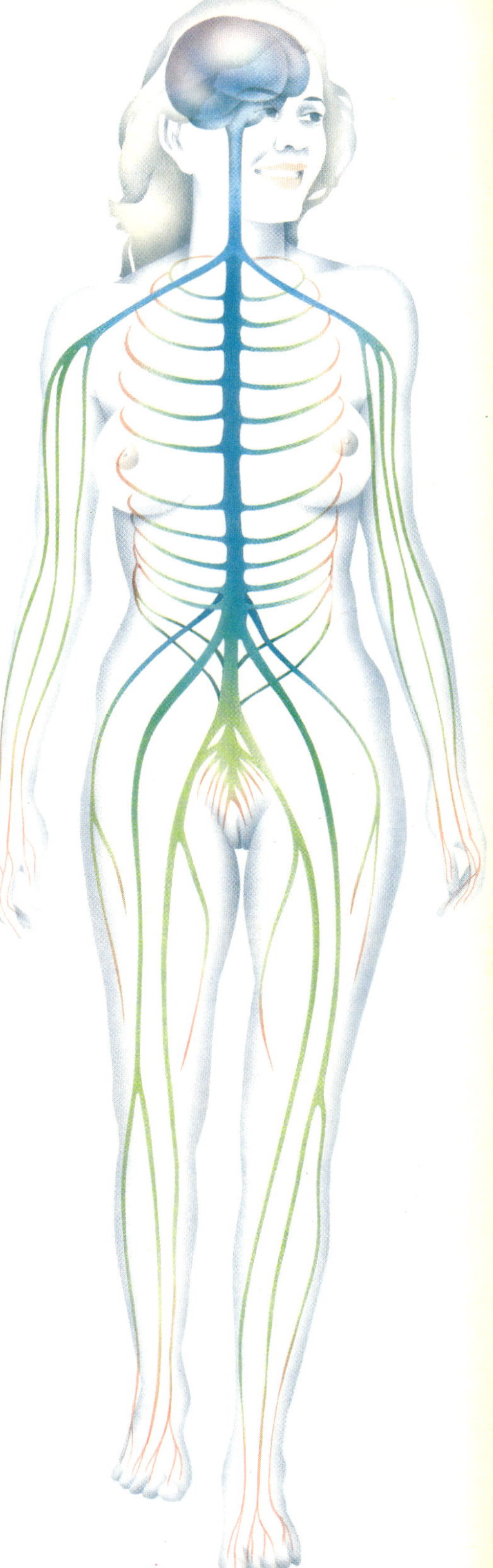

The central nervous system consists of the brain and the spinal cord. The brain sends and receives impulses along nerves.

collecting (have you never tried to check the texture of something too small to handle easily, by applying the tip of the tongue? Most of us have). The skin over the back and belly, on the other hand, is sparsely nerved; a light touch there may not actually be registered by the average person; fingertips feel more than palms, toes than heels, and so on.

The nerves which travel between body parts and the brain carry two kinds of fibres — sensory and motor. Sensory fibres bear messages to the cord and brain from the outlying body parts and motor fibres transmit back the instructions to work that the sensory messages suggest are needed.

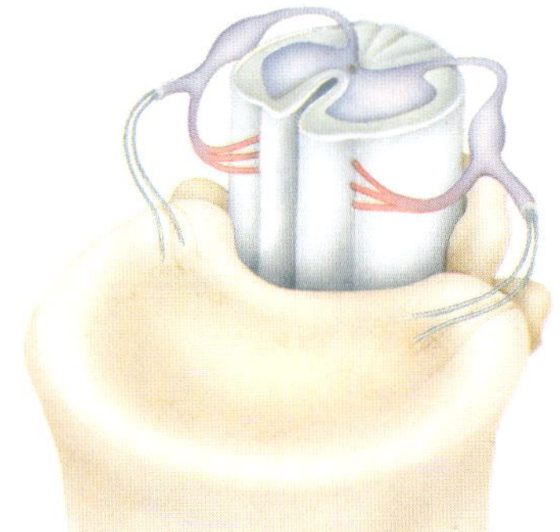

The spinal cord is the main nerve trunk to and from the brain. From here nerves branch to all parts of the body.

Thus, you step on a sharp piece of glass on the beach; the sensory nerves send an urgent message that damage is being done to cells, the motor message comes back, 'lift foot from glass,' and that is what happens. Together with several other reactions all of which emanate from the brain; you'll shout out an 'I'm hurt,' sound ('ouch!'), thus using the speech system; you'll hop about to maintain your balance (humans are not designed to stand on one leg) thus using the sense of balance based in the ears, and you'll rub the afflicted foot, thus using the voluntary muscles of the hand and arm to bring into play the stimulus which relieves pain (see page 147). All very complicated and unbelievably fast too, it can take less than a second to respond to the pain of glass-in-foot.

But there is more to the nervous system than these in-and-out message-carrying nerves that travel between brain and cord and other parts of the body. Look again at what happened when you stood on the glass. Your conscious brain registered the injury and instructed you to lift your leg, using your voluntary muscles, but as well as that happening, there were other mechanisms involved. The immediate removal of your foot from the glass was triggered off by the reflex arc — the message of pain got to the spinal cord and that activated the movement without involving the more distant brain. In addition, your autonomic nervous system came into play. This is the one that operates the parts of your body which are not under your conscious control; your heart, your blood vessels, your stomach and guts. It is this system, acting in concert with chemical messengers called hormones, which alerts the body as a whole to fight off danger.

It causes the heart rate to speed up (to send extra blood to distant muscles which may need added fuel to fight or fly from danger) the breathing rate to increase (to match the raised heartbeat and provide more oxygen for the hurrying blood to collect) the blood pressure to rise (as blood vessels change to accommodate the new demands made for a change in blood flow) pallor or redness depending on the nature of the threat (again caused by the changes in the blood distribution in the body) and so on and so on — all the familiar experiences we often recognize as 'being alarmed' or 'upset' or 'being nervous'.

Later on there will be more about how this system can be sent into action, and the effects it has — but none of it will make any real sense without an understanding of the chemical messengers which are so intimately involved with the autonomic nervous system.

Motor homunculus and sensory homunculus

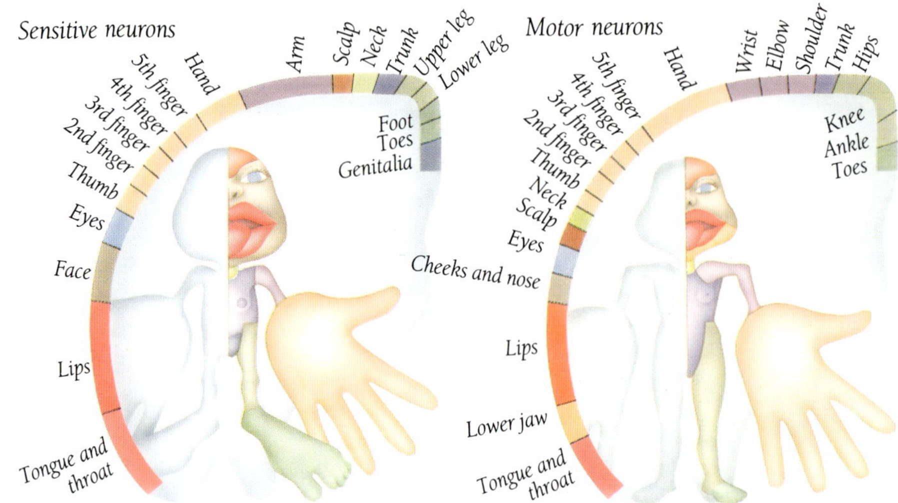

The left-hand side of the brain is shown here in cross-section.

Reflex arc

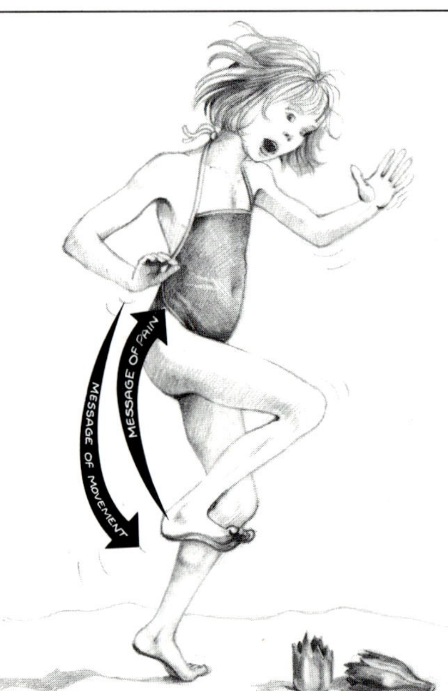

The reflex arc triggers the immediate removal of the foot from danger.

Hormones

Until this century no one really knew much about hormones. Some observant doctors had discovered that certain symptoms could be relieved by feeding patients certain substances; for example, a twelfth century physician called Roger of Palermo discovered that feeding burnt seaweed to people with swellings at the root of their necks made them better. He didn't know that the seaweed contained iodine essential for the thyroid gland to do its work and the lack of which caused the swelling, but the weed worked, and that was all that mattered. Beyond that ignorance was king.

Then, gradually, the different endocrine glands were identified and their functions worked out as the medical research explosion of the twentieth century gathered power. The glands were at first labelled 'ductless' because the anatomists couldn't see how they delivered whatever it was they made to the body. The liver is a gland too, but it has pipes — ducts — to deliver its goods to where they have to be. These odd glands did not.

It is now known that endocrine glands release their products directly into the blood, and this is why they can act as quickly as they do. When the adrenals, for example, which release adrenalin, among other substances, send a surge of their product out, the effects are felt in the whole body in a fraction of a second. If you've been badly frightened and your heart has 'missed a beat' it's because adrenalin has hit it — and the missing of the beat happened virtually as soon as the stimulus that caused the fear — it feels instantaneous.

We still don't know yet just how many hormones there are. They are constantly being identified and classified (the prostaglandins, for example, are newly described hormones) as medical research goes on digging deeper and deeper into human physiology. Nor can we be sure where all the hormonal sources are. There may be structures yet unidentified which are part of the endocrine system, but here are the ones we do know about.

Over and over again in these pages there will be accounts of hormones and what

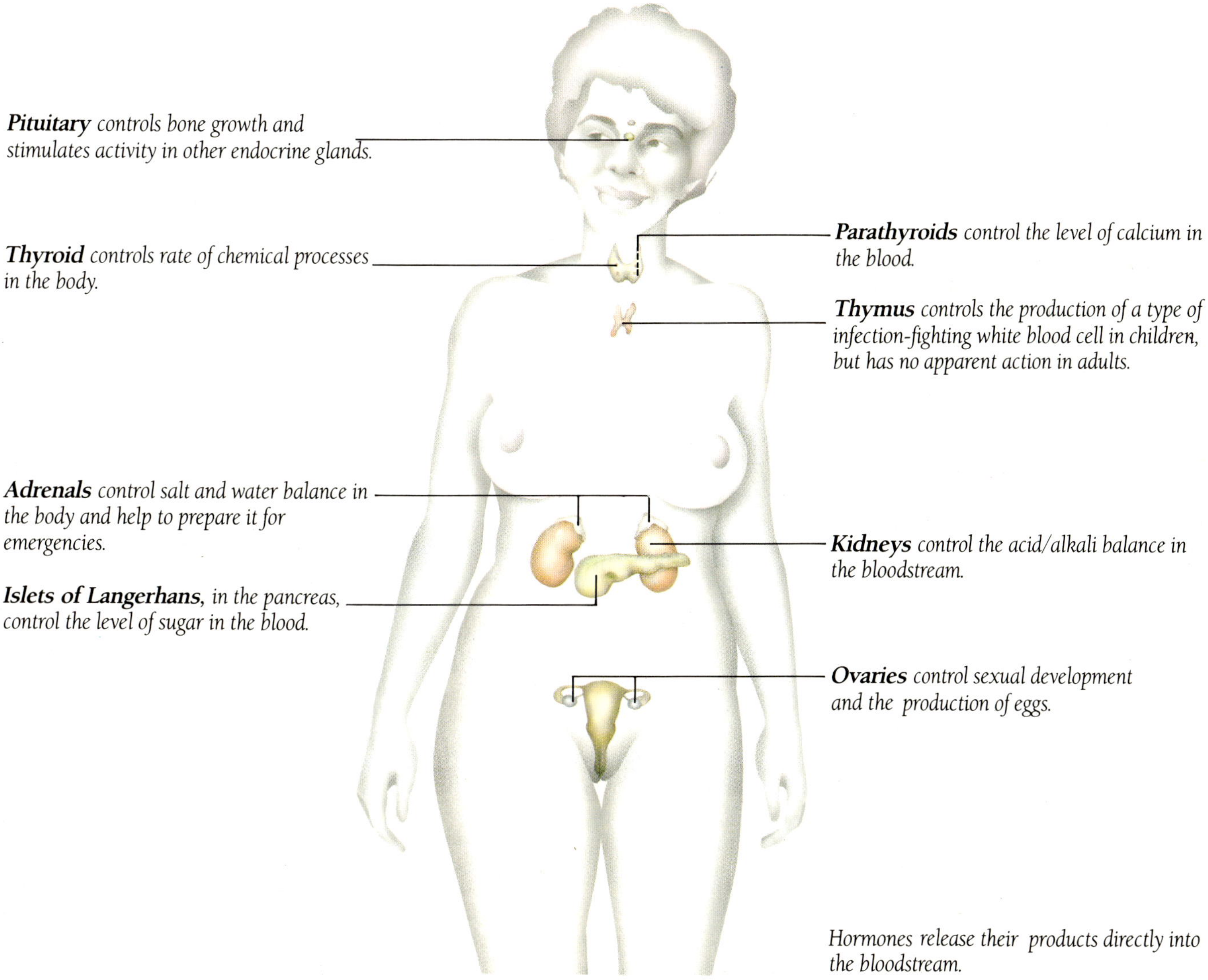

Hormones release their products directly into the bloodstream.

Interaction of the endocrine glands

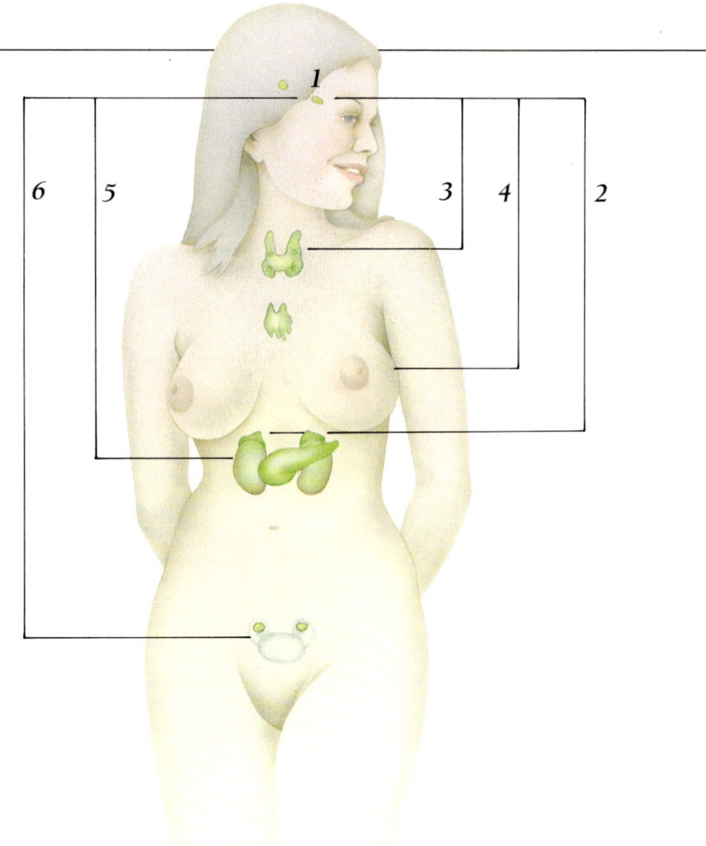

The endocrine glands secrete hormones and release them directly into the bloodstream. The body's master gland — the pituitary — is about the size of a pea and it regulates the activity of the other endocrine glands.

*The front of the pituitary secretes the growth hormone **1**, controls the production of steroids by the adrenal glands **2**, controls the thyroid gland **3**, controls the female reproductive organs and the breasts: the follicle stimulating hormone ripens the ovum, the luteinizing hormone controls the corpus luteum, and prolactin stimulates the production of milk by the mammary glands **4**.*

The middle part of the pituitary produces two hormones which are thought to affect body pigmentation.

*The rear part of the pituitary produces vasopressin which regulates the water absorbed by the kidneys **5**, and oxytocin which helps childbirth once labour starts **6**.*

they do, because these wondrous chemicals are the very stuff of life, and however much is said about them here, there will still be much left unsaid and much still to be discovered.

Here then is the small girl with the body that is so like her brother's, waiting for the metamorphosis that will transform her into a woman. She is already a wonderfully complex creation, a thinking, feeling, responsive creative person who is also a machine that operates mechanically, electrically, chemically. She will be even more complex when she changes into a woman and it isn't an easy change to make. A great deal has to happen to this small girl.

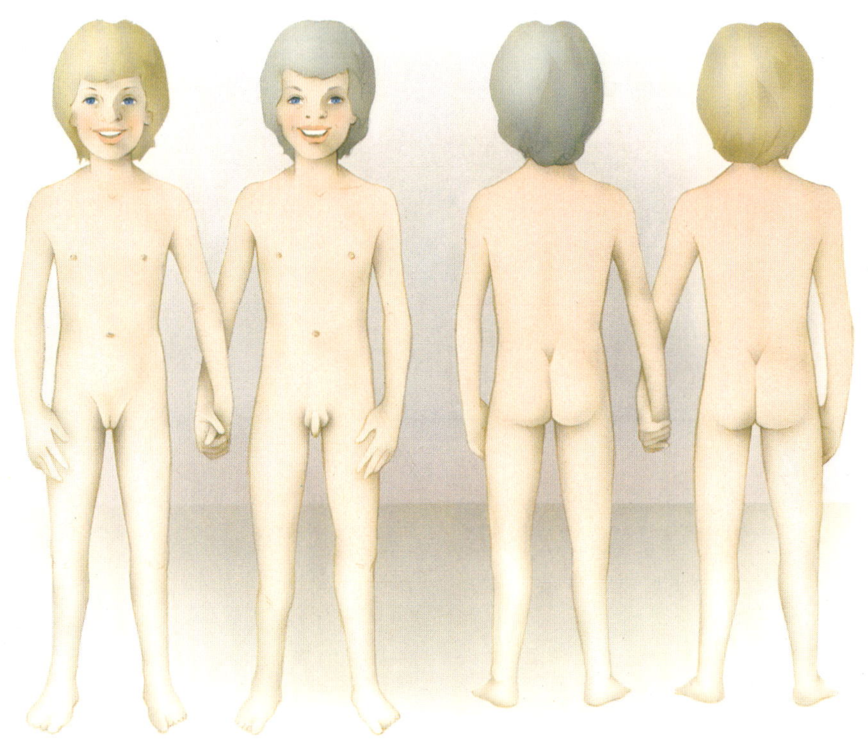

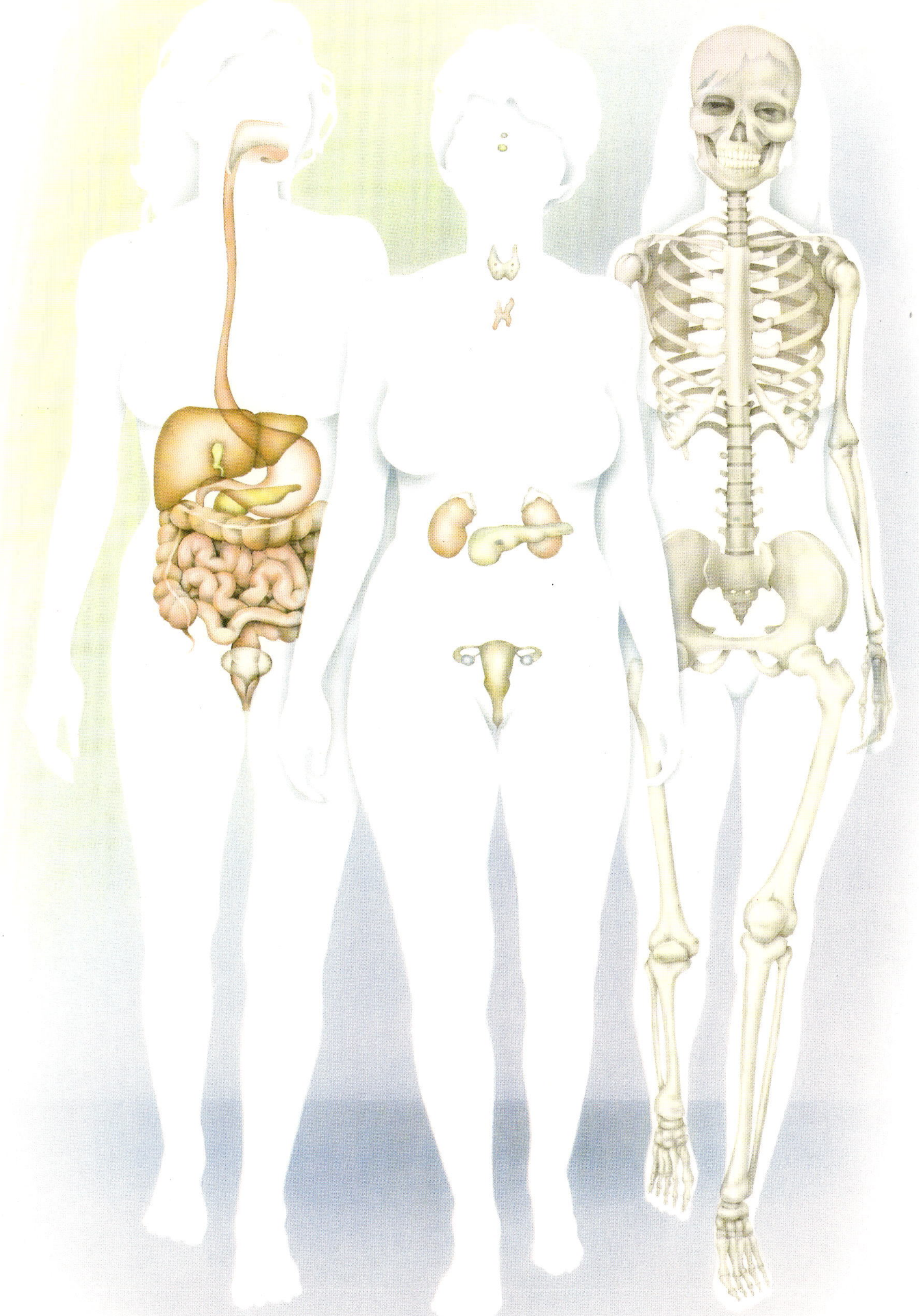

Nervous and digestive systems *Endocrine and circulatory systems* *Skeletal and muscular systems*

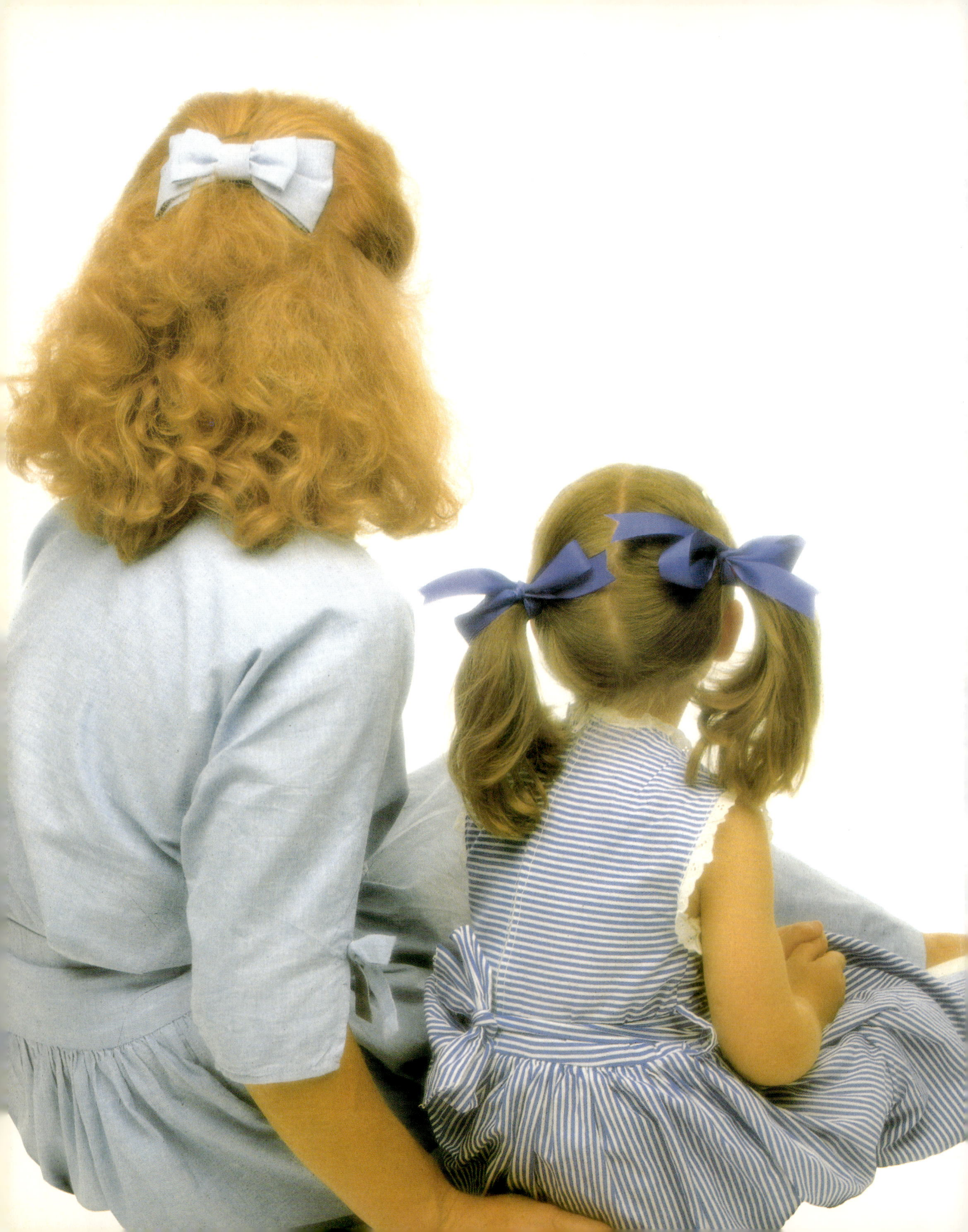

2
CHILD INTO WOMAN

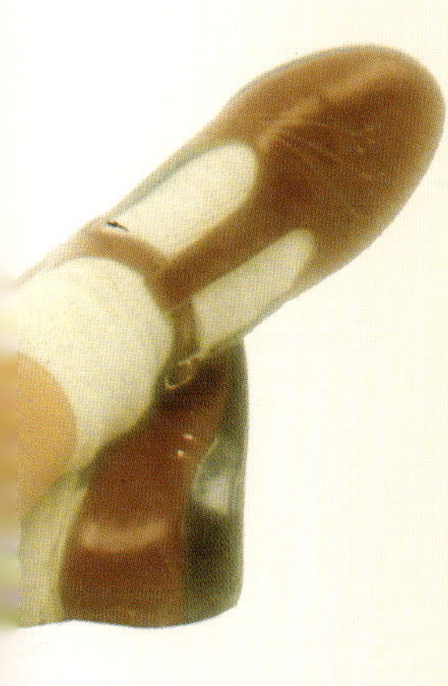

Listen to some present-day adults and you might get the impression that Difficult Teenagers are a modern invention. That in the past children became happy adults virtually overnight without any fuss and behaved like little angels all through the changeover time. That rebellious, ill mannered, promiscuous, anti-social young people are an invention of the late twentieth century.

The most remarkable thing about some of the people who hold these beliefs is their amnesia. Because, of course the period of change from dependent biddable child to independent capable and co-operative adult is today as it has always been; smooth sailing for a minority, choppy seas for most and a disaster for a few.

It's important to get labels clear before looking at what happens when children grow up, and why it can be so complicated and stormy an experience.

Adolescence is the total time of growing up in every sense – emotional and intellectual as well as physical. The label covers a period of around a decade, from nine to nineteen or so, and in some cases never seems to end; there are a number of people one meets in their thirties or even forties who display signs of the sort of immaturity of mind and spirit that can only be regarded as adolescent.

Puberty however describes a specific set of physical changes which take a child to sexual maturity. Puberty is complete when the child is capable of reproduction. Adolescence goes on for long after that.

Signs of puberty

It is difficult to say just when puberty starts. Boys get a gradual muscle development, penile enlargement, voice deepening and hair growth but the first nocturnal emissions of semen can happen without the boy actually realising and it does not have the same impact that the girl's major pubertal experience – the first period – has on her. This sign of girl's development is actually a late one; by the time it happens much of the growth of puberty has already taken place. It started around two years before the first period appears and since the average age for the first period is about thirteen, this means that in the average girl, puberty starts some time in the eleventh year.

But having said that, the point must be made that an average is only an average. It covers the many children who have their first period before they leave primary school, at the age of ten plus, and it also covers those in whom the vital sign is delayed till they are sixteen or even seventeen. So, some little girls of eight or so

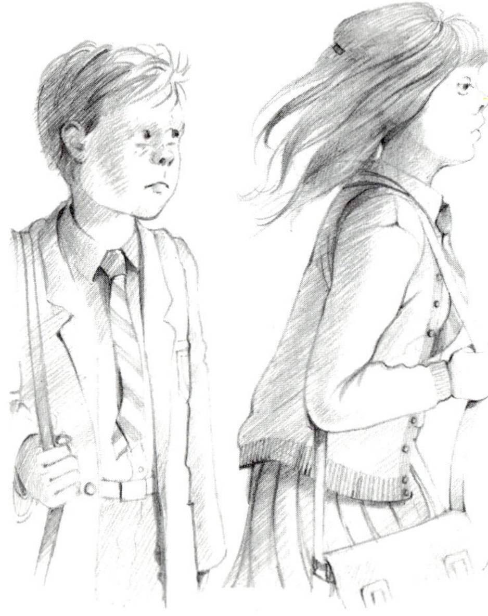

will be showing the first signs of puberty, while others remain straight up and down and as smooth as babies until they are fourteen or fifteen. This means that children in the same class at school can show an amazing range of maturity stages, and those who are in the minority group can have a rotten time of it; heaven help the little girl who 'hasn't started yet' if she's the only one in a class full of curvy young ladies or the busty eleven year-old in a class full of striplings.

(If it's any comfort, it can be much worse for boys who are expected to be macho – still! – and not show anxiety about their bodies or even any interest in them. Imagine being a shrimp of an undeveloped twelve year-old if the other boys with whom you share the rugger showers already have hair on their bodies.)

Girls usually start their pubertal changes two years earlier than boys and the physical changes together with the acceleration of other adolescent changes – in interests, in emotional capacity and in behaviour – have the effect of driving the sexes apart. The girls who once played happily with boys now dismiss them as 'boring' and begin to look towards boys of closer maturation age – that is, chaps of two or three years older – for their contacts with the male of the species.

Boys are also approached in a different way; the old familiar friendliness that was so appealing a part of nine year-old play becomes the more highly coloured and rather more ritualistic 'you're a boy' chatting up and giggling of eleven plus or so. It's a mistake to see this sort of behaviour as 'precocious' or regrettable. It isn't. It may appeal more to adults to see children as sexless and interested in each other only as playmates, but sooner or later they have to become aware of themselves as males and females, of equal worth and entitled to equality of opportunity and regard, but of different gender. That awareness starts in girls with the onset of puberty – and that, it must be repeated, can be early.

Good sex education should start early too, well before the first stirrings of sexual change are felt by the children. Talking to a seven year-old about sex and reproduction is no more exciting and dramatic to the child than talking about why the sky is up and the ground is down; it's as miraculous as everything else in their world. But talk about sex to a ten year-old in whom adult type hormones are beginning to be active, and such talk becomes difficult, even stilted, as the child's own emotions and sexuality become involved.

The child who copes best with puberty and its startling changes – and they do amaze the person they happen to, as those of us with long memories will know – is one who already has all the facts about what will happen and why it will happen as part of her collection of useful information. And, incidentally, it is not true that teaching children about sex and sexuality when they are young makes them 'forward' or 'dirty minded' or 'precocious' or any of the other accusations sometimes hurled at progressive teachers and parents. The fact is that children take in what they can cope with, and what they can't cope with they'll reject as something they don't understand; so they are at no risk from being taught about these adult matters, and may indeed be at more risk by being over-protected from reality. Children who are told how good adults behave can more easily learn to protect themselves against bad — that is, exploiting — ones.

Changes in puberty

Before any signs of the onset of puberty show on the surface, there are inner changes in the organs. What triggers them is uncertain. It could be body weight; it is known that underfed children experience delayed puberty, and in the well-fed West the age of puberty in both sexes is creeping steadily downwards as the general health and growth rates of children has risen. In Britain a hundred years ago the average age for the first period (also known as *menarche* — 'the onset of periods') was about fifteen, and eighteen or nineteen was far from uncommon. (But there's another odd fact — Shakespeare, writing four hundred years ago, invented a character of fourteen who had a very intense sexual relationship — and her experience wasn't unusual. He wrote of his Juliet 'Younger than she are happy mothers made' — so maybe the age of menarche used to be what it is now — or even younger — and then became later and is now falling again, for reasons we don't fully understand.)

It has been suggested that light may play a part in triggering the hormone production that starts puberty and girls living in Mediterranean and tropical countries where the sunlight is vivid are said to reach maturity younger, but the evidence for this is scanty.

Whatever the trigger, the activity of change starts in the pituitary gland which operates in concert with the section of the brain called the hypothalamus. The pituitary sends out several hormones, some of which trigger other endocrine glands — notably the adrenals — to produce some of their own. The thyroid and its metabolism-controlling hormone is also affected. This inter-linked system of growth and activity control by the endocrine glands is often described as being orchestral, with the thalamus-controlled pituitary gland being labelled the conductor of the orchestra. It isn't quite accurate because each gland, as well as acting reasonably harmoniously with the others and with the pituitary, has its own self-regulating mechanisms; but it's an elegant enough simile and does make it clear that the pituitary is indeed a very powerful gland, and that it acts under the direction of the brain, since it is physically so close to it and so responsive to its actions and reactions.

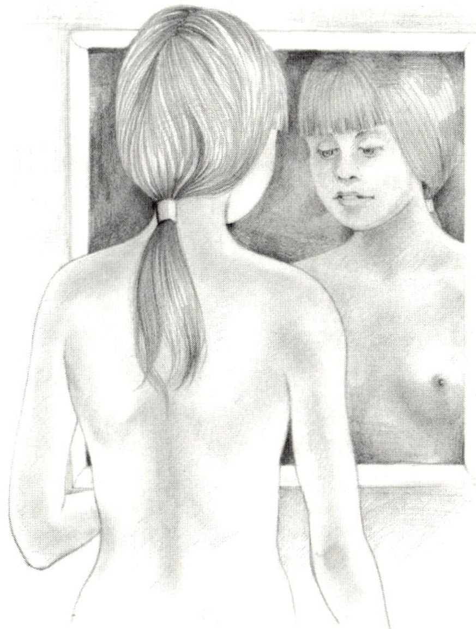

Among the pituitary hormones there are some that act directly on the undeveloped ovaries. When the little girl is born she already has in her tiny ovaries up to three hundred thousand ova — eggs — (some estimate less — around two hundred thousand — others estimate more — around four hundred thousand — but who could possibly count them all accurately?) Throughout her childhood these are merely potential eggs but now, as the pituitary hormones bombard the organ, it enlarges and begins to produce hormones of its own. These, estrogen and progesterone (you'll hear a lot more about these as the book continues) in their turn stimulate the adrenals which are perched over the kidneys, to produce androgens — literally 'man-making' hormones.

Androgens act on a number of body tissues. They control general growth, of bones and muscles and organs, and the result is a growth spurt. A girl can shoot up two or three inches or even four or five in a very short time. Suddenly none of her clothes fit and she keeps falling over her feet and dropping things as she learns to re-judge herself in relation to her environment. It can be a very disconcerting experience (as a person who put on seven inches in height in as many months at the age of eleven to twelve, I remember it well).

These growth hormones do not only affect bones and musles. They also affect the way fat is laid down in the body, and in girls they arrange for more fat to be settled than in boys. Generally boys have less under-the-skin fat than their sisters, so they at puberty tend to become lean — indeed, bony — whereas girls become rounder — and most especially so in some places. Extra fat is laid down over hips and thighs and buttocks and upper arms, and under the nipples of the breasts, and this helps to create the classic female shape of a swelling lower half and nipped in waist, and breasts, shoulders and arms rounded above it.

But, as usual, it has to be said that individuals vary. Some girls enter puberty and become skinny just as some boys enter their pubertal phase and develop so-called puppy-fat (it isn't; it's all too human). This is because, remember, both genders have male as well as female hormones, if in differing quantities. That is why some boys (about fifty per cent or more, it is estimated) develop enlargement of the nipples and sprout small breasts, much to their embarrassment, and why some girls develop male patterns of hair growth.

Because that is something else that changes. The down of the child becomes the true hair of the adult: thicker, less silky, more springy. It may lose its childish curl, and definitely becomes greasier as more sebum (skin oil) is produced. The change is most obvious on the head at first and then starts to affect the body. Hair appears on the new pad of fat that has been laid down over the pubis — the point where the bones of the pelvis unite at the base of the belly — and may also appear on the belly itself.

All the textbooks say that in girls pubic hair growth is in a triangular pattern and that in boys it is diamond shaped, but anyone who has seen enough bare bellies will know that both genders can have either pattern. It is not unusual for girls to grow belly hair, especially along the line that runs down from navel to pubis.

The average age for pubic hair to appear is around eleven, and hair under the arms starts to show a couple of years later. There may also be, in brunettes, some hair on the upper lip, in the moustache area, especially if this is a family pattern. People of Mediterranean stock – Italian, Greek, and so on – often show dark hair here. It's regarded as highly sexy in these cultures – and, indeed, so it is.

Androgens also affect the skin, thickening it and waking up the sebum-producing glands as well as the sweat glands. These latter often seem to become plugged and the result is that which afflicts something over eighty per cent of young people to some degree or other – acne, with blackheads and infected red angry pimples. Acne is so common it can hardly be called a disease, but it is if you have a bad go of it. Dermatologists spend large chunks of their working lives dealing with it and many people break their hearts over it; but it can be treated.

All sweat glands are affected by androgens, and that includes the special ones in armpits and round the sex organs, the apocrine glands. These are bigger than ordinary sweat glands and make a thicker sort of sweat which is acted on by bacteria in the air and broken down to smell in the way that has made a fortune for deodorant manufacturers. It is at puberty that decomposing sweat first starts to give off this adult odour – and also probably the less easily identified smells called pheremones, about which more later (see page 64). This can be a useful early signal that the growth of puberty has started in girls who show little else in the way of other changes.

Not only does the smell of sweat change; so does the smell of the vulva, the surface sex organs. Normally an agreeable smell in a healthy child, it becomes stronger and richer as the vulva shares in the general growth (see pages 35 to 36). This smell too is a part of the adult sexual signalling system (about which more in Section five).

There are other body parts affected by all this busy growth. The voice is one; the shrillness of the little girl which sounds much the same as the shrillness of the little boy becomes warmer as the larynx (voice box) grows, and the tone may deepen. The girl now sounds more womanly, though she'll be eighteen or so before her voice settles to its full adult timbre.

Bony growth also affects the hands and feet and the shape of the face. The girl who looked like a drawing by Mabel Lucy Atwell now develops visible cheekbones, a stronger nose, longer fingers and feet. She also develops a wider 'carrying angle' to her arms. That is, when she stands with her arms at her sides and her palms facing forwards (with thumbs to the outside) the lower part of the arm from the elbow makes a wider angle than it does in a male. This ensures that her arms clear easily her wider hips. Nature is as ever efficient in her planning and designing.

All these changes mean that it can be a startling experience for a pubertal child to look in a mirror. Sometimes it feels as if she's gazing at a stranger, she's changed so much. Yet it all happens over just twenty-four months or so, barely a hundred weeks. This growth and change will continue, of course, for some time. The girl will be twenty or more before she can feel she is a full-grown adult, but most major changes will show by the time her periods start; she is the woman she was born to become.

But growth and change will have affected not only the visible parts of the body, but also the hidden ones; the sexual organs in particular. In the next section there is a detailed account of the structure and working of the ovaries, tubes and uterus, the internal organs of reproduction, but here let's consider just the breasts and then the surface sex organs, the vulva, in which a great deal of change happens in the pubertal months.

The breasts

Not only is fat laid down under the nipples of the pubertal child; so is glandular tissue. It is the combination of both that create the shape of the breasts.

Breasts are generally said to be cone-shaped, but the variation in normal shape is really tremendous. Some women have tiptilted little breasts; others have large ones, some have heavy ones, some very small ones – and the difference shows fairly early in development.

There is also a great variation in the placing of the breasts on the chest wall. Some women are born to be high breasted, others to be low breasted; the positioning is an inherited factor, and it doesn't have to be passed on in the female line. Thus, a woman who is high breasted can have a daughter who develops low breasts because she inherited the tendency from her father (who got it from his parents) just as a woman with big breasts can produce a daughter with very tiny ones. All are normal, and all will function as they are designed to do, given the chance.

The nipples and the area around them – the areola – start to grow in puberty, and the effect at first may seem to a child to be rather odd. They look swollen and they change their shape from time to time; when the child is cold, for example, the nipples seem to shrink and the central portion rises into a harder section. This erection happens because the nipples are provided with numerous muscle fibres which react to various stimuli. Cold isn't the only one; simple friction can do it and sexual excitement also has this effect. It's a useful ability; it helps a breast feeding baby to get hold of the source of food more easily, and since the one and only function of the breast is to feed an infant (it is only incidentally a sexual toy) it is a vital part of the organ's structure and abilities.

When the nipple starts to develop it can itch a good deal, and many children find this tiresome and a little disturbing; when they scratch they may find there is some stimulation of sexual feeling, which can bewilder a child who doesn't realize what is happening. Once she is reassured it's normal and nothing to be ashamed of or upset about, she'll find it much easier to live with.

Breast growth tends not to be steady; there may be a time when the breasts seem to sprout a great deal and then nothing at all happens for a while. There may be uneven

Stages of puberty

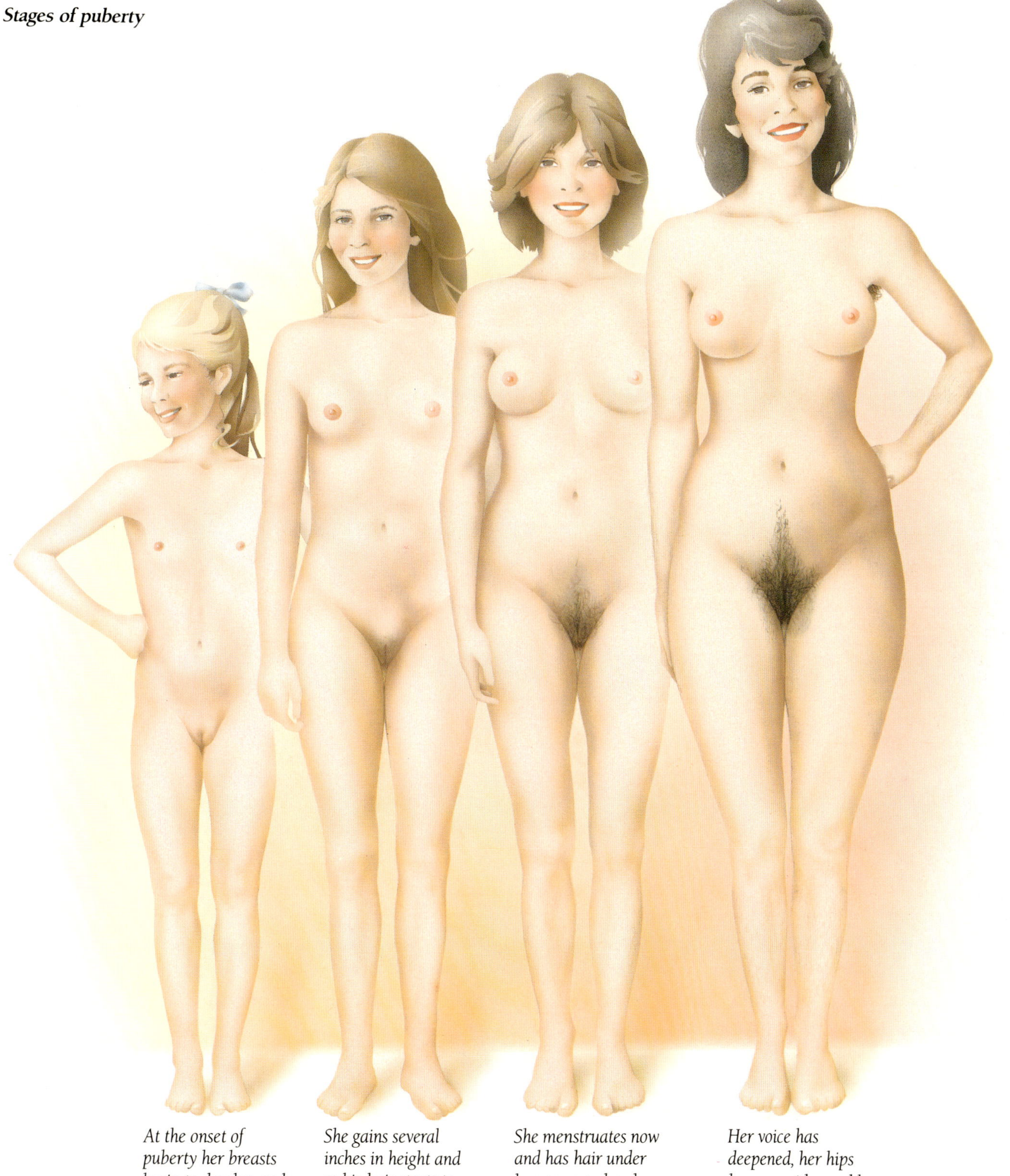

At the onset of puberty her breasts begin to develop and the nipples to darken. (Average age eight years old.)

She gains several inches in height and pubic hair starts to appear. (Average age eleven years old.)

She menstruates now and has hair under her arms and on her upper lip and belly. (Average age fourteen years old.)

Her voice has deepened, her hips become wider and her breasts more full. (Average age seventeen years old.)

Different shaped breasts

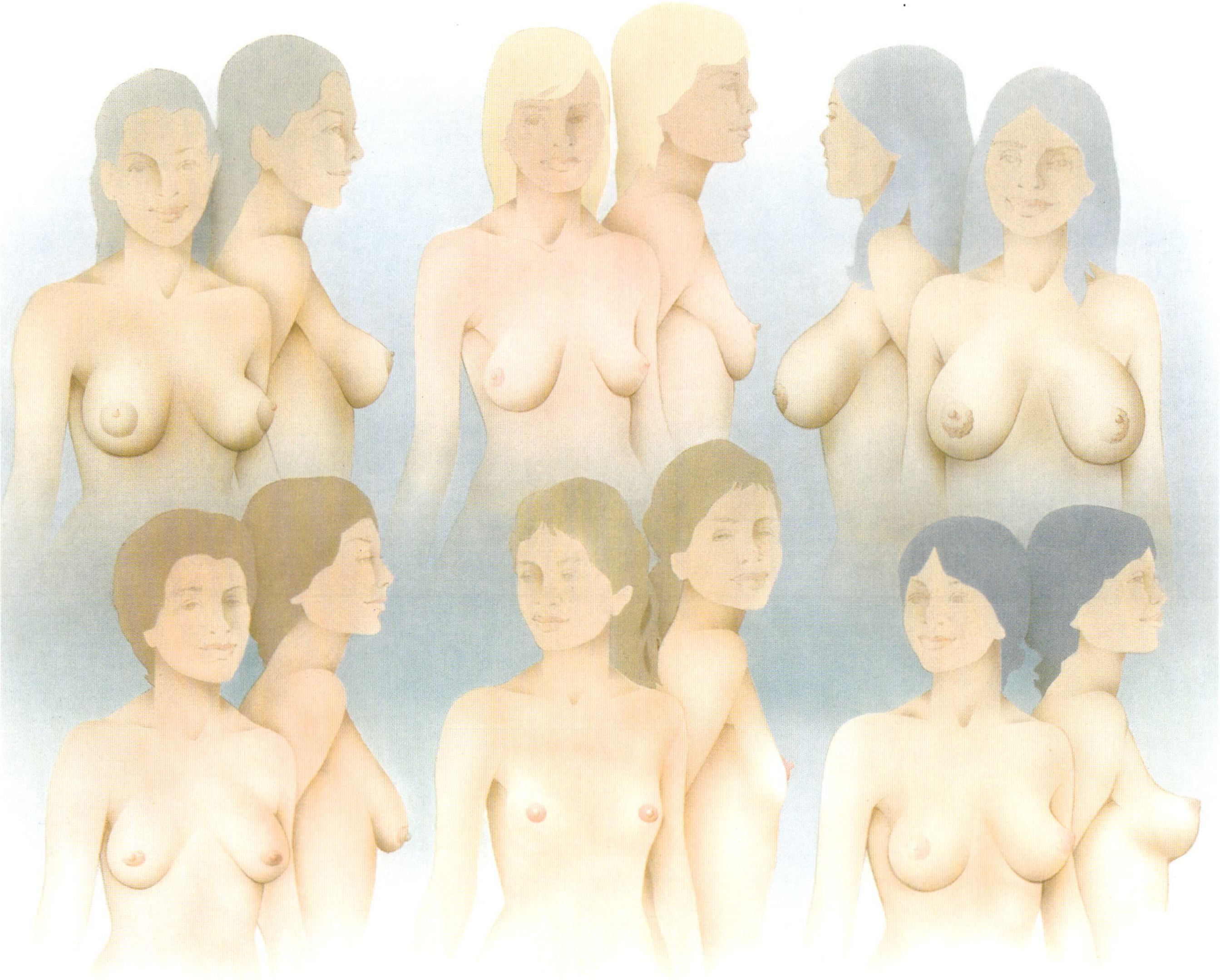

Different shaped nipples

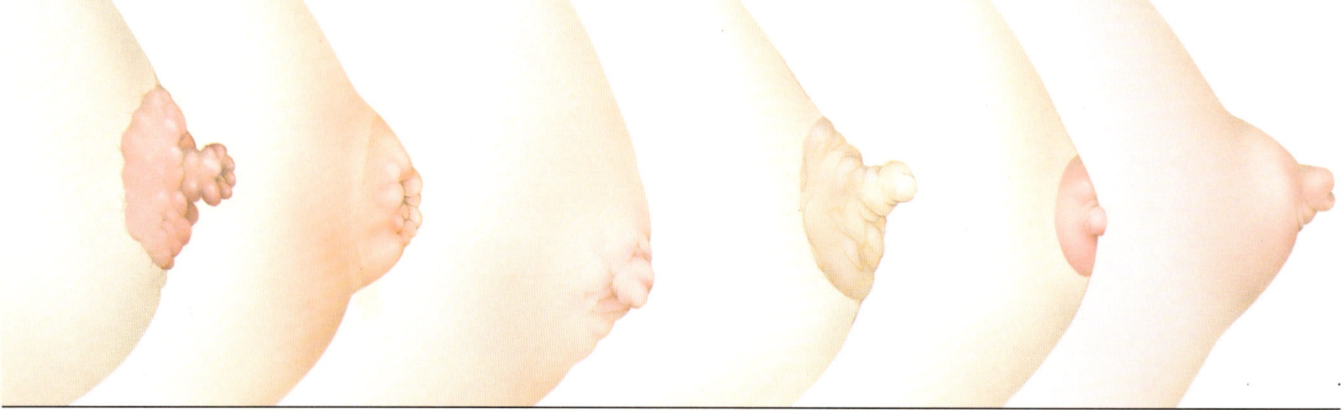

Nipple erection

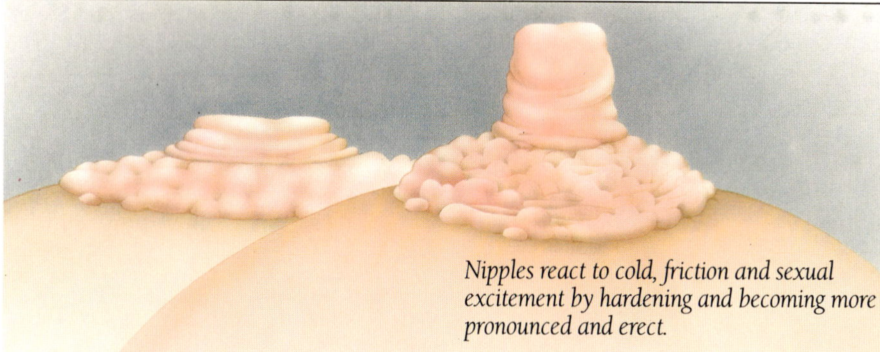

Nipples react to cold, friction and sexual excitement by hardening and becoming more pronounced and erect.

Breast structure

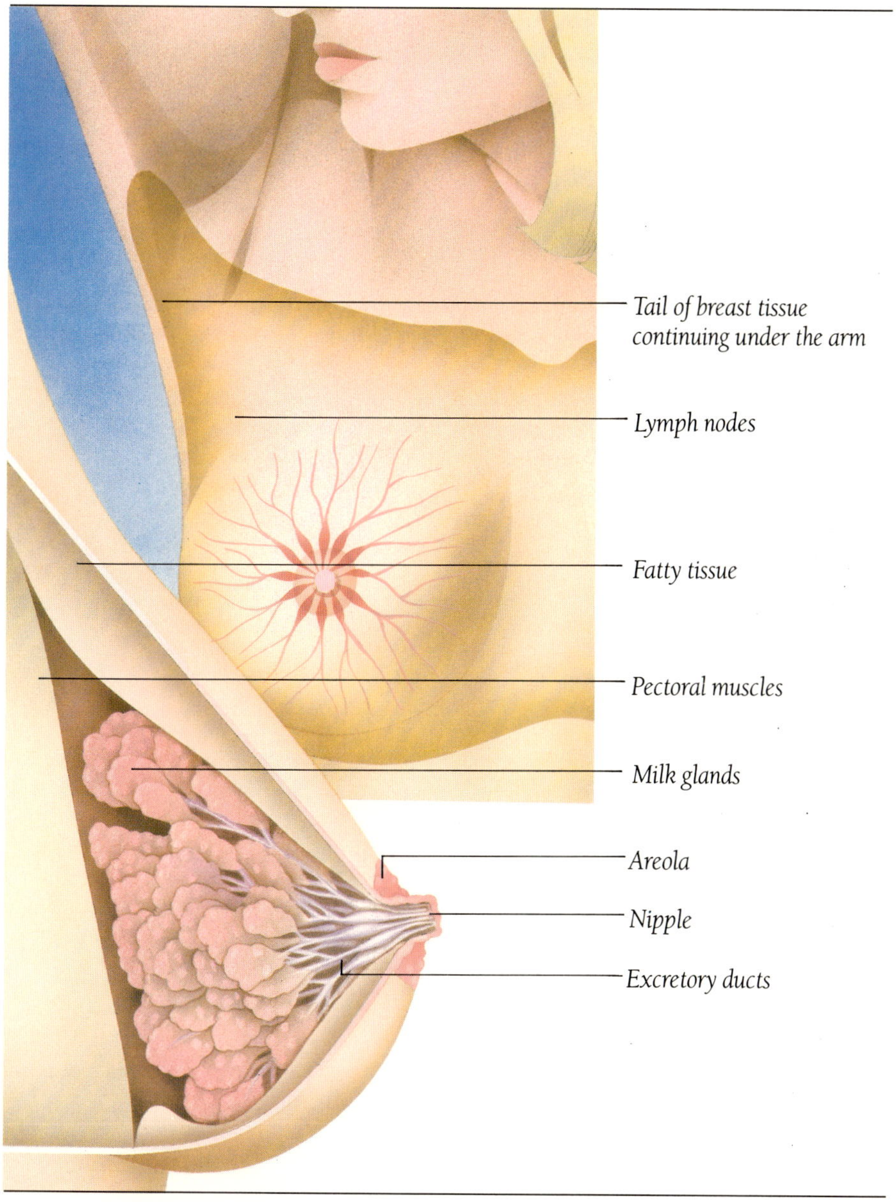

Tail of breast tissue continuing under the arm

Lymph nodes

Fatty tissue

Pectoral muscles

Milk glands

Areola

Nipple

Excretory ducts

Milk lines

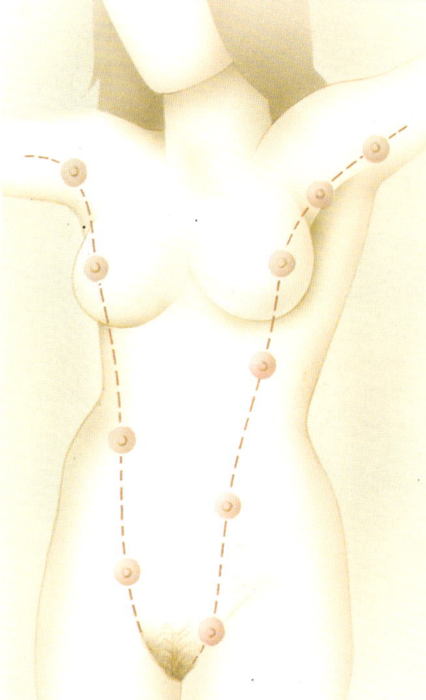

Women still have a pair of milk lines running from the underarm, down the chest and into the groins, where extra nipples can form.

Uneven breast development

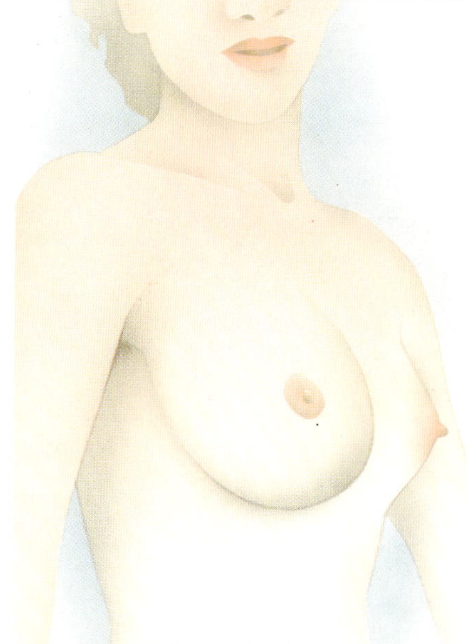

Sometimes one breast develops more quickly than the other, and it is rare for a pair to match exactly.

development with one breast growing much more than the other, with the second one catching up later on. Most people end up with two reasonably matched breasts, though it is rare for them to be an exact pair. Most of us have one that is slightly larger than the other.

In a few cases unfortunately only one breast grows as it should, and the other remains quiescent; in that case, all that can be done is to discuss the possibility of breast augmentation on one side with a surgeon — not an ideal remedy but better than nothing if the disparity is great and upsets its owner a lot.

There is one other very rare anomaly of breast development; extra ones. Like all mammals, we are designed to have rows of nipples. We don't need them, since generally we only produce one baby at a time (see Section six) but we still have a pair of 'milk lines' running from the underarm, down the chest and into the groins, one on each side. Extra nipples and even breasts can rarely appear along these lines. In modern women, the usual response is to have them removed surgically. In ancient times the unfortunate girls who developed them were regarded as witches equipped by Satan to suckle devils. Some of them were burned at the stake.

Breast growth

If the growing child touches her breasts, she will discover that beneath the growing nipple there is a section that feels hard; this is normal. Most people who don't own breasts think they must feel as they look — soft and yielding all the way through to the chest wall, but they are not like that. The glandular tissue inside is resilient to touch but firmer than the fat that surrounds it.

The glandular tissue isn't only beneath the nipple; in the majority of women there is a tail of it that goes up under the arm, which is why some girls at puberty complain of aching there. When the growing glandular tissue become tense and active under the stimulus of a hormone surge, as it often does, this will be felt all around the area, including the underarm.

Often the combination of growth of glandular tissue and the laying down of fat causes a very sudden enlargement of the breasts; within a matter of just a few months the flat chested child is very busty; she may then become aware of the appearance of stretch marks, running round the sides of the breasts and sometimes beneath the nipples, and she might think that this is

The breast growth of puberty

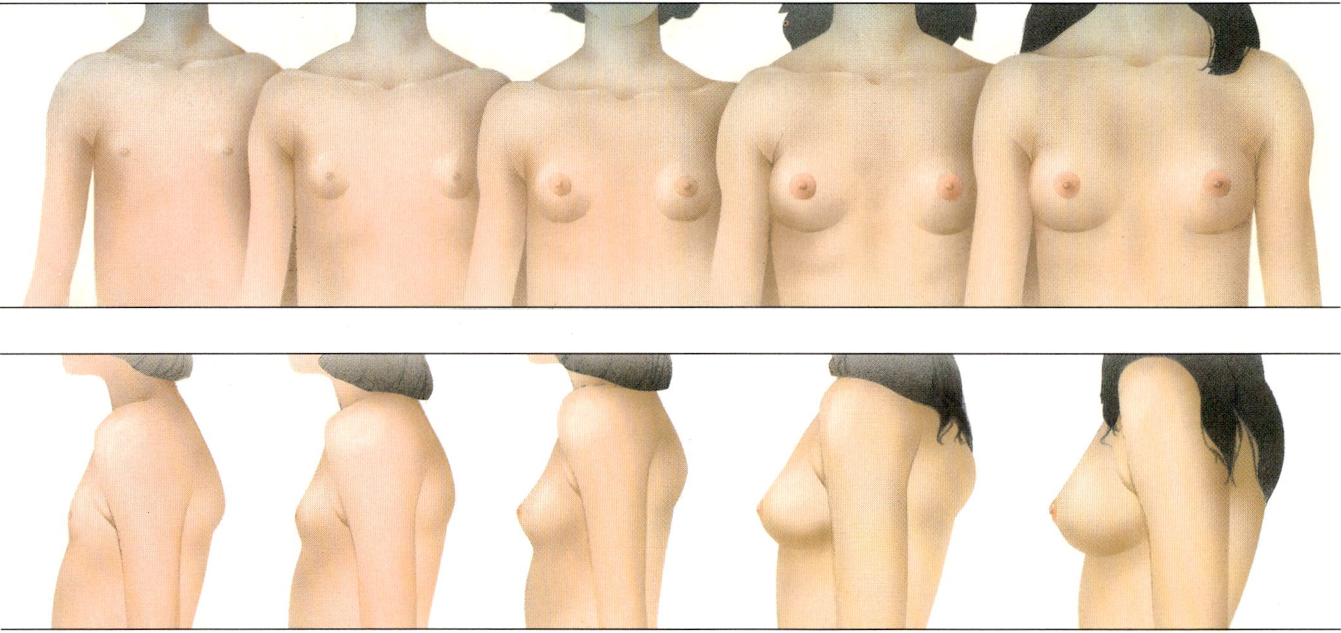

1 *Pre-adolescent elevation of the nipple only. There is no change in the colour of the nipple and its surroundings. There is no glandular tissue. The breasts remain flat.*

2 *The glandular tissue and the nipple start to grow, so that a mound projects from the chest.*

3 *More glandular tissue is formed, and the areola grows and begins to change colour. Everyone varies, but generally red headed girls have very pale pink nipples: blondes have darker pink nipples; brunettes brownish pink nipples, and dark brown and black women almost black nipples. The colour changes again later in life, during pregnancy (see Section six).*

4 *The nipple colour continues to deepen and glandular development goes on, but there is little fat in the breasts yet, so the nipple and areola form a mound on top of the smaller mound that is the underlying breast.*

5 *Fat rounds out the breast more and the nipple and areola come into the same plane as the rest of the breast. Rounding and enlarging can go on for some time yet.*

This whole process usually takes around six years or so.

because her breasts have grown 'too big'. They haven't. The stretch marks are there, not because of the size of the breasts stretching the skin – the skin can and does grow easily to accommodate the development – but because of the action of hormones on the deeper layer of the skin – the dermis. They can appear in girls with modest breast growth as well as in well-endowed ones. The marks can also appear over the buttocks and the thighs (see Section three).

An important fact here – nipples vary as much as breast shapes do. Some are the familiar simple flat-topped protrusion, but some look slightly twisted; some are pointed; some are fragmented; some are inverted (they look more like dimples than pimples) and some look like little knobs thicker at the top than at the place where they are joined to the breast. All these are normal and in no way damage the breasts or spoil the ability to feed a baby.

The vulva

Beneath the pad of fat that covers the meeting point of the bony girdle called the pelvis, at the base of the belly (it is called the *mons veneris*, by the way, the 'Mount of Venus' – rather pretty) lie a pair of soft 'lips'. They are called in Latin the *labia majora* 'the big lips' and when hair begins to grow on the *mons veneris* it grows on its outer surfaces too.

In little girls the *labia majora* lie close to each other, protecting what lies within, and so they create a slit (one little girl I know called hers her 'smiley' because she reckoned that was how it looked, tucked there between the upward pointing lines of her groins – a rather friendly name).

Another pair of lips lie within, the *labia minora* ('the little lips'). These are not covered with skin, and so no hair can grow on them (hair can grow only on skin). They are not fleshy either, being really more flaps of tissue than full soft structures like their big sister lips.

At the back, that is, towards the anus, the opening of the rectum, they open out and create a fairly wide gap on each side of the entry to the vagina, the pathway to the uterus inside; but at the front they meet at a tiny button of very sensitive tissue called the clitoris. Between the clitoris and the vaginal opening – usually nearer to the former than to the latter – there is the mouth of the tube that comes from the bladder, out of which the urine emerges. This is called the urethra.

So the opening to the vagina lies between the bladder in front and the rectum behind, a fact which made one dour Scottish gynaecologist comment sourly that he 'couldna' think what the Guid Lord was about to set the nursery between the sewers' – which may sound like a sexist comment but actually isn't. The sex organs are indeed intimately involved with the organs of excretion and this is a fact that sometimes makes sexual activity, pregnancy and giving birth a more complicated affair than it might be (see Section five).

The little lips and the inner sides of the big lips and the part that lies in front of the clitoris, between the little lips (called the *vestibule* since it lies adjacent to the opening to the vagina, and is the Latin for 'opening'; most of us know the word as meaning the lobby at the entrance of a building. It's always interesting to see how the old anatomists described the human body, isn't it?) – are all covered in mucous membrane. This is pink, damp and well provided with glands that create mucus, the clear slippery liquid that keeps it soft and moist. It's the same sort of tissue which lines the nose and mouth and parts of the lower gut and other areas of the body.

As well as plenty of mucus-producing glands, it also contains the openings of some other special glands (Bartholin's) which have the job of producing extra mucus when it is needed for lubrication during sexual intercourse (see Section five for more information on this).

There are other labels for other parts of the vulva which can be useful to know; like the hymen, or maidenhead. This is a thin fold of membrane which partially covers the opening of the vagina in the child. It is stretchy and has holes in it – sometimes

The vulva during childhood

The vulva after puberty

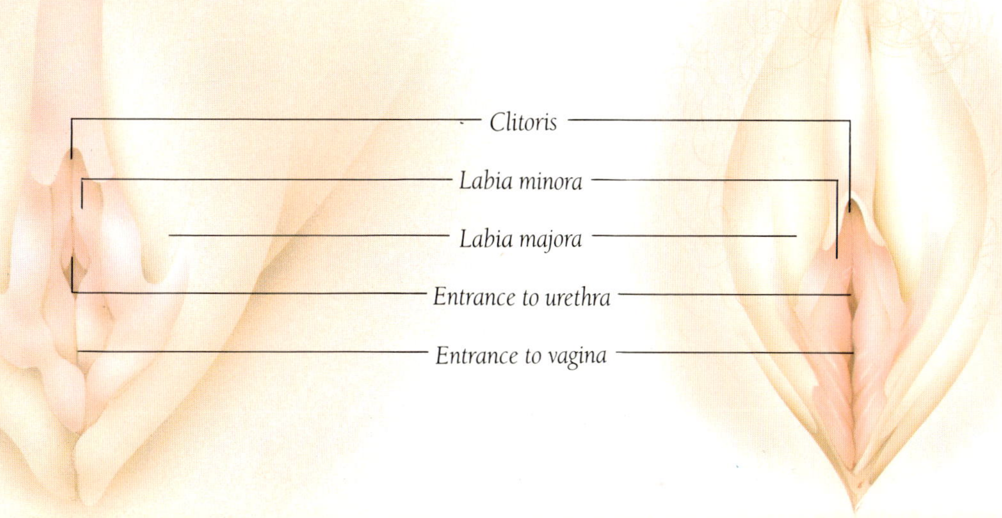

one, sometimes more. It has to have them, to allow the menstrual fluid to escape (see Section three). In the very rare cases in which it totally closes the vagina, the fluid can collect, harden and cause pressure and considerable discomfort. It then needs to be surgically opened, but it is well worth repeating that this is very unusual — almost as rare as hen's teeth.

More nonsense is talked about the hymen than any other part of a woman's body, since it has been for many years the symbol of virginity. It is widely believed that it is a tough protective barrier that has to be 'torn' or 'broken' during a woman's first experience of sexual intercourse, and that it always bleeds copiously and hurts horribly. This is not necessarily so; in fact in many a young woman it is so small a barrier that she feels no discomfort when she first has intercourse, because she is relaxed, eager and fully aroused. The practice of some societies to inspect the bedding of the newly married bride to make sure she bled properly, as evidence of her virginity and therefore fitness for marriage is not only a social insult (who ever checks on the men to make sure they are fit and virginal for their new wives?) but an anatomical one. Some girls can't bleed however virginal they are because their hymens create no barrier to the exploring penis.

Fortunately for the peace of mind of many such girls in these societies, older women tend to be well aware of the real facts of anatomy and send their daughters to bed for the first sexual encounter with their husbands equipped with a little bottle of animal blood to smear discreetly around as evidence, should they need it.

Incidentally it is not until the birth of the first baby that the hymen is likely finally to be lost, turning into tiny tags that fringe the vaginal opening. They're called *carunculae myrtiformes*, which is Latin for 'tiny bits of flesh'. It sounds more elegant in Latin.

More labels to conjure with — the furthest outpost of the vulva at the rear is the fourchette — fork, what else — where the skin joins to become the skin covered area that lies between the vulva and the opening of the anus. This is called the perineum, and it's a very important structure. It's a wedge-shaped piece of tissue made of muscle which separates the vagina and the rectum, and it has to stretch a great deal in childbirth. This can lead to damage (about which more in Section six).

There, then, is the structure of the surface sex organs and what happens to it all in puberty is considerable. The mucous membrane thickens and produces more mucus, so much that it can be felt by the child as a discharge. Not only does the vulva become more moist — so does the lining of the vagina and this can come away and stain a child's panties with a little whitish material. This is perfectly normal, but sometimes alarming when it first happens to a girl who has not been told of it. Equally the change in her body smell may surprise her. It is quite natural for women to enjoy their own clean and healthy smells — just as it is normal for men to enjoy them too (see Section five).

The appearance of vaginal moisture is an early sign of puberty and it is followed fairly soon by development of the tissues. The outer lips become thicker and fatter, and hairy, but more startling in some ways is the development of the inner lips.

They change from being tiny flaps into often very sizeable flaps indeed. Sometimes both grow long. Sometimes one does and the other remains fairly small. Often they start to protrude between the outer lips and chafe uncomfortably against the skin and underwear, and become very dry as they lose their protective mucus. The result is an itchy sometimes sore vulva which embarrasses its owner a good deal. It can also make her feel very worried and guilty, because one effect of all this growth — which includes the clitoris — is that she handles her own vulva more and finds she likes doing it.

All children explore their genitals with their fingers. That's what fingers are for, exploring the environment, and our own bodies are as much a part of our environment as anything else. Once puberty arrives, with all the new and sexually arousing hormones surging round the body, the simple exploratory handling of childhood start to become the more purposeful self-stimulation of puberty. The growing girl discovers that stroking her newly developed and now much more sensitive clitoris gives her very agreeable feelings. It is meant to, of course; women are designed to find pleasure in their own sexuality, and this early self-stimulation is necessary preparation for the time when it will be provided by a sexual partner.

But, often, young girls are not told this any more than they are told that their vulvae will grow and change. They learn it on their own, and unless they are fortunate enough to have relaxed and sensible parents and teachers who are unfussed about sex, are all too likely to get guilty feelings about it. It has been part of Western culture for many years to denigrate and fear women's sexuality, and it is almost inevitable that the uninformed girl exposed to such ideas will feel guilty shame about finding pleasure in her own body — and when she discovers that her *labia minora* are getting itchy, and are growing large and beginning to stick out beyond their outer lips, the result can be even greater guilt and shame. Many are the young girls who write frantic letters to the problem pages of magazines and newspapers begging to know how they can get secret operations to remove this dreadful damage they've done to themselves. All very sad, and so unnecessary.

All this will happen some time before the first period occurs. Once that happens, the girl is regarded by her elders as changed and in need of different treatment, which is an experience her brothers do not have. Their most obvious sign of sexual maturity is the first night-time emission of semen, but this can easily be hidden, and kept a secret by the boy who enjoys it (if he's aware it happened, that is. Not all boys are so aware at first). A girl can't so easily hide the fact that she has periods (though some do, amazingly, for a long time, coping incredibly well, in secret). In the West, often a girl who menstruates finds new controls are put on her comings and goings; when once she was happily allowed out to play, now parents want to know where she is and who with, and worry a good deal if boys are involved in the plans. In some societies she is not allowed to be with boys at all, and has to be chaperoned at all times; in rural Spain and Italy, Turkey and Greece, for example. In other parts of the world (and at other times in history) a girl's first period is marked by special ceremonies of initiation into adult society.

Some are rather bizarre to Western eyes, but why should they be? They do have the virtue of making the girl take pride and pleasure in her new status. In the 'civilized' world we tend to ignore this event and deny our girls their glory, which seems a pity to say the least. Some sort of celebration would be rather nice, wouldn't it?

Emotional effects of puberty

We are, of course, complete creations — minds and emotions as well as bodies — so the changes of puberty bring inevitable changes in our patterns of thinking and feeling and behaving. It's these that cause the upheavals that are part of adolescence, and it's because the development of emotions and intellectual maturity takes rather longer to complete than do the physical changes of puberty that adolescence lasts for so long.

The most important change of puberty is perhaps the sudden self-awareness it brings, an awareness that lasts all through adolescence. Children are, of course, intensely self-centred; the human infant is beyond doubt a most vociferous demander of immediate satisfaction of its own desires; but it has no self-awareness at all. Older children can be charmingly altruistic, showing warm concern for others' welfare but still making their own demands without thinking much at all about why they want what they want, or why they feel as they do, just reacting to their feelings as they are.

But the pubertal child starts to look inwards as the changes in her body make her ever more aware of herself. 'Who am I?' 'Why am I?' 'What do I want?' 'What will happen to me?' are all unspoken questions which clutter her mind and give rise to a great deal of introspection. The pubertal child, once happy to be in the centre of the family group, takes to sitting on her own in her room (if she's allowed to, and has the luxury of a room of her own, that is) or goes off to be by herself where she can't be found. She becomes secretive, needing to lock away her possessions, to prevent others from knowing what she has hidden and why. (This is often the sort of behaviour that most aggravates the rest of the family, who may well feel they are being silently accused of being nosy at best, potential robbers at worst.)

She may keep a diary, may compose poetry or music if she has gifts in that direction, or develop sudden interests in people, places or activities which may be dropped as suddenly as they were taken up. Yearning passions develop for people or animals or activities which, to the family's chagrin, become more important to her than anything else. The child who once loved nothing better than going on a family outing now refuses to budge because there is skating on television; the child who once seemed to care for her relations now seems to pour all her love into horses; the child who was once open to all sorts of interests now sneers at anything and everything — except, of course, her own particular pop group passion. Often her friend or friends become very obviously far more important in her life than her parents or her brothers or sisters.

All of which can obviously cause some spectacular family rows for which the child is blamed by all and sundry. But this is grossly unfair, because it isn't all her fault. Yes, pubertal children can seem headstrong, selfish and unpredictable, but to assume they are always deliberately so, or that they could by a mere act of will behave differently is to add sorely to their burdens. The child can no more help her swift changes of mind, her self-absorption and her bewildering switches from being her old sweet biddable childlike self to a prickly, arrogant, raucous almost-adult than she can help the way her body is changing. Living with a pubertal child can be exceedingly difficult for all the people involved, and in families where children are close in age, and two or even three sisters are going through their couple of years of storms at the same time because they overlap, domestic life can feel rather like a switchback ride.

But it's important that somehow adults do keep their heads when the ride is at its bumpiest; the pubertal and adolescent child is not only unpredictable but very vulnerable. Lack of patience at home can drive her out to seek her comforts and reassurance elsewhere; hence the alarming stories one hears of young people getting involved with glue sniffing, alcohol and drug abuse, premature sex and assorted forms of anti-social behaviour.

In saying, incidentally, that patience is needed, it is not being suggested that all restraints should be removed. The pubertal and early adolescent child needs a firm framework within which to do her growing up safely; she needs rules and regulations against which to kick, and the more she kicks the more she needs them because her emotional and intellectual muscle develops just as physical muscles do, by pushing against resistance; but it is possible for parents and teachers to provide that framework and to stand braced against the fury that may erupt with good humour and above all without anger and recriminations. It is possible to make it clear to a child who is struggling to grow up that you dislike some forms of her behaviour and won't tolerate them, without making her feel you dislike her. Too often in their attempts to control noisy teenagers adults fill them with a sense of self-disgust, convincing them they are worthless and unwanted people. Is it any wonder then that growing up successfully becomes even more difficult?

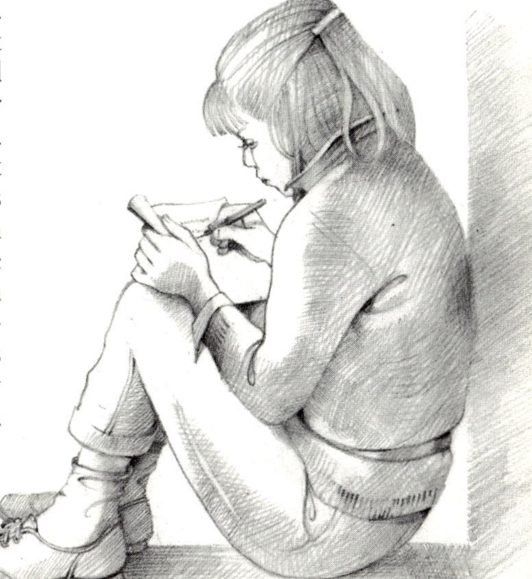

3
WOMAN'S RHYTHM

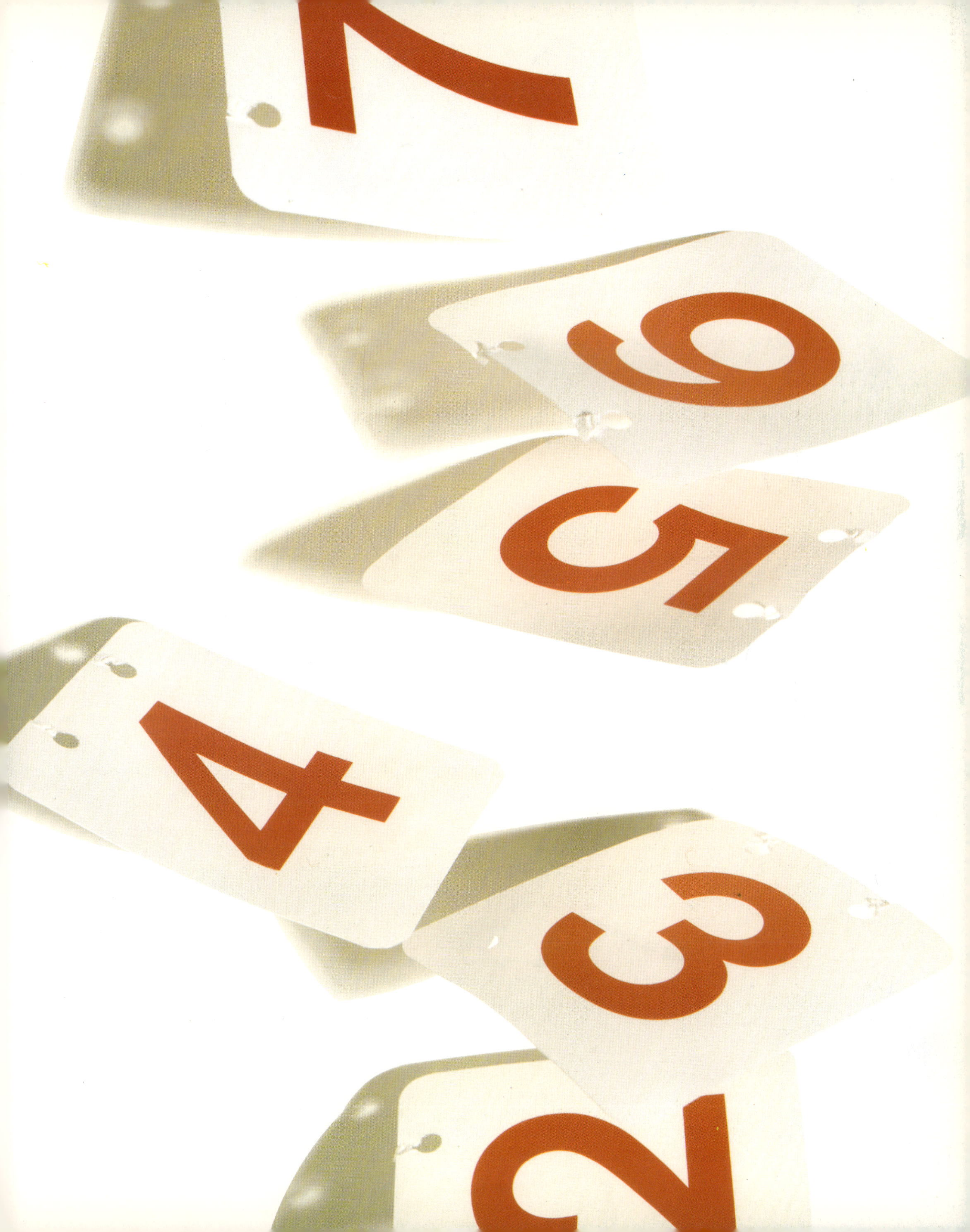

The one aspect of femininity that few women actually admit to enjoying is menstruation. They may take great pleasure in conceiving, carrying and giving birth to a baby, and may cheerfully devote many years of their lives to child caring and the invevitable domesticity that goes with it, but when it comes to periods, they regard them as an irritating inconvenience at best, a painful, wearing and debilitating burden at worst. And since the average woman who starts her periods at around the age of twelve or so and reaches her menopause at around fifty, having three children on the way, will menstruate some 450 times, that seems a pity to put it at its lowest.

It's hard to be sure just why menstruation should be regarded by so many as 'the curse' and as so unpleasant an experience. It doesn't happen every day, unlike the need to empty bladder and bowels — yet few people complain about that. They accept it as part of living, like breathing and eating, and occasionally as a source of pleasure; who hasn't spent a peaceful ten minutes in the lavatory reading a book while they sat and emptied their bowels, and found it a relaxing and satisfying experience? There can't be many. So why can't women experience their periods in this comfortable and enjoyable way?

For some there is undoubtedly a physical cause for pain, tension, sickness and debility; they are the ones for whom the hormonal control is not as smooth and easy as it should be, and for whom, therefore, periods become not just a normal physiological function but a form of illness (see Section four). But for many others there is no such hormonal disorder, yet still they dislike menstruating. Why?

Much of the dislike is, I believe, based on resentment of the female state, and women feel that resentment because they have been taught to do so. If you study the history of the relationship between the sexes you realise that male fear of female function started early in human society.

First of all primitive men gazed with awe on these fellow human beings who had the capacity to swell up and then produce new human beings; they saw it as magic. It seems that they did not understand the connection between sexual intercourse, engaged in purely for their own pleasure, and the appearance of an infant almost a year later.

Secondly they were puzzled by creatures who could bleed without being in any way injured and who did so in regular cycles;

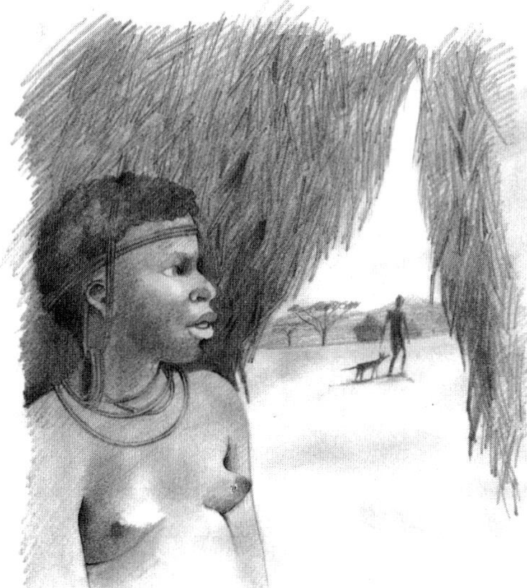

Separating menstruating women from their fellows is common practice in certain societies — even in the modern world.

this ability made women seem as mysterious and somehow remote as the moon in the sky which also behaved in a cyclical manner, appearing and disappearing, waxing and waning, seemingly at will.

Since the best way to deal with what frightens you was then, as it is now, to sneer at it, to try to control it, to subjugate it and thereby cut it down to a manageable size, the only way to handle women and their periods was to sneer at them and reject them while they were displaying their alarming abilities. That they did just that is undoubted; in many scattered groups around the world ceremonies evolved which separated the menstruating women from her fellows, and insisted that she behaved in a way that clearly demonstrated to all her 'uncleanness'. Under Mosaic law for example (which is obeyed to the letter among some orthodox Jews to this day) menstruating women may not cohabit with their husbands, may not serve food to them or handle kitchen utensils or sit in the same room with them. Only after the blood flow has ceased for a prescribed number of days and they have submitted to a ritual and very thorough submersion in water may they once more return to matrimonial closeness.

And it is not only in the marital relationship that they are spurned in this manner and regarded as 'the ultimate in corruption, a walking, suppurating, reeking pestilence' to quote one noted Jewish commentator; they may not attend certain communal religious activities — even funerals.

While the ancient taboos have generally lapsed in the modern world, there are undoubtedly lingering remnants still with us, and it is significant and sad that it is among women themselves that they are mostly to be found now. Far too many believe that they are 'unwell' when they have a period. Far too many believe that it is unhealthy to swim, exercise, go out in the cold/heat, wash their hair or have intercourse (all nonsense; you can do all of them, all at the same time if you can and you want to). Far too many regard the flow as a 'clearing out of impurities' when it is nothing of the sort.

Far too many are ashamed of the fact that they menstruate. They are literally terrified that they may in some way reveal to outsiders the fact that they are having a period. Sanitary towels must not show their outline under their clothes; there must be absolutely no odour of blood; there must never be any staining of clothing. Many are the manufacturers who have made considerable fortunes from marketing their goods by promising that their products will be discreet in use, and in seeming to soothe feminine fears by offering such items as deodorants, special small-sized pads and so on, they do of course feed the shame and fear that their customers already have. Excellent business, that!

Yet there is no need for this attitude. So what if the fact that you are wearing a sanitary pad can be detected? (And by the way isn't that an interesting euphemism? Why not call it what it is, a blood napkin, why should blood be considered unsanitary?) So what if people see a packet of tampons in your bag when you open it? (Most women hide them away in special little

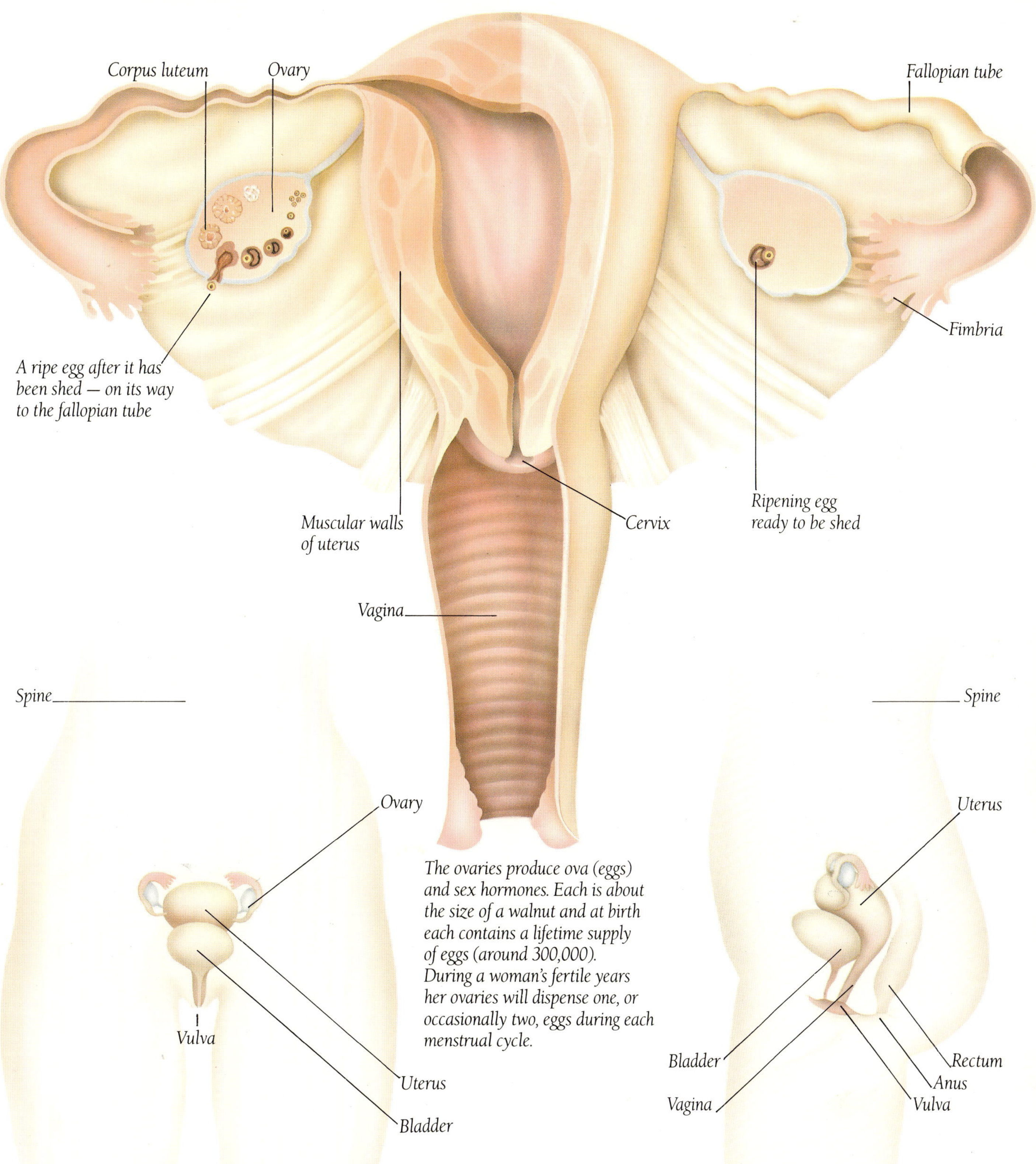

The ovaries produce ova (eggs) and sex hormones. Each is about the size of a walnut and at birth each contains a lifetime supply of eggs (around 300,000). During a woman's fertile years her ovaries will dispense one, or occasionally two, eggs during each menstrual cycle.

The internal sex organs consist of the vagina, the uterus and its neck the cervix, the fallopian tubes and the ovaries.

Side view of the sex organs supported by ligaments and muscles, encased protectively within the bones of the pelvic girdle.

containers) Menstruation is not an experience to be ashamed of — yet many women are ashamed of it, and feel it as painful and unpleasant as a result. Unfortunately anxiety and stress can cause menstrual disorders of various kinds, as will be seen in the next section.

Menstruation can and should be as comfortable as any other normal physical function, and every woman has the capacity, within herself, to make it just that. She can, of her own will, control discomfort by getting rid of the resentment she has been given of her own body. Her body is a beautiful superbly functioning structure and she should glory in its actions, not be afraid of or disgusted by them. Perhaps to help us to see it in that light we need to know more of how it is made and how it works.

The internal sex organs

These consist of the vagina — the pathway from the surface of the body at the vulva, to the uterus — the uterus itself with its neck, the cervix, which dips down into the vagina and the fallopian tubes which run from the upper 'corners' of the uterus to the ovaries, which lie on each side of the uterus. The whole group is supported on a series of ligaments and muscles which hold them comfortably in place, and which allow them the room for manoeuvre and growth which is vital for a successful pregnancy.

The uterus, which is the centre of the group, lies tilted slightly forwards, between bladder and rectum, and the top of it (called the fundus) lies below the level of the pelvic rim, which means that it is all well protected inside its bony cage. Not that it is a particularly fragile structure, quite the reverse. The uterus is one of the toughest and most remarkable organs; the only one in the human body that is capable of first growing and then ungrowing — that is, actually reducing its bulk (see Section six) and the muscle of its walls is about the strongest there is, after that of the heart. In an adult woman the uterus is a little smaller in size than her clenched fist, and it is made largely of that thick strong muscle. Inside there is a triangular shaped cavity, with the apex pointing downwards. There it meets the cervix, the opening of the uterus.

This is also made of strong muscle, in a ring shape, and it looks rather like your own small finger, clenched closed. In the middle there is a small hole; much too small to let in a finger or a tampon or a penis, but big enough to welcome in sperm, and to let out menstrual fluid.

The cervix dips down into the vagina, which is a bit like an empty toothpaste tube, in that it has a considerable capacity, but is usually collapsed so that the walls touch each other.

The vagina has its large capacity because it has ridged walls; these can be stretched out smooth creating a very large space indeed — big enough to allow a full grown infant, complete with its large head, to get through. That is why it is never true that a woman is 'too small' for comfortable sex. There was never a man alive with a penis so big or so erect that it could not be comfortably accommodated by an adult vagina; when there are difficulties and tightness it is because the muscles which guard the entrance to the vagina, and which are very powerful indeed, have tightened up to repel entry. This is called vaginismus and is dealt with in more detail in Section five on page 70.

The vagina is always moist, because like the vulva it is well supplied with mucus-making glands, but sometimes it is much more moist than at others. It produces copious quantities of lubricating fluid when a woman is sexually aroused, to make intercourse comfortable, but this is not the only source of fluid. The cervix also produces its own secretion, which varies in make-up at different stages of the menstrual and reproductive cycle (see also Section six, on conception and pregnancy) and which mixes with vaginal secretions to act as a guard system; the secretions have a certain acid level (called the pH) which enables it to destroy invading germs, and they also wash out debris such as dead cells and invading foreign bodies. This means the vagina is a very efficient self-cleansing organ and it needs no help to do its job. Using douches and chemicals and deodorants is not only totally unnecessary but actually damages vaginal health because it interferes with its ability to do what it is designed to do.

To return to the central triangular cavity of the uterus — the upper 'corners' run into the cavities which are in the centre of the fallopian tubes. These are a remarkable pair of organs too; they form the pathway from the ovaries at their other end into the uterus, but they are not just passive roads; their hollow centres are lined with tiny cilia: hairlike projections which wave from side to side and so waft the contents of the tube along. There are myriad tiny folds in the tubes and they are capable of muscular movement, so they play an active role in transporting their contents from one end of their four inch length to the other end. There, they open out into the fimbria, very pretty fronds which, like the cilia, wave about, and in so doing attract into the opening of the tube anything which is within their reach.

In fact they attract ova, the eggs produced by the ovary, and these are carried along the tubes' hollow centres. Each ovary is about the size of a walnut, in an adult, and each contains, when a little girl is born, a potential of up to three hundred thousand ova. The generosity of Nature is breathtaking.

Menstruation

All this starts to grow when a child starts puberty and also to change. The pituitary hormones, pushed into action by the releasing factors sent out by the thalamus, a part of the brain, start to act on the uterus, just as they do on the other parts of the body (see Section two) and eventually they stimulate the ovaries into action. There is no rule about which ovary is stimulated — probably both at the same time. They start to ripen between ten and twenty of the minute bubbles — follicles — on the surface of the organs in which the eggs lie, and as they ripen they release the hormone estrogen (that means 'egg making').

The estrogen gets into the blood, and so sends a feedback message to the hypothalamus which in turn instructs the pituitary on how much of its hormone (called FSH: follicle stimulating hormone) is needed. This prevents the ovaries from over-producing estrogen; it's a neat feedback loop system and one the body uses in many other functions too.

One of the up-to-twenty follicles which is ripening outstrips the others, and this leads to a peak of estrogen in the blood. That makes the pituitary change tack. It sends another hormone (LH, or luteinizing hormone) to the ripe follicle, which makes it burst, releasing the egg. This happens at about fourteen days after the follicle started to ripen. (In the very first follicle that appears before a child's first period, the ovum does not actually ripen fully — it could not be fertilized to grow into an infant — but the follicle behaves as though its ovum is ripe.)

The egg floats free for a while and then is drawn into the fallopian tube by the fimbria, to start its journey along the cavity, during which it is helped along by the cilia and the tube's muscular movements.

Meanwhile, back at the ovary, the work continues. The burst follicle becomes a yellowish scar called the *corpus luteum* ('yellow body' in Latin) and the LH — luteinizing, i.e. yellow-making — hormone encourages it to produce another hormone as well as the estrogen.

This is progesterone. The word means 'pregnancy-making' and it has the job of preparing the body to receive a fertilized ovum and nurture it. It makes the lining of the uterus, called the endometrium (literally 'inside the uterus') thicken and develop extra blood vessels which will be needed to carry food and oxygen-laden blood to the fertilized egg if it gets there. It also acts on the breasts, making their glandular tissue prepare to make milk in the future, and — working with the adrenal hormones — on the body's general levels of fluids, sugars and salt; it's all part of the preparation, like a good householder laying in supplies against the arrival of a much wanted guest.

It takes the egg around five days to travel along the fallopian tube to the uterus; if it is going to be successfully fertilized it must meet sperm in the outer third of the tube, and be fertilized there, but at this stage, we will assume no sperm are there (one hopes not, for a pubertal child!).

So, the egg reaches the uterus which, all through that five days, has been developing a thicker, warmer richer lining for its hopefully awaited guest. But this guest is not to stay; it is of no use to the body in its unfertilized state. So, seven or so days later — about twelve to fourteen days after the egg left the follicle — the ovary gives up making progesterone (it knows to do this because a fertilized egg produces its own hormone which signals back to the follicle it left that progesterone is needed; an unfertilized egg does not need progesterone, so the follicle just shuts up shop, as it were. This is another feedback loop.)

The result of the fall in progesterone levels is that the blood vessels which supply the newly thickened endometrium develop little kinks, so that less blood runs through them. This means that some of the surface cells of the endometrium are starved of supplies and die, and patches of dead tissue appear. Blood seeps from the damaged vessels behind the endometrium, and this peels it away from the muscular wall. It's a completely painless process usually, and leads to clotted blood and tissue scraps collecting in the cavity of the uterus.

These clots and tissue then dissolve and, with the uterus making gentle muscular contractions to help it on its way, the liquified blood and lining is pushed out through the little hole (called the os) in the cervix to emerge as menstrual blood in the vagina and eventually at the vulva.

The amount of the flow is variable, the quantity being estimated as being between 10 mls and 80 mls, with an average of 35 mls. (A teaspoon contains 5 mls, by the way, if you want to compare.)

The menstrual cycle

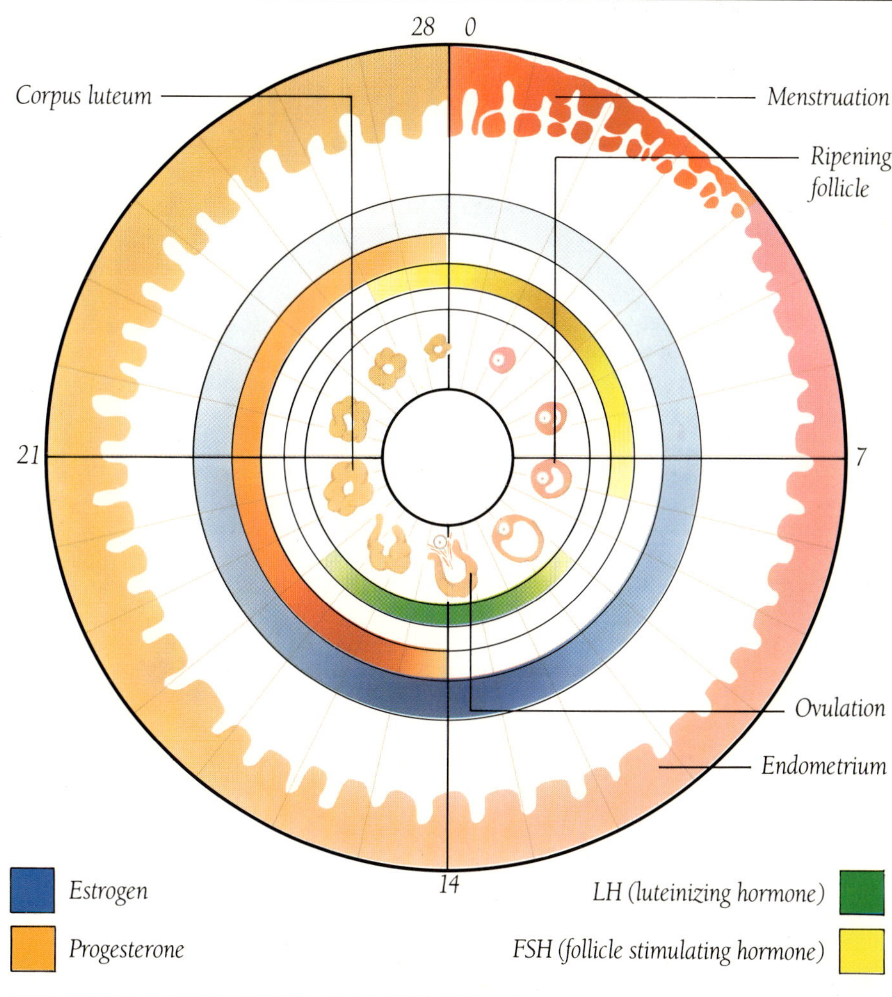

The flow lasts for around five days, so completing the cycle of twenty-eight days altogether. The length of the second half of the cycle — from ovulation to period — is constant, always fourteen days. The length of the first half — from period to ovulation — is not. This is the section that can vary greatly, a fact which has great bearing on the matter of planning when a conception should take place (see Section six).

Meanwhile back at the ovary , the pituitary hormones are once again busily stimulating the follicles to ripen, ensuring that estrogen is produced once more so that one follicle will ripen first and release its ovum, which will be collected by the fimbria and sent on its way, while the burst follicle it left behind starts making progesterone and so the cycle goes on and on and on, like an ever rolling wheel. It's a beautiful and elegant, if complex, system, and it goes on operating, month after month, year after year, all through a woman's reproductive life, which, remember, can last for up to forty years.

Timing

Having said that the menstrual cycle takes twenty-eight days, it is now necessary to make it very clear that this is only a textbook description. There are almost as many variations in a normal menstrual cycle as there are women; what is normal for one is not necessarily so for another.

There are some women who always have an erratic cycle; they may have a period twenty-eight days after the last one — and the next one may not appear for thirty-two days. Or they may have regular long gaps, menstruating every five weeks or even six weeks, just as some have their periods every three weeks. Studies have shown that the cycle is between twenty-four and thirty-five days in ninety-five per cent of women — and the five per cent who are different are usually just as healthy.

The flow can be very variable too; some women lose copious quantities of blood over seven or more days; others have but a scanty flow that lasts only three days. And they too can all be normal. Each woman has her own pattern and will soon learn to recognize it; it is changes in her own normal cycle which may indicate some sort of disorder or cause for anxiety, not the ways in which she differs from her friends.

But learning to recognize your own pattern can take time. The first cycle of the new woman, the girl who has just come through puberty, tends to be unpredictable. After the first period no more may appear for several months. One may be light, the next so copious that the child is alarmed if she hasn't been told this can happen, and thinks she's bleeding dangerously.

Generally the first few periods a girl has are anovulatory — follicles ripen and burst and the hormones swing into action, but no ripe egg is shed. They can also be, for some girls, rather uncomfortable, with cramps and headaches and a heavy flow, but this is by no means inevitable. A great deal depends on how the girl has been told about the workings of her own body, and how much pride and pleasure she is helped to take in it.

The girl who is made to feel she has reached a stage of her life that is to be greeted joyously, and regards her periods as a sort of status symbol — as indeed they are, marking as they do her arrival in the hopeful potentially exciting world of women — is much less likely to find her periods upset her. It is usually the girl who is fearful, ashamed and regretful to be growing up because she's afraid to be a woman who has trouble. Her body reacts to her fears via her endocrine system. Her anxiety pushes up her adrenalin levels which act, via the many feedback loops that operate the endocrine system, on her pituitary and ovaries and so affect her sex hormone levels. One effect of imbalance in estrogen and progesterone is contractions of uterine muscle — just as an action of adrenalin produces contractions of smooth muscle. The result is painful cramps. They can be accompanied by diarrhoea (due to adrenalin again, acting on gut muscles) with a resulting alteration in sugar and salt levels in the blood, as vital substances are lost in watery stools — and that can lead to headaches, nausea and faintness. So there are logical physical reasons why anxiety and fear should make people feel ill.

But it cannot be said too often that periods are not in themselves an illness. A girl is not 'unwell' when she menstruates, any more than she is unwell when she breathes.

Hormonal effects

Because hormones affect the whole body and not just the internal reproductive organs the entire body experiences effects from them. Estrogen as well as being the egg maker is the fat distributor; it is estrogen that ensures that fat desposits are laid down on hips, upper arms, thighs and breasts in such a way that the characteristic female shape is created. Interestingly another feedback loop comes into action here; estrogen is made not only in the ovaries but also in fat — it is a steroid, that is fatlike, chemical — and this can affect the way a woman experiences her menopause later in life. Those with more fat will have higher blood levels of estrogen than thin women (see Section nine).

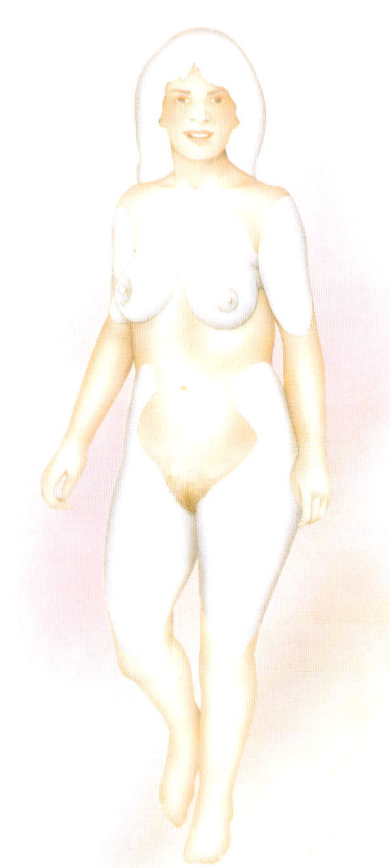

The coloured area shows where estrogen encourages fat deposits.

Estrogen also acts on skin and hair, and so does progesterone; so, at some stages in the cycle the skin and hair will be smooth and lustrous and meet with their owner's approval; at other times hair becomes lank and greasy as extra amounts of sebum are made, and skin develops infected spots. Many women find that the week before a period is due is the time when they get spots on nose, or forehead and more particularly chin, and sometimes on the upper chest at the front and on the back. Such spots seem to have a malevolent will of their own since they appear always on visible skin, but there is a reason for that happening. Skin that is normally covered by clothes is protected from the damage of the climate that makes it more likely to be infected, and is also of course protected from attack by bacteria in the air.

The rapid hormone changes of puberty cause the skin to change so rapidly that it loses some of its ability to keep itself clean and healthy. It will be remembered that as well as estrogen and progesterone the body is also producing androgens — the male type hormones — which act on the oil-producing glands in the skin. The cells which line the tiny duct that runs from each gland to the skin surface start to increase, so narrrowing the outlet. This can block the gland, which is already making extra oil, and so dam it back. Thus is a whitehead formed.

Sometimes the duct does not block, but narrows enough to slow down the escape of the oil. The result of this is that the gland swells to accommodate the extra oil, the oil starts to dry up, and the skin hardening substance called keratin moves into it. When keratin is exposed to air, it goes black. Thus is a blackhead formed.

Blackheads are less of a problem than whiteheads. They can be gently removed — and gentle is the key word; attacking blackheads with sharp nails or hard squeezing damages the skin and invites infection — but whiteheads are more of a problem. Their contents are attacked by a bacterium that inhabits the skin and the sebum — oil — is converted into an irritating fatty acid. Eventually there is so much there that the gland bursts, spraying its irritant contents on to the surrounding skin cells.

Skin changes

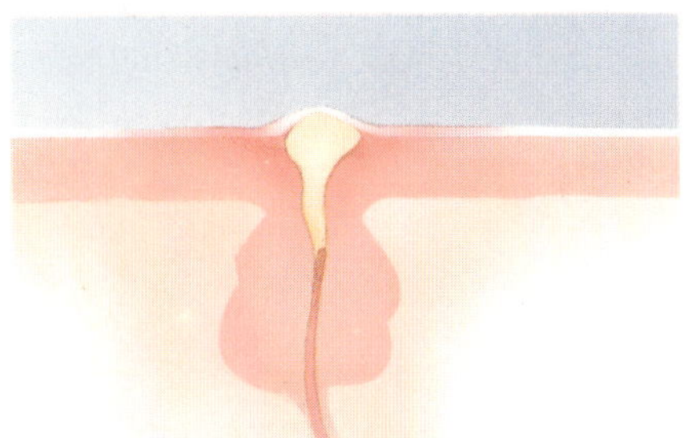

Whiteheads are formed when skin glands become blocked with oil and become thick, hard and white.

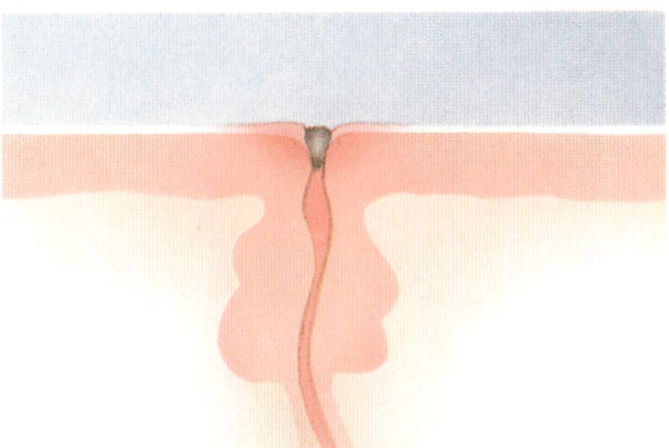

Blackheads are formed when oil seeps out to the skin surface and dries and hardens.

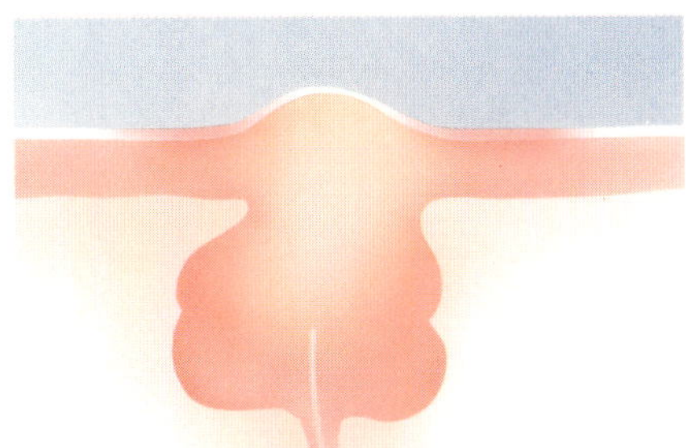

Acne is caused when the sebaceous gland ruptures and releases oil into the deeper layers of skin where it causes inflammation.

Stretch marks occur when progesterone, the pregnancy hormone, acts on connective tissue to ensure that the growing baby will have room to develop.

The result is the all too familiar hateful red and yellow pustule, or, if it's deeper in the skin, a tender inflamed area. As the burst gland heals the area is converted into hard scar tissue, and the result of that is the pits that can be seen on the skin in cases of burnt-out acne.

A certain amount of acne is, frankly, virtually unavoidable. Few are the young people who pass through puberty with never a spot to plague them. And few are the adults who don't have occasional flare ups of spots and/or blackheads.

Another effect hormones can have on skin is stretch marks. These are only rarely due to simple weight gain; the skin is really very elastic and capable of coping with considerable amounts of avoirdupois before showing the strain. But skin can be affected by progesterone, the pregnancy hormone.

One of its prime functions is to ensure that the growing baby will have enough room to develop, and also room to get out, and to this end it acts on connective tissue in the body to soften it. For example, it makes the cartilage between the sacrum (the broad part of the lower spine in the small of the back) and the pelvis become less firm and the result is that there can be more obvious movement of the hips when a woman walks. If you follow a mother or a pregnant woman you can generally see the swaying movement much more clearly than in the girl who has never had a baby (there will be more on the effect of progesterone on joints in Section six).

But progesterone can't be selective; it acts on all connective tissue including that in the deeper layers of the skin, and breaks down some areas of it. At puberty when there is a new flood of progesterone at the same time as the flood of estrogen which makes the breasts grow and the hips widen, the result can be visible marks showing through the upper layers. They are most common on the breasts, at the sides and sometimes underneath; on the hips and the buttocks and occasionally on the thighs.

It has to be said immediately that there is not a thing that can be done to prevent them. There are manufacturers who sell costly creams that are supposed to keep the skin supple, and no doubt they do a lot to soften the surface — that is, the dead — layer of the skin. But they can do nothing whatsoever for the deeper tissues and they certainly cannot avert the softening action of progesterone.

All that can be said to a girl on whom stretch marks have appeared is that eventually they will fade from the somewhat visible red marks they are when they first appear to become soft, white, slightly glistening threads that are far less noticeable. And secondly that they are all part of being a woman and are not in themselves ugly, unless you insist on regarding them as so. None of us was intended to be a smooth celluloid doll. We are breathing, moving, living women and that means we have some so-called imperfections about our persons. In some it is stretch marks on the skin. In others it is hair on the belly, thighs, breasts, chin or upper lip. Some of us are thin when we'd like to be plump, others are fat when we'd like to be thin — but the fact that we'd like to be different doesn't mean that the way we are is somehow despicable. Mere fashion shouldn't make us despise ourselves, surely?

There is yet another hormonal action that shows itself in puberty — that affecting the heat control mechanism.

The ability of the skin's blood vessels to tighten, and thus to force blood down from the surface to the deeper structures (which makes the skin pale and cold) and also to relax and expand, thus drawing blood to the surface (which makes the skin red and hot) is governed by both the autonomic nervous system and by hormones, particularly those made by the adrenals, the thyroid and the ovaries.

When we are threatened by danger and need to fight-or-fly the system whirls into rapid action — but this isn't the only time it happens. If we get cold and need to conserve heat, the system sends blood deep; if we get overheated the opposite happens and we not only turn red as blood comes to the surface to radiate its heat outwards, but also sweat to provide a water cooling system — as the sweat evaporates it takes excess heat away.

This system is at its most efficient in adults. Infants have a very inefficient system, which is why they need such special care to keep them at the right temperatures. While it is achieving the correct balance — estrogen and progesterone have a powerful role to play, along with adrenalin and thyroxine (the thyroid hormone) in controlling body heat — sometimes it goes out of kilter, and the result can be the very embarrassing violent blushes of early adolescence.

The tendency is exaggerated by the fact that so much of what happens to the pubertal child makes her anxious or embarrassed or frightened — life can be very complicated at this stage. These emotions have the same effects as fear or expectation of danger — they send the autonomic system and the endocrine system into fast action. So, a blush makes a child blush because she's so embarrassed by her blushing! This is one of the few situations when it's perhaps easier to be a pubertal girl than a pubertal boy. Blushing in girls is seen as rather charming; boys who do it are regarded as wimps. Fortunately for boys it is mainly adrenalin and thyroxine that are active when they blush, not high levels of estrogen.

It's difficult to find any evidence of an evolutionary reason for women's tendency to be generally hotter than men (they are) and to have a system able to radiate body heat more easily than men. Could it be a trait that developed because of the maternal need to keep the baby, with its inefficient heat regulating system, safe in cold conditions? A baby, held close to a hot maternal body, would be kept comfortably warm in quite severe chilly weather. It's a reasonable surmise, but that is all it can be; we've no proof that this is the reason. But we do know women have larger fat stores than men in order to victual their pregnancies, so it seems logical to suppose that they have a similar system for protecting their babies after birth as well as before.

Whatever the original cause for this readiness to redden it's tiresome for the girl to whom it happens; a sudden wash of heat on your face and neck makes you feel like a walking red torch. It's never as visible to others as it feels to the person it happened to, of course, but that is scant comfort. Reddening is a nuisance that affects not only girls at the start of their reproductive lives, but also women at the end of theirs (see Section nine). A few also have minor problems with heat control throughout their lives, linked with their periods. At some stages of their cycles — it varies from

Heat control

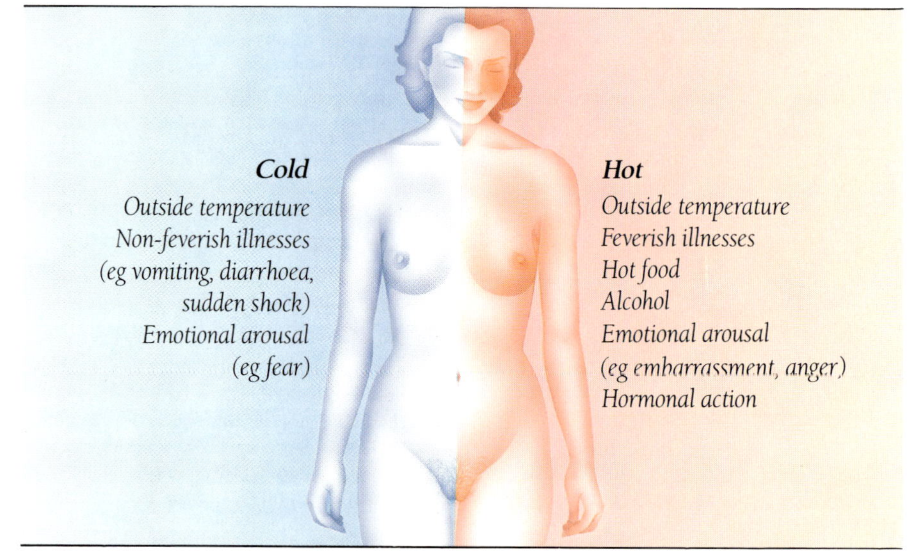

one woman to another — they find they cope better with cold, or with heat.

Others find that they have rather different problems at various stages of their cycle, problems connected with water balance.

One of the tasks that progesterone carries out is the conservation of body fluids. If pregnancy does start, the mother will need to make up to another two pints of blood to supply her developing baby, so in the stage of the menstrual cycle when progesterone is most active (after ovulation) all body cells retain more fluid than usual. Once menstruation starts and the tide of progesterone recedes, the water is no longer needed and the kidneys and bowels throw it out — which is why for many women the start of the menstrual period is marked by the production of much greater quantities of urine (some girls find this is the time that they have to get up in the night to pee) and also of some diarrhoea, as extra fluid is lost in stools. (In the next section there will be more discussion of the effects of water retention in some women — the condition known as the pre-menstrual syndrome.)

When fluid is retained in the body in this way it affects all body cells — fingers and feet can swell, and so can the face and the belly — but often it is most noticed in the breasts. These not only retain extra water in the fat cells; the gland tissue becomes more active too. Some women find that their breasts increase by as much as a couple of inches overall in the pre-menstrual and menstrual week. They may also find that their breasts are tender to the touch, and there may be some flaring up of the common problem of mastitis (see page 112 in Section eight).

These then are the basic facts about menstruation; others will emerge in succeeding pages. It is all a natural and healthy process and it can't be said too often that it need not cause distress. It can give a woman real pleasure in herself depending on her attitude to what happens to her body. Take the matter of breast enlargement and belly rounding in the pre-menstrual and menstrual weeks. One women might regard that as a nuisance, as uncomfortable and embarrassing, while one who values her essential femininity more positively could enjoy the changing sensations her hormones give her, and 'ride' them much as a surfer rides the big rolling waves. Her waves are inner ones, but as potentially exhilarating and enjoyable.

But of course sometimes there will be pains and penalties attached to this normal function, and knowing how to identify what is happening and why it is happening is one of the skills of being a woman.

Menstrual myths

Newly developed girls may be told all sorts of alarming tales about menstruation by women who should know better. Many of the things they are told are myths that have been passed down through the generations for many many years — but the longevity of the beliefs doesn't make them true.

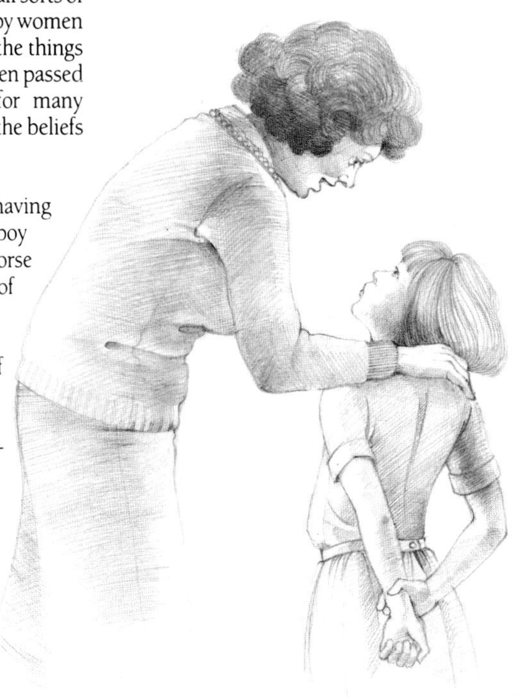

(I was told at the age of eleven and having my first period that 'if I ever let any boy know that I was "like that" and worse still ever let any boy see any sign of the blood, my face would "turn yellow"'. When I asked how my face would know to turn yellow, if I didn't know he'd seen a blood stain — perhaps I hadn't noticed it myself on the back of my dress — I was punished for being cheeky. That was in the nineteen forties. Recently a letter was sent to me by a twelve year-old who had been told exactly the same story, and was as puzzled by it as I had been.)

It is not true that...

Periods make you ill *You may get ill when you are having a period, but that doesn't mean one caused the other.*

Periods are dirty *There is nothing dirty about menstrual blood. Blood misplaced, like urine misplaced, could be regarded as dirt but that doesn't make the basic function dirty.*

Periods clean you out *Since the blood that is lost isn't dirty, there is no need to 'clear it out'. It is no more healthy to have a heavy flow than to have a light one. There are no 'impurities' to be disposed of. There is just the no-longer-needed preparation for a baby who is not to be born — 'the bloody tears of a disappointed womb' it's been called.*

Periods must be regular *They often are, but there is no rule that says they must fit man-made time — clocks and calenders.*

Periods make you smelly *They do not. Lack of washing and infrequent changes of clothes may create smells, as bacteria set to work to break down the substances your body creates, but it is their effects that cause the odour, not the body substances themselves.*

Periods make it dangerous to wash your hair *Not so. In fact it may be wiser to wash hair a little oftener when menstruating since the skin cells which produce sebum tend to be more active then. So, if your hair tends to be a bit oily, it will get oilier.*

Periods stop you from swimming or riding on bikes or on horses *Not so. Anything you can do when you aren't menstruating you can safely and happily do when you are. You may need to be a little more careful in arranging pads and/or tampons to be comfortable, but that is all.*

4
WOMAN'S PAINS

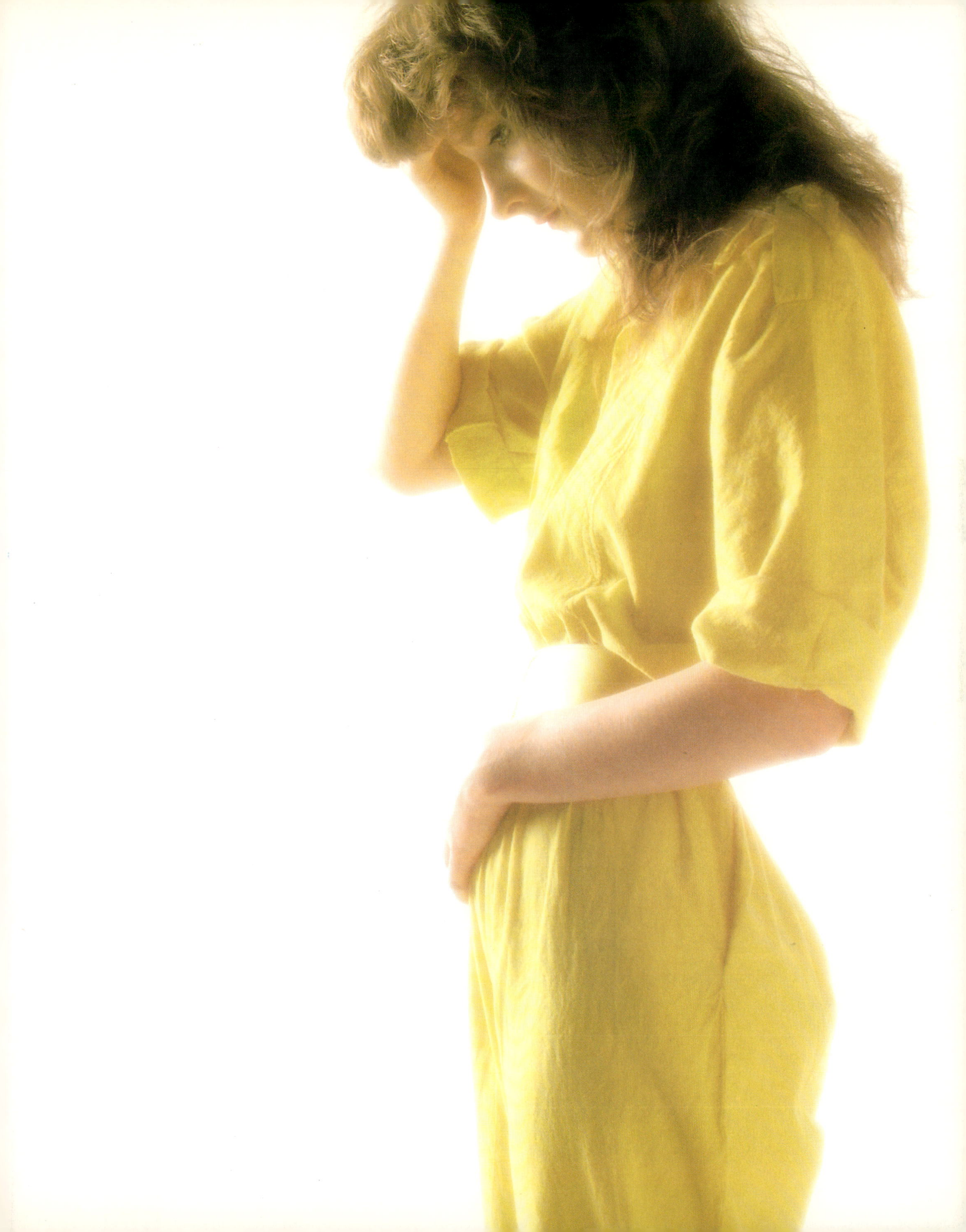

Perfect health does not mean thinking all the time, 'How well I am!' It is more of an unawareness of the workings of the body and mind — a complete release from body-consciousness — that will free the individual to think and feel and do and just be.

It should be the same for a woman and her periods; she should be unaware of her cycle except at times when it is important to her to be so (for example when she is trying either to have a baby or to avoid having one). So the girl who is not having an active sex life should hardly notice her rhythm, or the dates of her periods — just appreciate the reasonably pleasant sensations of actually having them.

But for some this blissful comfort just isn't possible, because they have disagreeable experiences associated with their periods. There are five main types of such problems.

Absence of periods

Known in the medical trade as amenorrhoea, the condition is subdivided into two — primary and secondary.

Primary amenorrhoea means periods have never happened at all. Because the range of normal is so wide, it is difficult to be sure when to label a girl as having this problem, but the usual rule-of-thumb is that if a girl hasn't menstruated by her seventeenth birthday, she should be checked by a doctor. If all her other sexual development is normal — change of shape, appearance of breasts, body hair and so on — there is a possibility that she has the rare problem of an imperforate hymen, and that she is in fact menstruating but the fluid can't escape (see page 52).

If she has no feminine development, then seeking advice a little earlier than the seventeenth birthday would be wise, remembering that puberty starts about two years before the first period happens. Most sensible mothers would want to get advice for their daughters if there were no such signs by the fifteenth birthday.

When medical checks are made, various causes may be identified. There may be disorders of the ovary, so that they fail to produce their hormones, or eggs, or both; there may be disorders of the pituitary so that they fail to trigger the ovarian hormones; or there may be disorders of other endocrine glands, such as thyroid or adrenals, so that their hormones interfere with the normal action of sex hormones. Many of these problems can be dealt with by giving hormones to balance up the body's own supply, or by surgery.

There is a condition called Stein Leventhal Syndrome, for example (also known as polycystic ovarian disease) in which the ovarian hormones are, for complex reasons, prevented from forming properly (they are converted into other types of hormones, the sort that have masculinizing effects). The ovaries fail to shed eggs, and so become covered with little cysts of unburst follicles and the woman becomes overweight, hairy and has no periods (though in some cases she may have occasional very scanty ones). If a surgeon cuts a wedge out of the ovaries it has the effect of making the organs work properly, though quite why the operation has this effect it's hard to say. Some people believe that hormone therapy is more effective in this case.

Secondary amenorrhoea is the label for the condition where periods have started but then stop.

The commonest physical cause is pregnancy, which is why the vast majority of doctors always ask a girl who seeks advice on absent periods whether this is possible. Unmarried girls who have strong religious or moral views about sex outside marriage may feel affronted at being asked the question, but one has to be fair to the doctors who ask it; it is a reasonable one.

The next common physical cause is marked and rapid weight loss and/or gain. Body weight seems to be closely involved with the functioning of the endocrine system, operating through its many feedback loops, and it has long been known that girls who are too thin and girls who are too fat may have difficulty in starting a pregnancy. There is an old country proverb, 'A thinning before a fattening', which suggests that plump girls who lose weight are very likely thereafter to get pregnant.

It is because weight loss leads to period loss that so often girls suffering from anorexia nervosa, the illness which may be totally psychological but which may have physical causes (some researchers think it may be due to lack of zinc in the diet, though this remains unproven) so often go to their doctors about their periods. They may not even realise that they are anorexic; as far as they are concerned they are just people who 'eat carefully' and who watch their figures. They have so distorted a view of their own bodies that they regard normal weight as fatness, and can't see that their exaggerated thinness is actually making them sick. But however warped their view of their body size may be they have a normal awareness of their periods, and may become very anxious when they disappear.

This is just as well, for often the only way a girl with anorexia nervosa can be helped by a doctor is when she seeks advice for her loss of periods and he realises that she is pathologically underweight. (Incidentally, sometimes such girls seek help for their hairiness, because the appearance of a lot of soft down on the body is also a side effect of excessive dieting.)

The treatment of the period problem is of course to treat the anorexia, and there are ways in which these sad girls can be helped to develop a more normal view of themselves and of food. It can take time, but their weight can be taken to acceptable levels and then the periods may start again, though it may be several months before full hormonal function is restored.

When the absence of periods is due to being severely overweight, again treatment of the obesity will solve the hormone problem, though it can take as long and be as difficult to get a large girl down to size as to get a skinny one up to her correct weight. Eating illnesses, whatever form they take, are distressing and hard to cope with for patients and doctors, unfortunately.

Another type of very thin girl whose periods may fail is the dancer or athlete. Ballet dancers in particular who are both very active and deliberately cut their food intake in order to be very slender, often experience absence of periods or sometimes erratic ones with very varying flows.

Athletes, especially those who start training before puberty, have a delayed menarche (first period). Research has shown that a group of girls who started their athletic training before puberty had, on average, their first period at the age of 15.1 years, while a matched group who started training after puberty had their first periods, on average, at the age of 12.8 years. It has been worked out that the onset of periods is delayed by 0.4 years with every athletically active year.

This effect can also be seen in women who aren't trained athletes, but who choose to take up a new strenuous activity. The recent fashionable status of 'workouts' and 'aerobic exercise' which made fortunes for writers of books urging women to over-exercise to the point of pain and beyond (very unhealthy; pain is there to warn you you are damaging yourself) and for track-suit and running shoes manufacturers, also had the effect of switching off (or rearranging) many women's periods.

Another interesting observation; girls who are vegetarians are more likely to miss their periods. One study of girls who were all runners, with some of them vegetarians too, showed that far more of the vegetarians than the meat eaters experienced amenorrhoea. The experts think that there are two possible reasons for this; one is that meat provides essential minerals such as zinc and iron, which are needed for healthy menstruation, and the other is that as some plants contain substances which are chemically similar to estrogen, it could be that vegetarians are actually getting a form of contraceptive from their plant-rich diet.

The next most common causes of amenorrhoea are the emotional ones. Because of the close link between the thinking part of the brain and the hypothalamus and the endocrine system, what we feel and what we believe and what we think about what happens to us has a decidedly physical effect on all the body cells. It's remarkable how often people try to deny this fact even though they know that it is perfectly true.

A woman may know for example that when she gets frightened her heart beats faster and she sweats and trembles — all very physical indeed. But tell her that being frightened can also make her hormones change their balance and thereby stop her periods, and she may refuse to believe it.

Yet there could be good evolutionary reasons for such an effect. Imagine prehistoric woman, living in a difficult environment, sometimes needing to run away from danger, sometimes needing to fight it. If she became pregnant at a time when danger threatened, her ability to fight or fly would be hampered. So her physiology protects her — and any child she may bear — by switching off the reproductive system temporarily under stress. (And also possibly when she had to be very physically active; perhaps on a forced trek to new hunting grounds. That would account for the loss of periods in athletic women.) And perhaps, also, Nature also ensured that underfed women couldn't get pregnant in order to protect them and their babies? It's an interesting idea.

The same system could still operate in us today; we may be almost twenty-first century sophisticates who know how to fly to the moon, but we still have our Stone Age bodies. So, fretting over modern stresses can have the same hormonal effect as being chased by a woolly mammoth or a sabre toothed tiger.

Yet too few women find themselves able to accept this effect of stress; many are those who have dismissed a doctor's diagnosis of anxiety-caused loss of periods and gone in search of another doctor who will give totally 'physical' reasons for the problem, and also physical treatments, such as hormone therapy.

There are plenty of doctors who will do that; the sort who see a girl who is anxious and tense, who has perhaps recently suffered a bereavement or changed her job or left college or had a disastrous love affair or marriage, and who is complaining of period loss — and promptly put her on the Pill. The Pill works by creating not periods but 'withdrawal bleeds' (see page 95 in Section nine for all details on how the Pill works). This may make the girl believe that she is menstruating again, but she isn't really; all that is happening is that her uterus is being tricked into bleeding. She isn't having a normal menstrual cycle, and she is unlikely to do so until her emotional upheaval has settled again, or she has been helped to deal with the dammed up feelings which are so distressing her by talking them out and learning the vital skill of relaxation (see page 154, Section ten).

Distress about absent periods can be particularly great in women who are worried about the possibility of pregnancy. The one who desperately wants to be pregnant may find her periods change their pattern, and may even disappear altogether (filling her with false hope) while the one who is fearful of an unwanted pregnancy may also find her periods fail, thus filling her with great terror. In both cases the only remedy — and just about the hardest to apply — is to relax and cease worrying. But until you do this the hormonal control of periods is going to be inefficient. (See also page 87, Section six.)

Uneven periods

Irregular periods worry many girls; they have perhaps three periods a year, or two or three close together and then none for several months. This can be a form of amenorrhoea, in that it can be due to the same basic causes — that is, faults in the hormonal control; being the wrong weight; being physically extra active.

There is one rather odd and fascinating observation that has been made about the regularity of periods; women who live closely with other women — say at college, in dormitories, or in nurses' training school residences, or in Army barracks — tend to find that their cycles change so that within a few months they are all menstruating at the same time. It's called menstrual synchrony, and it's thought to be caused by the effects of very minute quantities of pheremones, almost undetectable but very powerful scent messengers (see page 64 Section five). It has been noticed that there is often one 'dominant' woman in the group who exerts her pheremones — quite unconsciously, of course — on her sisters, and it is this that brings them into synchrony. The phenomenon was described by Mary McCarthy in her novel *The Group* and is well known to any woman who has ever lived the communal life. Ask a nun!

Excessive periods

The words used to label the variation in women's periods have a great rolling glory about them for all they are the very devil to spell. There is *menorrhagia* which means an excessive blood loss at period time, and *polymenorrhoea* which means very frequent periods, and *menostaxis* which means prolonged menstruation and then there is *metorrhagia* which means persistent and irregular bleeding.

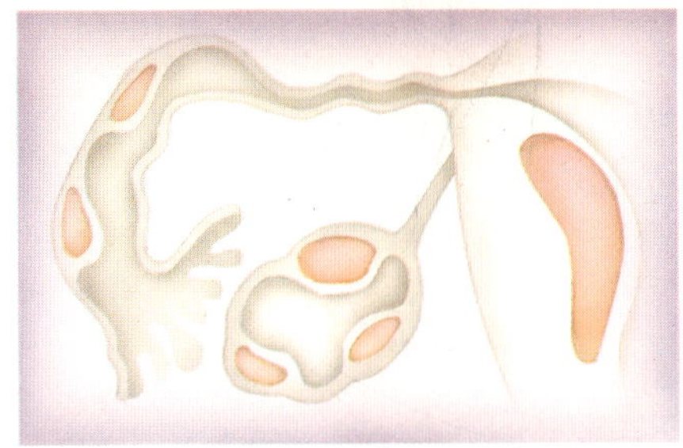

Endometriosis

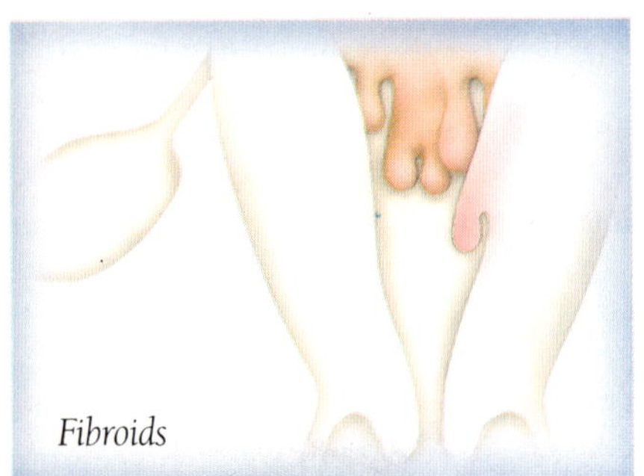

Fibroids

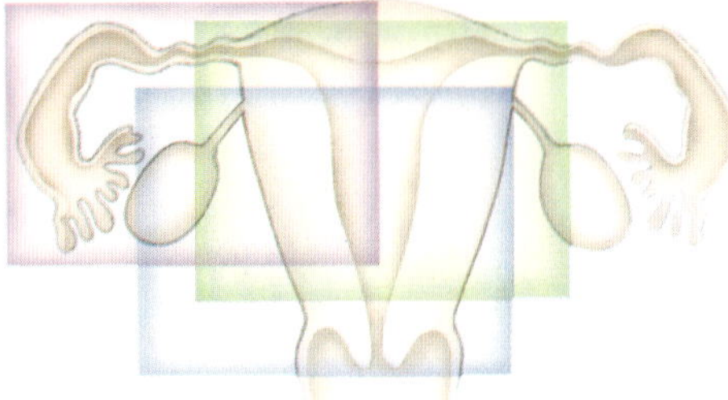

Uterus

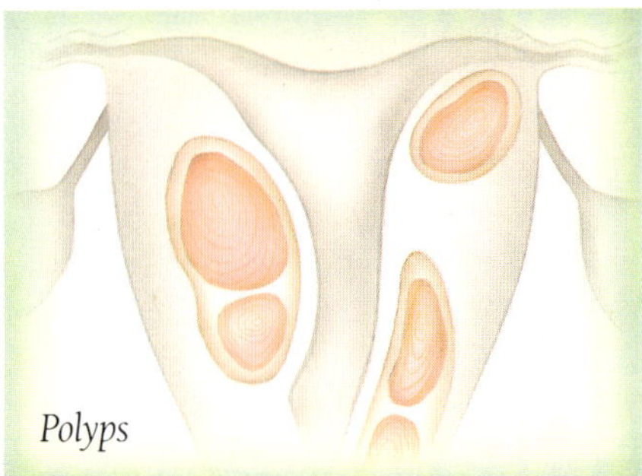

Polyps

Their causes can be various. Excessive blood loss at period time can be due to fibroids which are benign lumps which develop in the muscle of the uterus, and by pushing out into the cavity of the uterus increase its surface area. Since it is the lining of the surface area that is shed at period time, an increase in area means an increase in lining and therefore an increase in flow.

Another cause of heavy blood loss is endometriosis. The lining of the uterus, instead of developing neatly where it is meant to, goes to areas where it shouldn't. It may invade the muscle wall of the uterus. It may travel up the tubes and settle plaques of itself on them or on the ovaries, or by escaping into the belly cavity, from the other end of the tubes, can settle on other structures such as the outer walls of the gut, the bladder or the kidneys.

Wherever it goes, it is always under the influence of the ovarian hormones, so when they instruct it to thicken and develop more blood vessels, lo and behold, it does. The woman who has the condition may get pain and swelling in the belly, or severe cramps and heavy bleeding at period time and often has difficulty in conceiving. She may also develop 'chocolate cysts'. These are areas of bleeding endometrium which are so deeply embedded in the wrong place that the shed blood can't escape — as it can from the uterus, of course — so the areas become large and swollen as each month passes and the blood gets thicker and thicker and darker and darker until it resembles chocolate. Women with endometriosis can suffer chocolate cysts in any site, but the most common is the ovary.

Endometriosis can be a very unpleasant condition and difficult to treat. Some women respond to a course of hormone therapy; they are given hormones in such a way that the body is tricked into thinking itself permanently pregnant. This prevents menstruation and so stops the swellings and the bleeding and the pain. Alternatively, the woman may be given a drug that is a synthetic male hormone (Danazol) which leads to a drug-induced menopause, by stopping the pituitary from stimulating the ovaries.

Both remedies can have side effects, such as increased hairiness, weight gain and changes in breast size, and of course prevent a real pregnancy, but if the pain and misery of the condition are bad enough, most sufferers feel that the side effects are worth tolerating.

Sadly, one effect of endometriosis is subfertility; although if a patient does manage to conceive, often she finds her problem is resolved afterwards. And it is interesting that in countries where early marriage and motherhood are usual, the condition is quite rare. In Western countries where women are tending to delay motherhood till their thirties it seems to be increasing.

Heavy blood loss can also be caused during and between periods by diseases of the vagina and the cervix. Cancers in these sites bleed when touched so any episode of bleeding after intercourse must always be reported and medically checked. Cancer of the body of the uterus can also cause heavy bleeding during a period, which is another reason why the symptom should always be taken seriously.

But it is not only cancerous growths which bleed; so do benign ones. Polyps are little outgrowths of the mucous membrane which bleed easily, and when they occur on the cervix can cause a copious and alarming loss. Then there are the fairly uncommon but tiresome varices of the vagina — varicose veins of the area which bulge and easily break down and bleed. Varicose veins happen in other parts of the body too; the legs, the anus — where they are called haemorrhoids or piles — the oesophagus, or gullet. They bulge because the valves which are supposed to ensure that blood doesn't go backwards down the vein fail to do their job, and there is a certain amount of 'pooling' of blood inside the vein. The walls become less elastic and therefore more likely to break down.

Infection of the walls of the vagina — it's called vaginitis — can make the area tender and likely to bleed when touched. This sort of bleeding is most common in older women, after the menopause (see page 127 in Section nine).

Sometimes what appears to be bleeding between periods isn't — it comes from somewhere else, for example the urethra, the opening from the bladder. This can develop a caruncle, a pouting outwards of some of the mucous membrane which is tender to touch and bleeds on contact. Similarly, vulvitis, inflammation of the vulva, the surface sex organs, can lead to bleeding, but most women will know when their blood comes from the surface and when it comes from inside.

One other cause of bleeding between periods is 'breakthrough bleeding'. Women having hormone therapy, either for treatment of a disorder or in the form of the contraceptive Pill, may find that the control is less secure than it should be and the effect is occasional spotting of blood between the times when a withdrawal bleed, which mimics a period, is expected. (See page 95, effects of the Pill.)

Something similar can happen to women who are not on the Pill or any hormones, but whose own hormonal control slips at ovulation time; when the shift in production levels between estrogen and progesterone happens there may be very slight bleeding. It must always be checked with a doctor, just to be sure there is no other more sinister cause, but once a woman has been assured her bleeding is ovulatory she can ignore it. It's harmless. It might be a little uncomfortable, though, if it's associated with pain. Some women regularly get a niggling pain on one or other or even both sides of the belly approximately half-way between periods. It's called *mittelschmerz* — German makes an agreeable change from Latin — a word which means literally 'middle pain'. Again it's nothing to fret about. It's harmless, if irritating. It affects about ten per cent of women and many of them find it a useful indicator. It tells them they are at their fertile, ovulatory, stage, and can behave accordingly, should they want — or not want — a pregnancy.

And once again, uneven bleeding between periods, like absence of periods or excessively heavy periods, can be due to emotional stress. All such bleeding is lumped together under the heading 'dysfunctional bleeding' and doctors offer various treatments for it (see Section eight). Once women are given an explanation of why their periods may be heavy, uneven or absent and offered a remedy, most of them are able to cope with the problems. It is less easy, however, to be phlegmatic about regularly recurring pain with periods.

Painful periods

Some of the conditions already described, fibroids, for example, and endometriosis, can cause pain during the period's flow. It's called dysmenorrhoea (any word with 'dys' in front of it means painful and/or difficult) and is usually subdivided into primary and secondary.

Primary means that the girl suffers it without having any demonstrable underlying disorder. In this form it is commonest among girls who have just started their periods, and there seem to be two main reasons for it.

One is the time the child's body needs to settle to an adult pattern. In the early cycles the production of hormone may be uneven, and in some cases rather excessive. So, the early periods can be copious and accompanied by strong contractions of the uterine muscle. These crampy pains may have the effect of sending pain waves through the groins and down the legs and through to the lower back, and are often accompanied by nausea and sometimes vomiting, as well as diarrhoea — and all of it together can make a girl feel very sweaty and headachy and altogether wretched.

There has been a good deal of research into why this should happen, and it is a difficult knot to unravel. After all, menstruation isn't an illness — it's a normal physiological function. Why should it hurt, and rob a girl of her comfort and peace of mind one week in every four?

The reasons are, as is so often the case, probably both physical and emotional. Girls who get agitated and distressed about their new femininity may cause their hypothalamuses to push their pituitaries into over-action, and this very physical effect reacts on the muscle of the uterus, so causing the pain and other symptoms. Similarly girls who are not in the best of health — living on junk food, suffering from constipation because of a lack of fibre in their diet, low on sleep and exercise and fresh air — may find even a normal period is just too much to cope with, and experience it as painful and unpleasant.

The purely physical causes — if they can be so described, seeing that we are all made up as an inextricable combination of body and mind — are rooted in the action of prostaglandins, which are recently discovered (in the last thirty years or so) body chemicals that are very similar to hormones, but which come from as yet unidentified sources in the body.

One in particular, known as prostaglandin F2 alpha seems to be involved in painful periods. Research into frequent sufferers shows they have raised blood levels of the substance. It acts on all smooth muscle, including that in the gut, which would account for the diarrhoea which so often accompanies dysmenorrhoea. (Another note about words — those which end in 'rrhoea' mean 'a flow' — rhinorrhoea, for example, is a runny nose). It is likely that prostaglandin F2 alpha is a necessary part of the menstrual system; it is the tool the body uses to push out the menstrual flow, and to encourage the gut to hurry waste food along and so send excess fluids that have built up since ovulation out of the body. It's just that the girl with primary dysmenorrhoea has too much of it.

The remedy is therefore obvious; find a drug that inhibits the prostaglandin F2 alpha — and we have several. The most efficient is one that we all know well; aspirin. It is more than a painkiller; it reduces the body temperature (that's why it's so useful for fevers) reduces the tendency of the blood to clot (which is useful when there is a heavy menstrual flow which needs to be kept liquid and is finding difficulty in doing so because there is so much of it) and does all this by controlling the body's own supply of prostaglandins. Taking half a tablet a day also protects the middle aged from coronary thrombosis. The only bad news about it is that it has some potentially damaging effects; any drug that is efficient will have them; only drugs that are so bland that they do no good can do no harm. In the case of aspirin these include gastric irritation, so those people with a tendency to indigestion shouldn't take it. In heavy dosages it can also cause ringing in the ears, dizziness, sweating, nausea, confusion, a tendency to overbreathe (see Section eight for more on the latter, by the way) and several other nasty experiences. So it is a drug to be used with cautious respect, however commonplace it may seem.

There are other drugs that can be used to relieve the pain of dysmenorrhoea. One contains hormones, and is the well-known contraceptive Pill used as the combined pill which prevents ovulation, see page 95. Some doctors regard this as ideal, others are more wary with their younger patients, being unhappy about giving hormones to untried systems; they fear the possibility of delaying the normal settling down process of the body, left to itself, and point out that the Pill is a potentially dangerous drug and that there are other methods of helping the young girl.

The alternatives do exist. There are some drugs normally used to treat inflammatory conditions like rheumatoid arthritis, and which act rather as aspirin does and which give relief from period pains. They include flufenamic acid (marketed in the UK as Meralen), mefanamic acid (Ponstan), naproxen (Naprosyn) and ibuprofen (of which several brands are available) and they can give great relief. Their drawback is that they may possibly have a teratogenic effect; that is, they can damage the unborn baby in the uterus (another Latin word that makes excellent sense when you know its roots — it means 'monstermaking'). So, they can't be used by a girl who is having an active sex life and who may become pregnant while she is taking the drugs.

One comfort; if a girl does learn to live with her recurring discomfort and discovers how to use relaxation techniques to calm her excessive hormone production (see Section eight) her hormone balance will sort itself out in time and the pain will fade away. The classic remedy that doctors used to recommend was, 'have a baby, my dear', and it is true that a pregnancy does often have the effect of finally getting rid of recurrent pain in periods; but it seems a pretty bad reason to create a new human being. A baby surely should be wanted as a person, not as a sort of aspirin tablet. What having a baby does to relieve dysmenorrhoea, incidentally, is to stretch the cervix. It has been found that such stretching helps a good deal; the very common operation of D and C (dilation and curetage, see also Section eight) seems to give relief in many cases. This is odd because no one has ever found that there is any significant narrowing of the cervical canal in afflicted women.

For secondary dysmenorrhoea, the sort that starts after there have been quite comfortable easy periods, the obvious answer is to seek for the underlying cause, and treat that. Dealing with the fibroids, or the endometriosis, or whatever, will be the same as dealing with the dysmenorrhoea.

Both kinds of dysmenorrhoea have sometimes in the past been dismissed as being due to 'women's neuroticism' and this has made many women justifiably annoyed and justifiably suspicious of the sort of male doctor who makes such a judgement. But women doctors may say it too, and even if they are saying it clumsily, they are in fact expressing an underlying truth which is the one that I have tried to express on these pages — that once a woman accepts herself and her femininity in all aspects, and glories in it rather than regarding it as making her of less value than a man, then she has a much better chance of experiencing her body's functions painlessly and pleasantly.

The pre-menstrual syndrome

Thirty or so years ago, no one talked much about the pre-menstrual syndrome (and, incidentally, the word syndrome means 'a cluster of symptoms'). Now it's a phrase everyone knows. Does this mean that it is a newly invented/discovered disorder? Or is it, as some doctors maintain with some heat, a non-existent condition which some women use as an excuse for unhappiness and to describe normal life experiences?

Certainly it exists; women everywhere know that they may experience changes in themselves the week or so before their period is due and these can be at the very least disagreeable and at the worst make them feel very ill indeed. They report that the symptoms disappear dramatically once the menstrual flow is established, and that they dread the onset of the next pre-menstrual week when the discomfort will all return. Just what are the symptoms? What causes them? And above all what can be done to relieve them?

Physical symptoms

• Bloatedness — a feeling of being abnormally heavy with excess fluid. Clothes, rings, shoes feel extra tight, and the weight actually increases.

• Tender breasts which feel heavy, tense and sore to the touch.

• Acne type spots start to appear.

• Greasy hair which is hard to manage and needs constant washing.

• Increased hair growth on chin, upper lip, breasts and so on.

• Appetite changes with, in particular, craving for sweet foods, which can eventually lead to steady increase in weight.

• Changes in sleep patterns with excessive daytime sleepiness, or attacks of night-time insomnia.

• Fatigue becomes a problem.

• Muscular aches and pains.

• Headaches especially of the migrainous type, that is, affecting half the head, and sometimes accompanied by flashing lights and other visual disturbances.

• Nausea and sometimes vomiting especially in connection with a migraine.

Psychological symptoms

These can upset the sufferer even more than the physical sensations, and include:

• Irritability often to the point of uncontrolled temper outbreaks, and heightened aggressiveness.

• Depression often accompanied by bouts of tearfulness.

• Loss of sex drive or, paradoxically, a marked rise in sex drive.

• Memory lapses which affect work patterns, and can cause considerable stress to schoolgirls, especially at examination time.

• Dreaminess in waking hours, often this is matched by very vivid and sometimes alarming night-time dreams (a progesterone effect, it is thought).

• Clumsiness of movement which may lead to accidents. (There is a statistical increase in accidents on the road, at work and in the home affecting pre-menstrual and menstrual women.)

Added together, these lists add up to a formidable amount of feminine misery, but there are two important points to be made.

The first is that by no means all women experience all of these symptoms. Some may have one regularly — say the bloatedness — but nothing else. Others may have just the migraines and these only two or three times a year, and yet others may get irritable and tearful but have no physical symptoms at all. The possible permutations are many.

The second important point is that nowhere in either list of symptoms is one labelled 'criminal tendencies'. There have been cases in courts around the world where women charged with acts of violence and even murder have pleaded diminished responsibility on the grounds of pre-menstrual tension at the time of the act of which they are accused.

Cases from the past have been evoked such as that involving Lizzie Borden, the New England woman who in the late nineteenth century murdered her parents. (Remember the old rhyme? 'Lizzie Borden took an axe and gave her mother forty whacks. When she saw what she had done she gave her father forty one.') Because she was said to have been in the first days of her period at the time she committed her murders, some modern day commentators have said she was suffering from pre-menstrual tension and therefore should be forgiven. Many women today (including me!) find the suggestion that periods make women lose all sense of proper social behaviour abhorrent. Yes, women can find some aspects of their menstrual cycle difficult to cope with, in some cases, but women are no more at the mercy of their hormones than men are at the mercy of theirs.

To suggest that a woman should be regarded as unable to control herself because of the stage of her menstrual cycle is to suggest that men must always be forgiven if they are violent, on the grounds that their levels of testosterone — the male hormone which contributes to male aggressiveness — are always high. Surely, whatever our hormones are doing, we are thinking people and as capable of self-control as any man. To believe otherwise is to put us, as women, back into the closet out of which so many of us have been trying so hard to escape.

Causes of PMT

There are two distinct schools of thought about the source of this complex of symptoms. There is the 'this-is-all-physical' school which says that women feel as they do because their progesterone levels ensure that too much fluid is retained in the body. The resulting bloating accounts for all the symptoms, both physical and emotional, and the sense of wellbeing that accompanies the onset of the flow and increased peeing and therefore loss of fluid, is evidence that this is so.

There is another school that says, however, 'this-is-all-social', and that women when they are bad tempered, angry and aggressive are not so just because of their hormones but because they are at this time of the month allowing their guard to slip and behaving as they want to, instead of in the socially accepted ways women have always been made to behave when under the control of men.

It seems reasonable to suggest that the truth, as is so often the case, is an amalgam of both views. Yes, the raised fluid levels of the second half of the menstrual cycle can contribute heavily to the way a woman feels; and yes, the external pressures that are put on women to conform to a stereotype of passive subservience do exist. It could be that a woman's ability to control her own feelings is a little eroded by the high fluid levels in her cells, and this is how the two sets of causes interact. But the actual mechanism of course doesn't really matter so much as finding out how to deal with the discomfort and get rid of the symptoms.

Dealing with PMT

The first stage of any self help system has to be identification. You need to know whether in fact your symptoms are cyclical and whether their cycle matches your periods. So, charting is needed.

On the following page there is a system to help you keep a record. You will need to chart your experiences for at least three months before you can see any sort of real pattern, but once you have you will know whether you really have a PMS (Pre-menstrual syndrome) problem or whether your main difficulty is external pressure from relationships, work, housing, money and so on. Maybe your problems coincide with your, or your partner's, shifts at work or visits from disliked relations, or the day the rent is due — all these can be part of the stress that can make people feel lousy.

If you believe that your symptoms are undoubtedly linked with periods then the first stage of your self treatment is to see just how you can help yourself feel better.

Lifestyle

It could be that changes in your lifestyle are all you need to get back on an even keel. Perhaps a different shift at work or getting a different more rewarding job altogether is the answer (if one is available). Maybe you're in a relationship that you know is a less than happy one, but you hang on to it out of fear of loneliness, out of habit, out of guilt, out of sheer apathy. Three weeks in the month you can cope — but on the fourth it gets to you. Moving out of the relationship could make you feel that all the month is worth living.

How to use this chart

This chart will enable you to trace the pattern of your menstrual cycle. Note in the appropriate squares any symptoms or factors connected with PMT. Use the letters suggested here as a code and indicate on the female figure the areas involved (as shown in the sample square on the right). The tiny square at the top corner of each square should be coloured in to indicate which days you have your periods.

G Good mood
B Bad mood
S Sex
T Tired
C Cravings
A Acne

Headache
P
Period
B
Bad mood
Breast tenderness
T
Tired
Stomach pains
98·6
Temperature
(or 36°C)

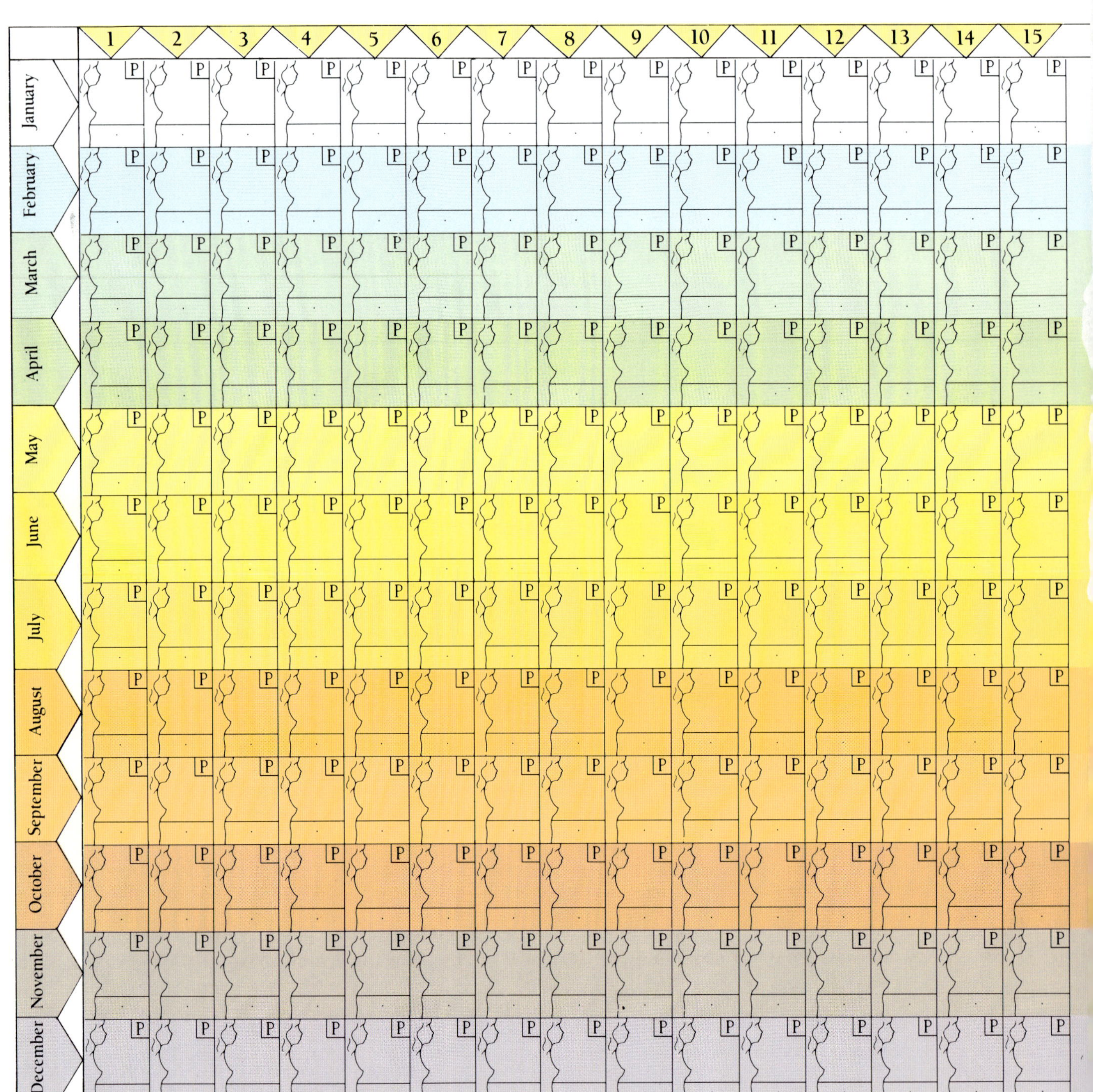

Calculating your fertile period

The bottom of each square can be used to keep a record of your daily temperature. This normally varies from 96-99°F (36-37°C) but ovulation, when the monthly egg is produced, is heralded by a sharp rise in temperature (this will remain quite high until your period begins). So taking your temperature at the same time each day — perhaps before you get out of bed — is a helpful way to find out when you are most likely to conceive a baby.

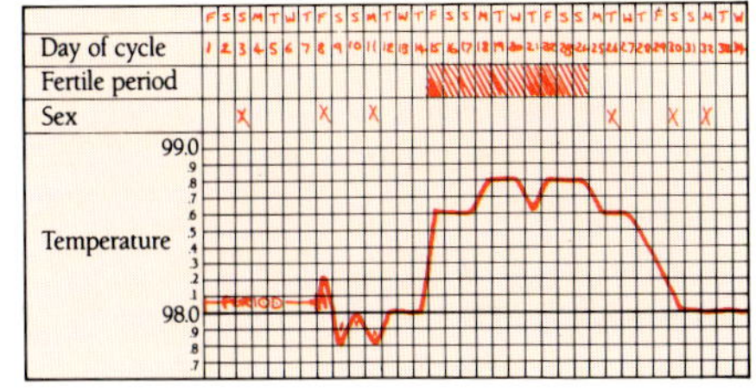

Regular temperature rise = ovulation beginning = fertile period.

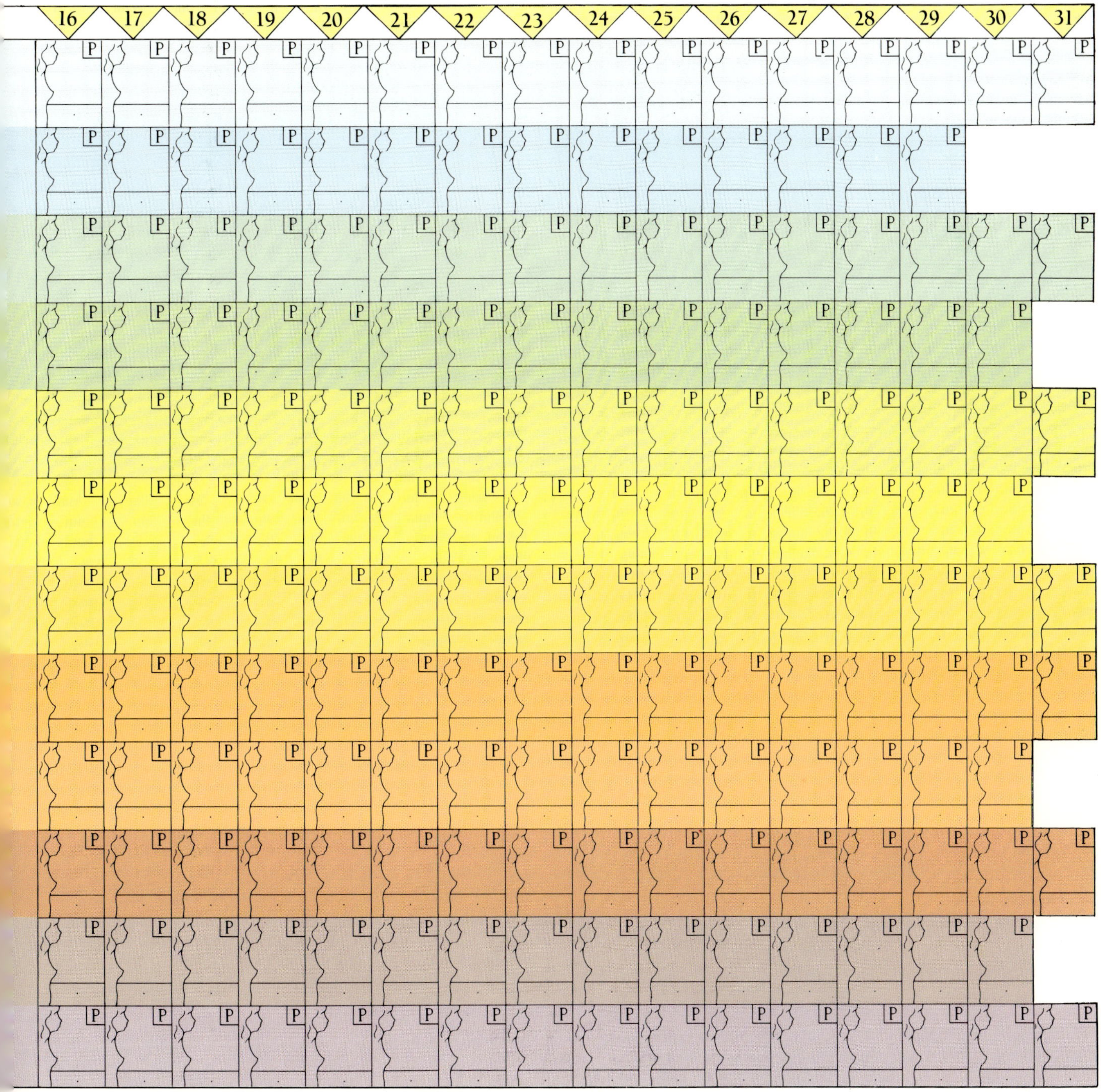

16	17	18	19	20	21	22	23	24	25	26	27	28	29	30	31
P	P	P	P	P	P	P	P	P	P	P	P	P	P	P	P
P	P	P	P	P	P	P	P	P	P	P	P	P	P		
P	P	P	P	P	P	P	P	P	P	P	P	P	P	P	P
P	P	P	P	P	P	P	P	P	P	P	P	P	P	P	
P	P	P	P	P	P	P	P	P	P	P	P	P	P	P	P
P	P	P	P	P	P	P	P	P	P	P	P	P	P	P	
P	P	P	P	P	P	P	P	P	P	P	P	P	P	P	P
P	P	P	P	P	P	P	P	P	P	P	P	P	P	P	P
P	P	P	P	P	P	P	P	P	P	P	P	P	P	P	
P	P	P	P	P	P	P	P	P	P	P	P	P	P	P	P
P	P	P	P	P	P	P	P	P	P	P	P	P	P	P	
P	P	P	P	P	P	P	P	P	P	P	P	P	P	P	P

Diet

For some women changes in diet are all they need to feel better. Many of us eat far too much salt which encourages fluid to stay in body cells (and also could in some vulnerable people push up the blood pressure). Many eat far too little fresh raw unprocessed food. Nutritionists are still studying the quality of the human diet, but there has been a great deal uncovered in recent years, enough to lead to an extraordinary change in the Western diet.

More and more people find they feel better on high fibre, low animal fat and low sugar regimes, and over and over again women who have made such a dietary change on a permanent basis (and not just as a two-week-wonder crash diet) report that they feel much better and have fewer pre-menstrual symptoms.

Quite why this should be is hard to say; perhaps the diet ensures that some trace elements and minerals that they were not getting in their earlier diet of highly refined foods are replaced; perhaps they get more of the vitamins and other nutrients they need. But whatever it is that makes people feel good on this modern sensible diet, it's a pleasant one, not too expensive, certainly can't do any harm, and might well relieve PMS symptoms. (The diet is discussed in detail on pages 144 and 145, Section ten.)

Associated with dietary changes are new drinking habits. Many women drink large quantities of caffeine rich drinks — coffee, tea, colas — and there is a possibility that the use of this particular stimulant can have an effect on PMS. Drinking less of such beverages will not only cut down on caffeine — it will also cut down on fluid intake in general — because no one ever drinks as much of water as they do of flavoured fluids — and that can have a beneficial effect. The less you drink, the less likely you are to retain excess fluid.

Relaxation

Allied with all this there are changes in relaxation patterns that can help a lot. Many of us who live in the urban West get into a style of living that is constant rush and excitement; it's as though we are hooked on our own adrenalin, and we rush from work to play to home to work and everywhere else at a rate of knots. People sit in traffic jams behind the wheels of their cars, cursing and aggressive inside, showing a calm exterior on the surface — because that is how women in particular ought to behave — and naturally the stress hormone levels rise and rise.

The answer has to be to use techniques that stop the stress hormones from rising high enough to upset the balance of other hormones, including those which govern the menstrual cycle.

Women who learn to be tranquil and who use their inner peace — and it is in there somewhere — often find that PMS symptoms just fade away. So classes in keep-fit or regular exercise, or swimming or walking, all of which burn off stress hormones very effectively, may be useful.

Much of the interest in exercise regimes and aerobics and 'working out' and all the other fashionable sweat-scented activities of the past few years could well be based not so much on the fact that they improve the shape of the body by tightening and enlarging muscles as on the way they affect hormones and create a sense of wellbeing (see Section ten).

There are other benefits of course; for some women it's a comfortable social experience, in a setting where it is 'permissible' to enjoy the company of other women. There are women who feel uneasy if they don't have men around; they are the sort who define themselves always in relation to men. Having a man on your arm is regarded as having an essential accessory.

Never mind if you love him, or even like him; having him is what matters. Yet what such women find when they get together with the girls at the gym is that it's remarkable how relaxing and agreeable the company is.

But conscious relaxation helps too, and on pages 149, 150 and 151 there is a system of relaxing. You could also try joining a yoga class (which mixes exercise and relaxation very cunningly), or meditation.

Medication

If despite all this there are still symptoms of PMS the next stage is to try medication. There is no harm in using drugs as long as they are used sensibly.

Simple diuretics, which are medicines you can buy over the counter or which a doctor can prescribe to encourage the kidneys to throw out more liquid, can be very effective. However, they must be used carefully. Overuse (and particularly continuous use) of diuretics can lead to excessive water loss — dehydration — and with it loss of essential substances in the urine. Even a desirable fluid loss may be accompanied by such chemical deprivation, and certain foods added to the diet may help to prevent that. Potassium is a case in point; eating dried raw fruits such as figs, currants and dates, or fresh bananas, can keep potassium levels up. Alternatively a doctor can prescribe a drug which prevents the loss of potassium — it's called spironolactone — (Aldactone) but this should not be used if there is any possibility you are pregnant — it might be teratogenic. (See food lists on pages 144 and 145).

If diuretics taken in the days before the symptoms are expected don't work, the use of Vitamin B6, also known as pyridoxine may be helpful. This vitamin has been used in some formulations of the Pill, because it has been found to prevent the depression that some Pill users experience as a side effect, and it has been tried in a number of studies for PMS, notably at St Thomas's Hospital in London. The dosage they recommend for B6 in PMS is as follows:

Mild adult cases (with few symptoms) and children aged twelve to sixteen years may respond to one 20 mg tablet at breakfast and another 20 mg tablet with the evening meal, or just before bedtime. People experiencing more than mild symptoms should try an increase in this basic dosage; start with two 20 mg tablets at breakfast time and two 20 mg tablets with the evening meal, or just before bedtime. If this dose is not sufficiently helpful, the dose should be increased to one 50 mg tablet at breakfast and one 50 mg tablet in the evening. If this is still not helpful, the dose may be increased to 60 or 75 mg twice a day.

Exceptionally, 100 mg twice a day may be needed, but this dose should not be exceeded as it can cause unpleasant gastric acidity. (If it does, reducing the dose gets rid of the problem.)

The tablets should be started three days before the expected start of any of the symptoms of PMS. This is most important if full relief is to be experienced. At the time that PMS symptons would normally disappear, i.e. one or two days after the start of the period, the tablets can be stopped until just before the start of the symptoms in the next month. (Keeping the chart filled in will help you pin-point the time.) Where a smaller dose has been used initially, the dose can be increased by one tablet each day if symptoms become more severe just before the time of the period (i.e. three instead of two per day, or four instead of three per day).

Approximately seventy-five to eighty per cent of PMS sufferers are helped by this treatment once the correct dose for the individual is worked out. However, if little or no relief is found, specialized advice or investigation may be necessary and you should ask your doctor for further help. Vitamin B6 (pyridoxine) is on prescription, or it can be obtained in the UK from chemists under various trade names such as Benadon (Roche Products Ltd) and Complement (a 100 mg long-acting tablet, Napp Laboratories Ltd) or in most health food shops simply as Vitamin B6.

Some women have found considerable comfort from taking foods rich in gamma-linolenic acid. This is an essential fatty acid which is needed to make various body substances, including prostaglandins. Usually we get it from a common fatty acid called gamma-linoleic acid (it sounds very similar, but the different spellings are significant — they are different substances). Gamma-linoleic acid is present in many ordinary foods, but it isn't always easily converted in the body from one form to the other. The ability to make the conversion seems to be limited by our cholesterol-rich Western diet, and ageing seems to reduce the ability to make it too. But it — that is gamma-linol*en*ic acid — can be tapped from other sources, and considerable claims have been made for its efficacy in a wide range of disorders involving prostaglandin action, from high blood pressure to arthritis and multiple sclerosis as well as PMS. Once again, the substance has been tested at St Thomas's Hospital and early reports suggest that this can be a very effective answer for some PMS sufferers. It is most easily obtained either as oil of evening primrose which is marketed under various names, and oil of blackcurrant seeds, and is usually stocked in health food shops as well as pharmacies. The recommended dosage is to start with 250 mg a day (usually that is one capsule of oil) and if this doesn't help to increase to 250 mg twice daily. The dosage can be increased by one capsule increments up to 500 mg three times a day. If that doesn't help then this obviously isn't the remedy for you. At the time of writing it's rather an expensive method, unfortunately, but shopping around for different brands may help reduce the costs.

If none of these help, then hormone therapy may be the answer. It has been suggested that the cause of PMS is a relative shortage of progesterone in the second half of the cycle and some women have been treated by being given sizeable doses of it, either as a progestogen, or as the pure progesterone which can't be swallowed (it would be destroyed in the acidulous stomach) and has to be given as a vaginal or rectal pessary. The wax base in the pessary dissolves and is then thrown out in the normal process of excretion, and the hormone suspended in it is absorbed through the mucous membrane.

There are doctors who do not believe that progesterone used this way is the right remedy and others who swear by it. Never think that medicine is an exact science; it is as much an art as anything, with different practitioners using different methods. What matters is finding a doctor who is sympathetic to your needs and who is willing to try various remedies to find one that suits you.

It may be that one woman needs not so much drugs that relate directly to her hormone levels, as anti-depressants to deal with an underlying depression that flares up at period times. These drugs are not like the much talked of tranquillizers (which were once seen as the answer to all sorts of anxiety symptoms and which are now known to cause as many problems as they cure, if they are over-used) but specific answers to the all too common disorder of clinical depression. They can be very effective for PMS symptoms which turn out to be depressive symptoms in disguise — but of course a definite diagnosis of depression must be made by a doctor.

It may be that some women will respond best of all to the so-called 'fringe' methods of acupuncture, naturopathy, herbalism, hypnotherapy and so on. That's fine it it's fine for them. It's never wise to abandon all orthodox medical care, however, in favour of the unorthodox. Sometimes symptoms are misdiagnosed by a patient herself, and potentially severe illnesses which need the expert care of a medically qualified doctor with a broad base of experience are missed.

It may seem there is some contradiction on the last few pages since in describing the menstrual cycle I have put so much emphasis on the normality and easiness of it in a healthy woman, and then have gone on to concentrate so heavily on the problems that seem far from normal and easy. But never forget that these problems affect only some people, and then only some of the time. Periods, I must repeat, need not be a burden. Those problems that do arise from them can usually be relieved considerably, given enough understanding of what is going on in your body.

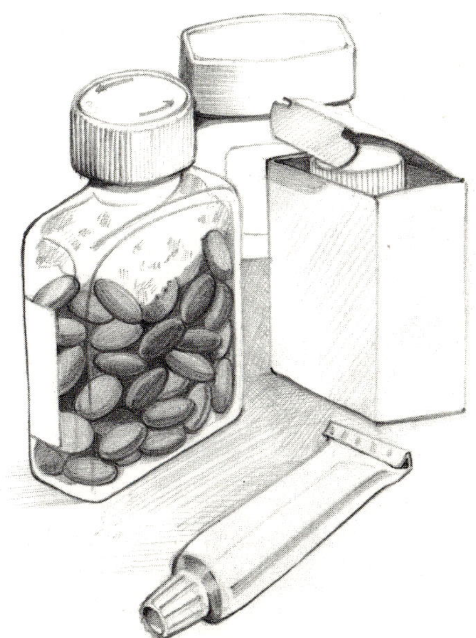

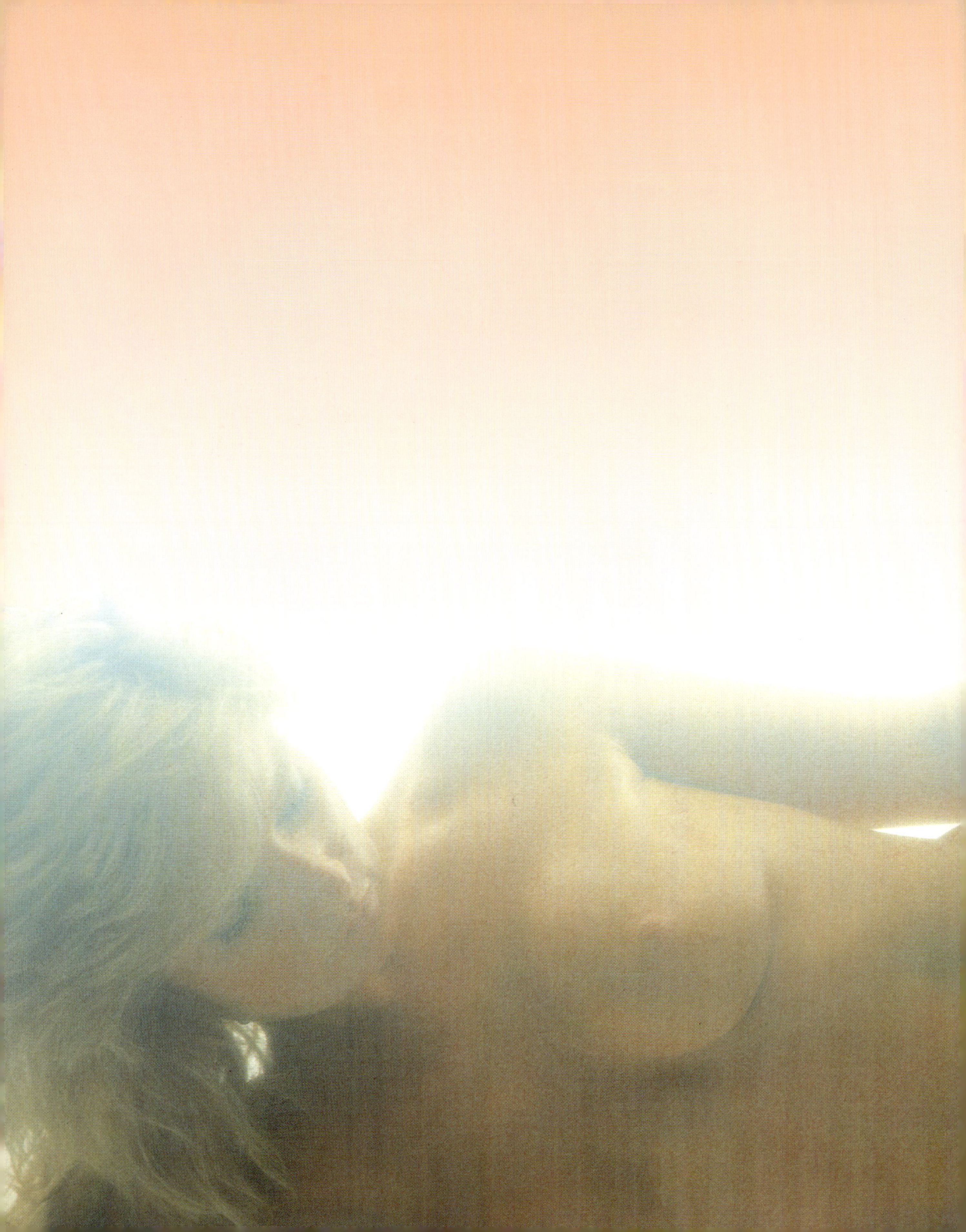

5

WOMAN'S SEXUALITY

Sex is the best fun you can have without laughing and the worst misery you can have without dying — it's an old joke, but it's true. Sex drives people to remarkable creative heights as the source of inspiration for music, poetry and painting, yet also to the most appalling acts of cruelty and violence. It makes people fearful, hopeful, happy, sad, angry, compassionate; there isn't a human emotion or intellectual response that isn't to some extent modified by an individual's attitudes to sexuality — her own and other people's.

Women's sexuality poses some particular problems in understanding. It has always been seen as different from that of men; in ancient times menstruation was a puzzlement and a threat (see Section three) and still is for some people. There are modern men who shun the menstruating woman and modern women who fear their own periods. Similarly, women's sexual appetite has long been regarded by men as puzzling and therefore potentially dangerous. Women don't have an obvious sign of sexual arousal as men do (though there are signs there to be read, by those who know where to look, as will be seen) and women seem able — as far as men can tell — to do without sexual gratification in a way they themselves can't. Women can have babies, and that seems to male onlookers, deprived of the experience, to be sexually satisfying (it is — see next section) and that confuses and alarms them, making them feel inferior to a woman. They need her so much more than she seems to need them.

In the past this male response to women's sexuality made them try to control women. They used violence, they used political methods, they used every and any weapon they could to trammel this terrifying female ability to attract them and please them. The Judaeo-Christian tradition (and its offshoot, Islam) was strongly tilted against women (reading some sections of the Bible and the writings of St. Paul and his supporters and apologists makes many intelligent women today seethe with rage) and even some of the more humane and sensible of the Eastern religions — Buddhism, Taoism, Hinduism — incorporated anti-female sentiments into their teachings. Women are a Snare and a Delusion, men have shouted to each other down the centuries. It's their fault we rape them and beat them — they make us do it — control them — they are evil.

How much of this male confusion and fear has affected women's own view of their reactions and needs, it is hard to tell. It seems likely that many of us have had our perceptions of what we want and what we feel in a sexual way altered by what we're told by men we ought to feel. In Victorian times, for example, a very famous English doctor, William Acton MRCS, wrote a book called *The Functions and Disorders of the Reproduction Organs in Childhood, Youth, Adult Age and Advanced Life, Considering their Physiological, Social and Moral Relations* which became a classic and ran to several editions and powerfully influenced the thinking of a whole generation, both medical and lay. His views on normal male sexuality were startling enough (his dark and dire warnings about the appalling effects of masturbation froze large numbers of nineteenth century men into sexual immobility and fears of this normal, enjoyable and highly educational form of sexual activity still bedevil young men to this day) but his opinion of what was normal for women was even more surprising to modern readers.

'The majority of women (happily for society) are not very much troubled with sexual feeling of any kind. What men are habitually, women are only exceptionally. As the divorce court shows there are some few women who have sexual desires so strong that they surpass those of men and shock public feeling by their consequences. It is from these erroneous notions that so many unmarried men imagine that the marital duties they will have to undertake are beyond their exhausted strength.

Married men, medical men, or women themselves, would, if appealed to, tell a very different tale, and vindicate female nature from the vile aspersions on it by the abandoned conduct and ungoverned lusts of a few of its worst examples. I am ready to maintain that there are many females who never feel any excitement whatever. As a general rule, a modest woman seldom desires any sexual gratification for herself. She submits to her husband's embraces, but principally to gratify him.'

People believed this, even to the point of assuming that there were two kinds of women, in physiological terms; 'normal' 'good ones', who became wives, and 'abnormal' 'bad ones' who became prostitutes. In London alone at that time there were some 20,000 prostitutes, and there was also a very lively market in pornography, but this seems not to have fazed society one bit. All those prostitutes were abnormal — end of discussion. And, of course, no discussion of the normality of the men who used them was considered necessary.

Acton's influence stretched well into the twentieth century. In the nineteen twenties a highly educated young woman (she was a paleantologist) discovered from reading a book she had found in a library that her marriage was unconsummated; until then she had had no idea what sexual intercourse was or what she could expect to experience. The result of that discovery by Marie Stopes not only made her seek personal sexual satisfaction in a new marriage (which she found) but also led her to help other women to find theirs. She wrote several excellent books which had a volcanic effect on women's views of their own sexual potential (one called *Married Love* was a great bestseller and still has much to offer) and when she discovered how large a role fear of unwanted pregnancy played in women's sexual relations, Marie Stopes pushed the idea of free availability of birth control to lengths which appalled respectable British society at the time. Women today still owe a great deal to this irascible, difficult, often pretentious, high handed and marvellous woman (her biographies make absorbing reading).

She led the way towards what has been labelled the Sexual Revolution — the nineteen sixties explosion of free sexual activity by women released from the fear of their own reproductive functions by the Pill (that was invented in 1952). This was the era when glossy magazines announced in ringing tones that women were just the same as men, sexually speaking, with the same ability to enjoy casual sex in a promiscuous way, and the same rights to do so, because women had sexual appetites that were as voracious as any man's. By and large, ran the message trumpeted at all women everywhere, sex for women was a

Very Good Thing. And all this was much aided by a string of reports on human sexuality which stunned everyone with the revelations of what people actually did when they romped — from the Kinsey Report to Masters' and Johnson's *Human Sexual Response* and beyond.

The result, far from being true sexual emancipation for women, was for many a new kind of sexual enslavement. Now it was incumbent upon all women to be as randy as goats. If a young woman in the sixties didn't have her first sexual experience almost as soon as she was into her teens, didn't explode into multiple orgasms on every single occasion and didn't come up smiling and eager for more, she was a failure, a wimp, a non-sixties woman. Many were the sad girls who wrote to the same glossy magazines that were assuring them that the world was their sexual oyster asking plaintively for the address of the Permissive Society so that they could take out a subscription.

Side by side with this, feminism was rising like a tide. Women were told by a number of their angry sisters that marriage was the real snare and delusion, a way of making women into chattels, and that it was absurd to expect one woman to love one man all her adult life — and that there was no way the men were behaving so.

Married men were being as promiscuous as ever, women were told, while trying to control their wives with financial sanctions and threats to take their children away from them. The only real love for women, some of these sisters said, was lesbian love. That was the pure, the real and the sensitive kind. All male sexual love was exploitative.

All of which made commentators in the popular press gloom over the death of marriage, the end of the family and the terrible effects of this social breakdown — all because of the intransigent behaviour of modern women — which was the ruination of The Family, and therefore the End of Civilization As We Know It.

Stirring stuff, all of it — but what are the facts? From our vantage point of the late eighties in the twentieth century, what do we know now about female sexuality?

Not a lot more than our foremothers did, quite honestly. We do have far more understanding of the nuts and bolts of our bodies and of the physiology that makes those physical parts work and react, but it is doubtful we are any nearer a global understanding of woman's sexuality than Eve was. And for a very simple reason. Because there is no such thing as a global woman. We are all different.

This sounds so obvious a thing to say, but sadly the obvious is frequently ignored, and that lack of observation can lead to great distress. In the nineteenth century women who were born to be as randy as goats had a dreadful time, racked with guilt and shame as well as frustration; in the nineteen sixties women who had low sex drives and small sexual appetites had as bad a time, racked with guilt and shame as well as a sense of failure; *plus ça change, plus c'est la même chose* — the more things change, the more they stay the same.

If we have achieved anything from the sexual revolution, it surely ought to be the right to be ourselves, whatever 'ourselves' happens to be. No woman should be harangued into believing that sexual love for a man is wrong, any more than she should be made to feel peculiar because she happens to prefer to love members of her own sex. No woman should be made to feel less of a woman because she happens not to be particularly interested in sexual activity any more than another should be sneered at because she happens to enjoy it a great deal and engages in it whenever she can. The only true freedom is surely freedom to behave as seems best for the individual, in a manner which does no harm to other individuals and their freedoms.

There is a vital ingredient to exercising such a freedom — and that is knowledge. Unless a woman understands how her own body is made and how it works she can't make the right decisions about how to use and enjoy it. And that applies as much to sexual function as to any other.

In the following descriptions of how a woman's sexuality operates, I will be dealing with the heterosexual response. It isn't all that different from the homosexual one (except that when it comes to sharing sex, there is no penetration of the vagina by a penis and no emission into the vagina of semen) and the basic facts are much the same. No judgement is implied of the importance or otherwise of homosexual behaviour by describing women's sexuality in these pages in heterosexual terms. It's simply that heterosexuality is the choice of the majority as far as we can tell.

The female sexual response

The parts of the body most affected by sexual response are the endocrine glands, the vulva, the vagina, the uterus and its appendages, and the breasts, but they are by no means the only parts. The skin, the heart, the lungs, the brain, the blood vessels, indeed, virtually the whole organism takes part. The sexual response is a highly organized and very logical sequence of events in both sexes, and very similar in both, too. The sequence is aimed entirely at successful impregnation of the female by the male; humans may be deeply interested in the recreation provided by sex; Nature is concerned only with creation. Sex was invented by Nature to ensure the birth of a new generation which will be made up of inherited material from both parents, so a response from both parents is needed.

If the act of intercourse is to be fully successful in physiological terms, the genitals of each partner must undergo changes in shape and function; but it must be said that it is possible for impregnation to occur even if a woman is totally unaroused. It is not possible for a man to engage in sexual intercourse unless he is eager to do so, and has an erect penis — the result of arousal in him — and is able to achieve orgasm with the emission of semen. It is, however, possible for a woman to conceive even if she is totally unconscious at the time a man has intercourse with her, and shows no response at all in consequence. It won't be easy, and it may damage her tissues, but a pregnancy could be started. But we will assume for the purposes of this description that the woman is interested in engaging in sexual intercourse, and is co-operative. What are the processes involved?

The origins of arousal are hard to pin-point. In some women, it may be due entirely to the level of sex hormones in the blood. It is known that where there are high levels, sexual desire is likely; when there are low blood levels, it may be absent. However, this is by no means the whole picture, because it is possible for women with normal or even high blood hormone levels to be without desire at all and those with low hormone levels to feel very eager.

The more important input seems to be from the mind. A woman who has an emotional attachment to the man she is with is more likely to be responsive than one who is with a stranger. A woman with a stranger she regards as attractive is more likely to respond than one with a man she regards as ugly or repulsive in any way. A woman who sees, hears, or smells things she associates with sexual arousal may be responsive, while another exposed to stimuli other people regard as sexy may be switched off by it. That is why for some women watching a pornographic film is exciting while another, who regards such films as 'bad' will be repelled. There are many other cultural and social elements involved in what women regard as sexy; a woman from India, say, could be turned on by rich scents which an occidental woman might find cloying; a deeply religious woman could become aroused by reading 'The Song of Solomon' or attending a revivalist meeting; an ambitious woman could be keyed up and eager for sex after a successful business meeting, while another may need to sit around indolently for several hours in order to be receptive. The trigger varies as much as women do.

Once the trigger has been applied, there are four stages to sexual arousal and response.

The excitement phase

As awareness of sex comes into the woman's mind, from whatever trigger, there is a generalized increase in her body's muscle tone, accompanied by deeper breathing, increased heart rate and raised blood pressure. There may be a slight increase in the surface temperature of the body, with some associated flushing of the skin. All this is due to changes in the way the blood vessels tighten and relax to control the body's blood supply, a process governed by a very complex interaction of hormonal and other body chemicals. There is particularly an increase in the blood supply to the genital organs as the blood vessels serving them relax and allow more blood through, and those taking blood away tighten. This leads to local congestion (it is this congestion that in the male causes an erection). The vulva becomes a deeper red in colour and swells, especially the outer lips. These, because they are plumper, move away a little from the vagina they guard, pulling the inner lips (which also swell) with them, so allowing access to the opening.

In some women there is an associated enlargement of the clitoris, the small sensitive structure at the front of the vulva where the inner lips meet (see Section two). This is made of spongy erectile tissue, which means it can collect and hold blood in its inner spaces, and so become firm and larger. Not all women experience this, but those who do will find that the little organ becomes erect and moves forward a little so that it protrudes from the hood that usually covers and protects it.

More important than this is the lubrication response. As the deeper tissues of the vagina become more and more engorged, the pressure on the walls of the vagina leads to the appearance of droplets of liquid. This can be sparse in some women, but in others it is so copious that it runs out of the vagina and wets clothing or bedding. This lubrication (it's known vulgarly as 'love juice' — a rather charming expression) appears within ten to thirty seconds of the start of arousal, and for some women is the first physical sign of their feelings. For others there is an awareness of the pleasant engorgement of the vulva and vagina, felt as an agreeable mild ache.

As arousal goes on, the vagina begins to balloon, becoming less of a potential tube and more like a real one, and the uterus, sharing in the general congestion, enlarges and begins to rise from its resting position on the pelvic floor.

Concurrent with all this reaction in the pelvic sex organs there are reactions in the breasts in some women, though by no means all. They may enlarge as they too become congested, as do the nipples which, like the clitoris, are made of erectile tissue. They harden and the surrounding tinted area, the areola, becomes wrinkled and firm and smaller in area. There may be some mottling of the skin and the eyes may begin to look darker as the iris, the central section, enlarges.

(An interesting sidelight; one of the triggers to a man's sexual arousal is awareness of arousal in a woman. So, in the past, women tried to make themselves more attractive to men by making themselves look aroused when they were not. The use of reddening agents for the skin and lips, to mimic the mottling of sexual arousal was one method — and the use of the drug atropine put in the eyes as drops was another. This relaxes the irises and makes the eyes look very large and dark. For a very long time therefore atropine — which derives, incidentally, from the deadly nightshade plant and is a potent poison — was known as belladonna: beautiful lady.)

An additional reaction is increased sweating, particularly in the apocrine glands in the armpit and round the vulva. It is this sweat which carries pheremones,those hormone-like substances which act as powerful scent stimulants. It is pheremones which entirely govern the way many insects and some animals mate, and there remains in humans an ability to respond vigorously to scent stimulation. When a great deal of pheremone is produced during sexual arousal it contributes to the unmistakeable smell of sex — a musky richness which many men find extremely arousing and which many women too find a potent trigger.

It is possibly because of pheremones that some forms of love play — the mutual sexual stimulation a couple use to arouse each other and themselves — are so popular. Kissing is an obvious example, especially when tongues as well as lips are used. This brings the lover in closer proximity to the source of smells that arouse him/her and also to substances called semiochemicals (semio is Greek for signalling — the chemicals signal sexual arousal). It is also thought by some researchers that there are other components in saliva which add to sexual arousal when passed from one partner to the other.

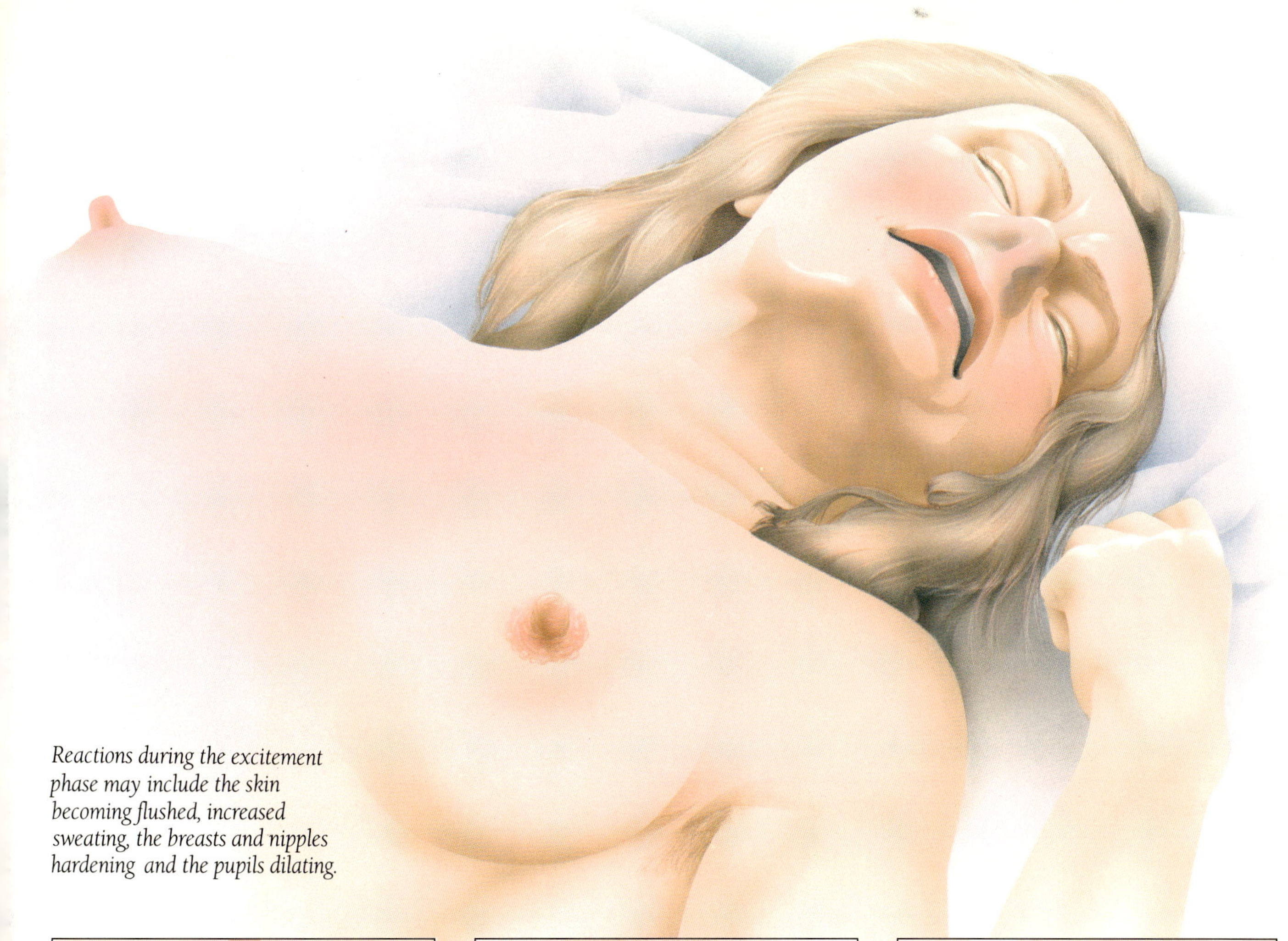

Reactions during the excitement phase may include the skin becoming flushed, increased sweating, the breasts and nipples hardening and the pupils dilating.

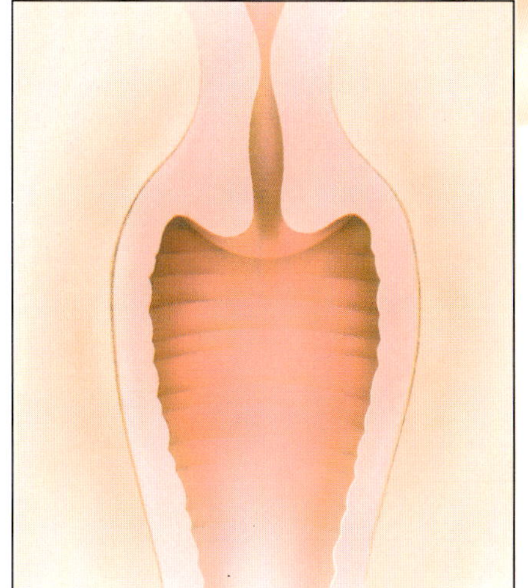

The vagina begins to balloon and assumes a more tubular shape.

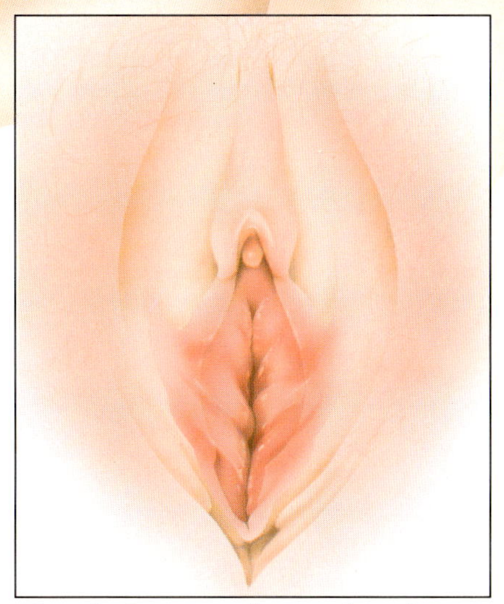

The vulva becomes a deeper red in colour and the outer and inner lips move away from the vaginal opening. The clitoris becomes firm and larger and lubrication occurs inside the vagina.

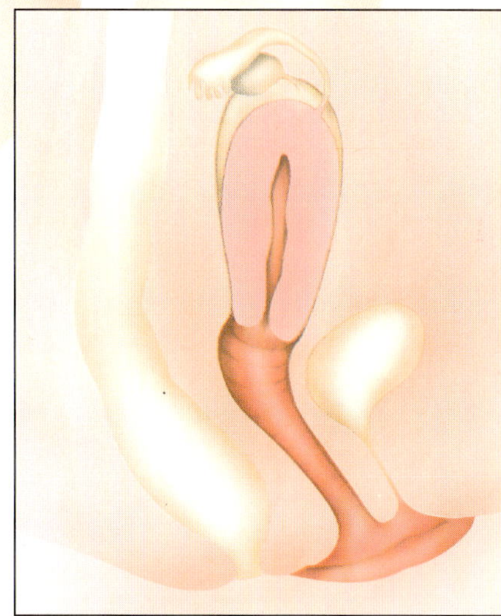

The uterus enlarges and begins to rise from its resting position on the pelvic floor.

Kissing of the genitals — oral sex — is another way in which to provide a powerful stimulation via the sense of smell. This sense is the most immediate we have; the other senses send their messages to the cortex, the thinking part of the brain, via other brain structures, to be interpreted and responded to. The sense of smell, on the other hand, feeds in its information directly, and for this reason acts far more rapidly than any other. This is why a smell can immediately change your mood, or trigger a very old memory with a speed that nothing you see or hear or touch ever could. And in the sexual context, smell is exceedingly important especially in this first excitement phase.

The excitement phase can be maintained for a long time, with occasional rests to allow the level of arousal to subside, thus giving the lovers more pleasure from their encounter. It would be possible to go into great detail about how to make love at this stage, with lingering descriptions of ear-nibbling and belly and buttock stroking, and thigh-trembling and heaven knows what else, but that would be of small value (apart perhaps from being sexually arousing reading, which can be agreeable and a useful preliminary to lovemaking). The most assiduous mapping of erogenous zones — the parts of a woman's body which are particularly responsive to touch and caress — would not be accurate for all women, as individuals. To make that sort of body map, every inch of it would have to be included, because of the wide range of individual responses. Sufficient to say that kissing, licking, sucking, stroking, caressing, talking, laughing, shouting and everything else you like are part of normal lovemaking and contribute to the excitement phase of the female sexual response.

The plateau phase

This is really not a separate stage at all; it is more an intensification of the excitement phase. All the reactions already described reach their peak. Skin mottling increases, and the skin over the vulva — the 'sex skin' — changes as the small inner lips swell, and they alter colour to a marked degree in some women (hardly at all in others — never forget the differences there are in individuals). The swelling creates a sort of 'platform' just in front of the vaginal opening, which at this stage is now at its most ballooned and open. The colour of the small lips, which can range from a dusky pink to the deepest of burgundy, could be a remnant of our primitive past, when the male needed a visual sign to tell him that penetration would not only be possible but welcome. (In face to face sex, this sign is less important, unless the woman is tipped high on her pelvis and has her knees spread very wide, but in rear-approach sex it would be very visible.)

At this stage, the woman is eager to respond with orgasm, and she may find she does so very soon. Others find it possible to maintain the plateau level for some time, thus prolonging pleasure, though it takes an experienced pair of lovers to do this. But some do manage it, moving backwards and forwards from plateau to excitement and back again for some time. But there eventually comes a point, just before orgasm is imminent, when the clitoris (if it has been prominent) seems to withdraw. In fact it turns up at an angle of 180 degrees and tucks itself in under the arch of the pelvis (the symphysis pubis).

The orgasm phase

This is the peak of sexual excitement and the most pleasurable. It is this phase that gives rise to much of the poetry about sex and a lot of the fear, because it involves not only intensely pleasurable physical sensations but also an abandonment of self control that some people find alarming. The French have labelled it *la petite morte* — the little death — and there is some reason in that.

In purely physical terms what happens is that the muscles that surround the vagina and those in the perineum (the skin covered area between vulva and anus) go into rhythmic contractions which involve the whole area, and which create intensely enjoyable sensations. It is probably this feeling that rewards intercourse which encourages people to involve themselves in the activity at all. Without pleasure it would all be rather uncomfortable, not to say absurd. (Lord Chesterfield is said to have told his son that 'the cost is exorbitant, the pleasure momentary, and the posture ridiculous'.)

The contractions happen at intervals of 0.8 of a second, and the number of them is variable — for some women there are a great many, for others only a few. The intensity of feeling is very variable too, from woman to woman and from time to time in the same woman. Sometimes there may be an associated twitching of other body muscles — the toes may curl and the belly muscles may tighten. The uterine muscles also contract and the opening of the uterus — the cervix — gapes. This is to enable semen deposited at the end of the vagina to enter the uterus; the uterine contractions create suction, which draws the sperm inside (incidentally, when Marie Stopes guessed that this happened and said so in one of her books, she was laughed to scorn by medical men. Now Masters and Johnson have proven that it does happen).

None of the described reactions are obligatory. There are women who read verbal accounts of what an orgasm is and become very upset because although they have a pleasurable experience and enjoy it, what happens for them doesn't seem to match the words. They never notice that they flush or mottle; they don't twitch, or they don't arch their backs and grimace and shout out aloud (some do, and there are vivid descriptions of such reactions in a number of sex manuals). But it cannot be said too often that comparison with others' descriptions is pointless. It is your own experience that matters; if you are happy with it then that is fine. If not, then help may be needed — but it is never needed simply because you don't 'go by the book'.

There are some women for whom the plateau/orgasm phase is so prolonged that they are able to have several orgasms, one after the other. Masters and Johnson in their research reported such responses and this created a storm of interest and anxiety all over the world. Women told each other that because some of the subjects in Masters' and Johnson's research reacted so, they ought to as well.

But since all women vary in appetite and response, this is a silly thing to suggest. It is probable that the women who were the subjects of Masters' and Johnson's research were of a particular physiological, cultural and emotional type. It is surely reasonable to suggest that the majority of women would find it difficult to enjoy engaging in sexual activity while being observed. It goes deeply against our inherent self-protective instincts, after all; the animal that copulates while available for observation could be the animal that is killed while doing it.

The women who volunteered for the Masters and Johnson programme were particularly relaxed about their sexuality, so what was true for them may not therefore be true for all. It is no failure in any woman if she does not have multiple orgasms, and to set out to have them because of a sense of 'ought to' rather than 'I need to' seems to be a search fraught with the risk of failure. All that is likely to happen is anxiety sufficient to block off the normal orgasmic response altogether.

The resolution phase

This final stage takes the woman back to her pre-arousal state. The general reaction is often a sense of deep relaxation and deep desire for sleep. There are people who use sex mainly as a way of inducing sleep, and that most people see sleep as a natural follow on to enjoyable sex is seen in the common euphemism for intercourse; 'to sleep with someone'.

Physiologically the heart rate, breathing rates, blood pressure and blood vessels return to normal within a matter of minutes after orgasm. The clitoris returns to its normal position five to ten seconds after orgasm is completed and there is rapid loss of congestion in the vulva which regains its normal colour within ten to fifteen seconds. The vagina, however, may take up to ten or fifteen minutes to return to its usual pale and relaxed state, and the cervix too may take its time to return to normal, continuing to gape for up to half an hour after orgasm, by which time the uterus too has returned to its usual resting place on the pelvic floor. During this time it is still possible for sperm to enter the uterus, even though the contractions are not actually sucking it in.

Sexual questions

That, then is the 'normal' process of response but it can be greatly modified not only by an individual woman's temperament and constitution, but by her worries. Fear, and its first cousin, anxiety, can, as has already been said many times, cause a large number of physical reactions, and many of these reactions profoundly affect the sexual response. And because the sex drive is so powerful, and so potentially pleasurable, it always has been a rich source of anxiety. Women worry a great deal about a great many sexual matters, and ask a lot of questions.

Q *'I used to play with myself when I was a child. Will this damage my ability to have normal sex and babies?'*

We have to thank people like Dr Acton for the notion that masturbation — 'playing with yourself' or 'self abuse' as it has been most outrageously labelled — is abnormal. It most certainly is not. The vast majority of young people of both sexes discover, as part of their normal self exploration during their growing years, that handling their genitals can give them pleasure. Many of them go on to discover that with the right sort of manipulation they can create an orgasm, and enjoy it very much. This is an essential part of any person's sexual development. How can a person learn to share her body enjoyably with another person if she's never learned to enjoy it for herself?

While it would be wrong to tell women that they were in some way lacking if they didn't masturbate at some time or other (it would be as bad as telling them that it causes acne, hairy palms and feet, weakness and an early death, as Dr Acton used to declare) it is reasonable to say that most girls will learn to do so and enjoy doing so, as long as they haven't been filled with a horror of touching themselves, or a fear of their own healthy sexuality. It is harder for therapists to help women who seek assistance because they are having sexual difficulties if they have never masturbated. They have to be taught this first, before they can learn to share sex.

So there is never any need to fear that an orgasm, whether given to you by someone else or by yourself is in any way harmful. It's a gift, whoever the donor may be.

Q *'My man wants to do things when we make love that I think are peculiar. Like kissing me all over — and I mean all over — and dressing up and acting out games. And he wants to do it so often, too — what is the normal frequency?'*

There is no sort of sex play between humans that hasn't been invented by millions in the past, isn't being tried by millions in the present, and won't be enjoyed by millions yet unborn. We have a huge capacity for inventiveness and playfulness, and keep on, in every generation, discovering the many ways there are to amuse and arouse ourselves.

And it can be said as an axiom that there is no form of sexual play that is wrong if both partners desire and enjoy it, and neither is harmed by it. Sexual immorality is, surely, the use of force of any kind to make one person do something they dislike or fear in order to satisfy another's pleasure. The force can be physical, social, emotional or financial — whatever form it takes, it must be wrong to use it in the sexual context (or any context, come to that).

Fantasy — dressing up and acting games — is for many people a vital part of sexual pleasure. The majority of us start to learn about sex by masturbating, and virtually always masturbation is accompanied by fantasy; it would be a wicked waste of our rich imaginations not to use them in this way. Even after fantasy is no longer apparently needed, because there is a flesh and blood partner, it can still go on being of value. Many women, however loving they feel towards their partners, need to fantasize during lovemaking in order to increase their arousal (remembering that the mind's input to the physiology of arousal is at least as important as the hormonal one, and often much more so) and many men do as well. They may imagine themselves in a romantic scene on a beach, or in incredible luxury, or with the real beloved who has been magically transformed to be like an ideal cinema heart-throb.

But, because, by and large, men seem to be less gifted at imagining scenarios (women have an inbuilt gift for using words and making images with them) they tend to like their fantasy acted out to make them more 'real'. Hence the delight many of them take in seeing a partner in sheer underwear, high heeled shoes and nothing else (the foot has long been a fetish — that is, sexually arousing — for men, rarely for women) and other 'sexy' items.

There are women who find this worrying. They believe that men who want them to dress up are devaluing them; that their bodies 'aren't enough' and that the men are using them as sex objects. This may be true in some cases, where the man feels no emotional involvement with his partner, but it isn't always necessarily so. A man can love his partner very deeply and yet enjoy — indeed, need — fetish stimulation to accompany his lovemaking.

This doesn't mean that his love is failing, or that his partner is insufficiently attractive to him. It means simply that his ability to use his own mind to vary and freshen his experience (and we all, men and women, have a very low boredom threshold and need constant new stimulation to keep us alert and interested) is limited.

This is not an attempt to excuse pornography or the use of images of women's bodies or part of them for commercial gain. That is a political issue that deserves thorough addressing and this is not the place to do so. But it is unrealistic to believe that a particular man who is, in other ways, caring and affectionate, is unloving, uncaring, or exploitative simply because his imagination and ability to turn himself on need a boost. It's a lack in him, not a sin.

Another way in which some women are unrealistic is in their expectations of their ability to arouse a man. Too many seem to feel they should be the be-all and end-all in the life of the person they love; they ask for repeated expressions of undying devotion and constant reassurance that they, and they alone, are enough to provide him with all his sexual needs.

Some of these ideas have been fed into women by a certain sort of romantic fiction; both sexes are prone to be dazzled by the stories they are told; there are men who believe because of the fiction they read that they 'ought' to be forever randy and forever capable of instant masterful sex, which is absolute nonsense; every man has times when he can't, or doesn't want to, or would rather have a nice cup of tea, thank you, just as women do.

All of us are at risk of having our responses warped and anxieties created because we believe in the stereotypes sold to us. We'd all be much happier looking clearly at ourselves and each other, rather than darkly through the glass of other people's notions of what is 'right' and what is 'normal'. If it's right and normal for you and you enjoy it, then why not? How can it be wrong? And if you can't always be seen by your partner as the ultimate in female allure, it doesn't mean there is anything wrong with you. It means only that you are being somewhat unreasonable in expecting to be so.

There are, however, some provisos about the normality and morality of our love play. There are some forms that might do damage. Penetration by the penis of the anus rather than the vagina can cause damage and pain, and the man who insists on this in spite of his partner's objections is being immoral. However, some women enjoy it, because the bed of spongy tissue which lies between the rear wall of the vagina and the rectum, and which fills with blood as part of the excitement phase, is particularly responsive in them. (See page 74.) And if they enjoy it there is no moral reason why they should not do so.

However, there may be health reasons why they should not; there is some evidence that the disease AIDS is spread more easily by this mode (see Page 104) and this possibility is one both partners must consider.

Similarly, the use of bondage or sado-masochistic fantasy — with one partner inflicting pain on the other — can misfire and lead to damage, and in some cases has led to death. It has been said that a relationship between a sadist, who enjoys inflicting pain, and a masochist, who enjoys experiencing it, is a joyous marriage of true minds; and so it might be — but it can still lead to damage, if control is lost at any time.

On the question of normal frequency — there is no such thing. For one couple it may be normal to have intercourse three times a day, for another three times a year; it is only if there is a marked imbalance between the appetites of a regular couple who are tied together by more than just shared sexual pleasure that there may be a need to seek help. It is often possible to use psychotherapy to uncover reasons for both the inability to share sex as often as a partner wants to, and for demanding it more often than a partner wants to, and also techniques people can learn to increase — or limit — their appetite if the imbalance is causing problems.

Q *'I really only like making love if I can be on top. I feel more comfortable that way, but I can't help thinking there is something wrong with me, because most of my friends prefer the normal way, on their backs.'*

The answer to this is the same, basically, as the answer to the previous worry. Whatever suits both partners and distresses neither is fine.

And whoever said that there is only one normal position for intercourse?

Actually it is true, according to some surveys, that most women prefer the so-called missionary position — woman below, man above. (It got its name from the meddling behaviour or Victorian missionaries who told South Sea Islanders that it was wrong to have sex as they enjoyed it, 'like animals' with a rear approach, and insisted they do as the British did — how was that for arrogance?) But many more much prefer the woman-superior approach because they are able to control the movements of intercourse in a way that ensures they achieve the sort of clitoral stimulation that they need to reach orgasm. It can happen with inexperienced couples that they fail to provide each other with enough continuous stimulation to pass from plateau stage to orgasm stage, and it is usually the woman who has the most difficulty. If she is on top of her partner she can guide her body as she needs in a way she couldn't when crushed by his weight.

Other women prefer the rear approach, which enables their partners to reach round and use their hands to give them manual stimulation of the clitoris during intercourse, while others like to lie on their sides. The possibilities are many, though there aren't quite as many positions as some of the more athletic sex manuals would suggest (incidentally, the use of the term 'sixty-nine' or *'soixante-neuf'*, does not imply that there are that number of different positions possible for intercourse. It is a label used to describe the top-to-tail position used by couples who want to kiss each other's genitals — a figure six is a figure nine upside down and vice versa.

Illustrated are a few of the most practised sexual positions, but there are many more — just use your imagination!)

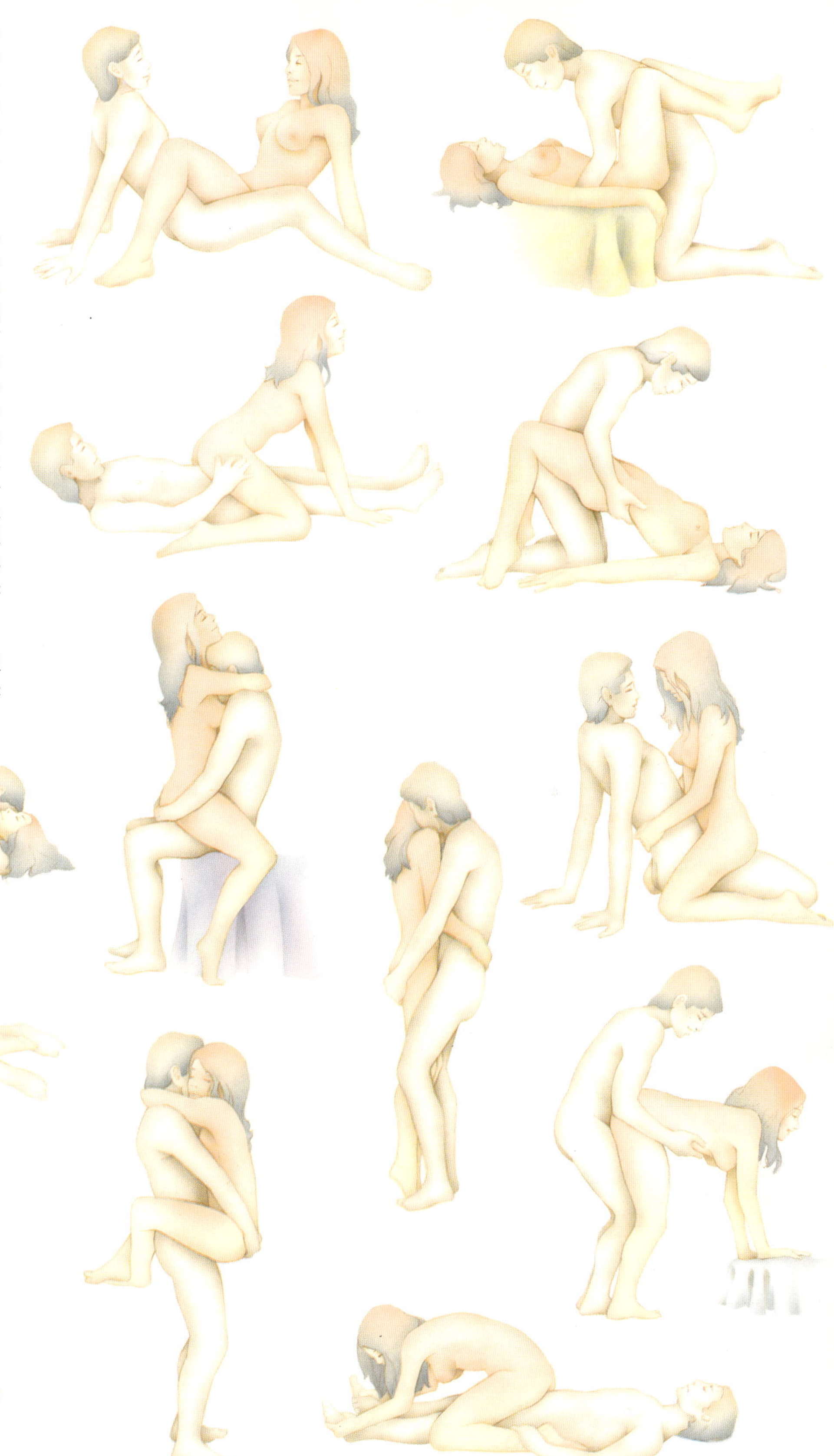

Q *'I tried to make love to my fiance but we failed. He is a very tall big man while I am petite and I was just too small for him. It hurt dreadfully — I know the first time is supposed to be painful and that you bleed but this was unbelievable agony.'*

There are two myths here to be dispelled. One, that a woman who is small in height and build has a tiny vagina and, two, that first time intercourse has to be (literally) bloody agony.

The vagina in any adult woman is designed to allow the passage of a full grown infant with its disproportionately large head. That is why the vagina has walls with folds in them — to allow the great expansion that is needed. No man anywhere, however large in build or in penis, can ever produce an erection that will be larger than an infant's head. It is impossible for a vagina to be 'too small'.

However, it is possible for a woman to have deep anxieties about sex which make it difficult for her to achieve full arousal and excitement, and which make any attempt to enter the vagina react on the muscles of the area and send them into tight spasm so that they snap shut. It is as though the muscles are guarding the entrance and will not permit any invasion. Some women are able to become excited enough to feel, on a conscious level, that they are ready for penetration, but at a much deeper level there is fear — so the muscles act against the excitement and prevent entry. Any attempt to force past this barrier is exceedingly painful.

This state is called vaginismus. Sometimes it is a temporary state, in a virgin who isn't sure about what will happen to her. Once she feels safe and sure with her partner and can relax enough to allow some penetration she may well be able to complete the first act of intercourse in comfort. Others may need several attempts before they can be really comfortable.

For others the problem is that they have so hazy a notion of how their bodies are made they fear that the vagina cannot cope with the penis. Study of the pictures in this book should help dispel that particular anxiety. Others have been reared with the idea that sex is dirty, damaging, painful and so react against it, however hard they consciously try to enjoy it. Yet others are comfortable in the early days of a sexual relationship, and then later, possibly because of an unhappy relationship or unhappy birth experience, develop vaginismus.

In some cases, the woman consistently refuses intercourse (though she may allow sex play, with manual stimulation to the clitoris, to reach orgasm) and there are marriages which have been unconsummated for many years for this reason. In situations like this the answer is sex therapy, the chance to talk in some depth with a trained sympathetic doctor who will explain and reassure and teach a girl to explore her own vagina painlessly, so that she can, eventually, allow her partner to do so.

Now, the second myth — that first intercourse is always painful (and that it causes bleeding). In some cases, indeed, a first intercourse may be painful:

Because the girl is unsure of her own readiness for it; because she has a partner who does not understand when she is excited enough to be ready for penetration and tries to hurry her; because the couple are in circumstances where real relaxation is impossible, say in the back seat of a car or in a parent's living room while they are out and expected back at any moment.

But, if none of these or similar problems exist and the couple have enough knowledge (and that isn't, by the way, the same as experience; a man may have had sex with hundreds of girls and still be an inept and selfish lover, while a man who is a virgin can be very successful in making his partner feel relaxed and happy because he is informed, concerned and sensitive to her needs and her signals) then the experience can be painless, bloodless, and enjoyable.

It is rarely true that the hymen, the so-called maidenhead, is tough and has to be 'torn' or 'broken' at first intercourse. It is, remember, a fold of membrane rather than a true barrier; it may need some stretching, but this can be comfortable and easy in a relaxed and excited woman. In a few cases it is a true barrier and needs surgical attention, but these are really very rare indeed. (See Section two.)

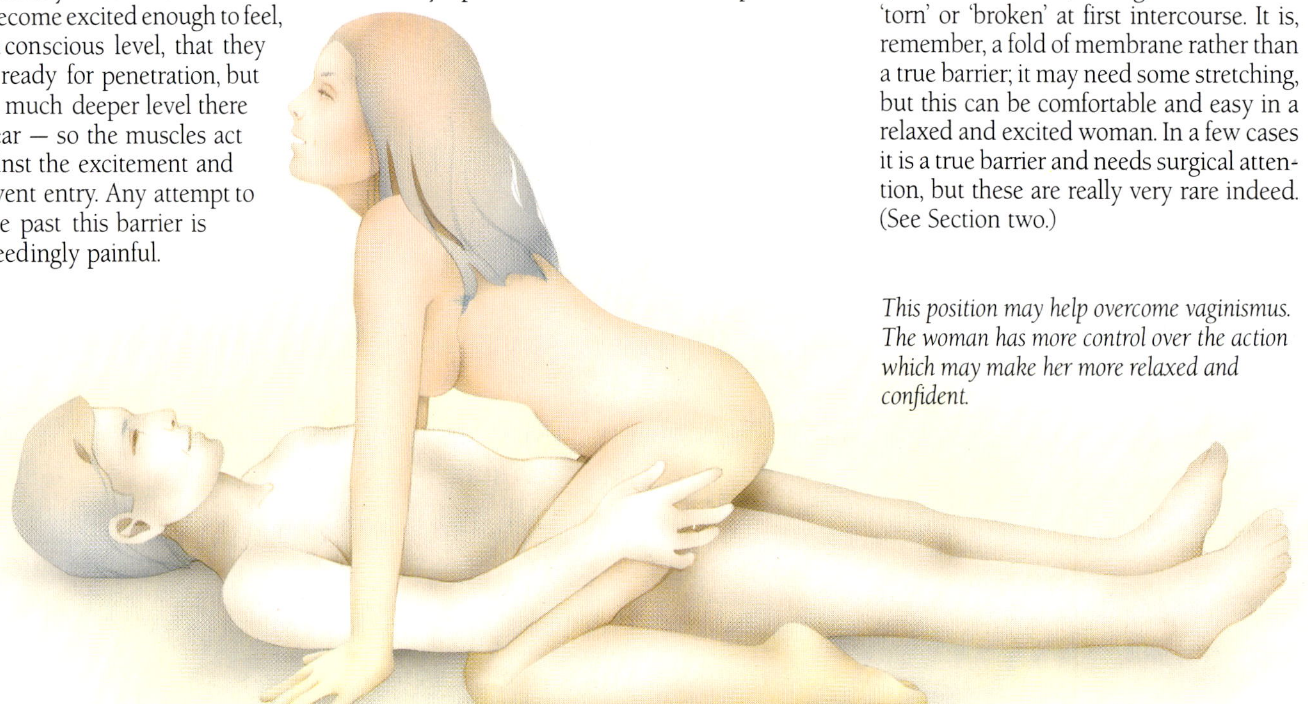

This position may help overcome vaginismus. The woman has more control over the action which may make her more relaxed and confident.

Q *'I have had two children, and now I have left my husband and have a new lover. He says my vagina has been so stretched by the children that he can't feel anything. Can I have an operation to put it right?'*

Just as the vagina is capable of great stretching to allow a baby to pass through, so it is capable of great elasticity — it can return to its normal size very rapidly. It is rare that a woman's vagina is so lax that her partner cannot feel his penis inside her. If she had prolonged and difficult labours and has therefore weakened pelvic floor muscles, then there may be some weakness, but not usually enough to affect intercourse.

It is sometimes possible for there to have been inadequate stitching of a tear suffered during childbirth or after an episiotomy (see next section) which can greatly widen the opening to the vagina, but even then, the muscles can easily be contracted to hold the penis firmly and comfortably. It is possible for a woman to have surgery to repair a badly stitched introitus (vaginal opening) if it is really very ragged, and if there is enough prolapse of the uterus due to weakened muscles this too can be operated on (see Section eight). But most surgeons would need more evidence for an operation than a man's complaints.

One form of evidence is the occurrence of 'vaginal wind'. If the muscles are very lax, it may happen in some intercourse positions — for example, when the woman kneels with her buttocks raised high, for the rear approach — that the thrusting penis pushes air into her, which later escapes, slowly. Surgical tightening of the muscles could help prevent this, though it seems an extreme remedy. It is no disaster if there is a noisy air escape after intercourse; people don't usually have operations to prevent air leaving the gut, so why have them to prevent it leaving the vagina? 'Vaginal wind' isn't even offensive in smell.

The most likely reason for a man's complaints about a lax vagina is a failure to understand exactly what happens inside a woman's body when she is sexually roused. In the excitement and plateau stages, it will be remembered, the vagina balloons in order to accommodate the penis. If a particular woman is so aroused that this is a marked feature, the man may find he feels less of her vagina round his penis. The answer may be, if she is willing, to start intercourse before the plateau stage is reached, to enable him to feel a little more of the tighter vagina — but he must realise that once she does reach plateau, then her vagina will balloon more.

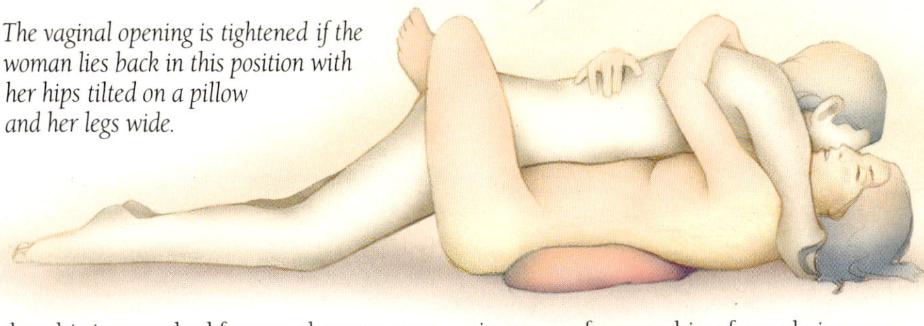

The vaginal opening is tightened if the woman lies back in this position with her hips tilted on a pillow and her legs wide.

Changes in posture may help both partners. If a woman lies on her back with her hips tilted on a pillow and her legs wide, the vaginal opening will be narrowed and the vagina too may seem tighter.

Another possible cause of such male complaints is misdirected resentment of the woman's previous sexual partner. There are men who have great difficulty in accepting that a woman they care for has ever 'belonged' to someone else (thinking in terms of ownership of people is repugnant to many women, but there it is — there are people who feel this way and can't be made to lose their feelings by being told to). The children she has borne are unavoidable evidence of this previous liaison, and may become objects of his resentment. Or, if he can't express his feelings directly to her about her ex-partner and about the children, he may complain about what happened to her when she bore the children. Thus he is able to deal with his feelings by making her feel inadequate.

The answer for a woman in this situation is not to submit herself to surgery or to feel guilt (that is, surely never necessary). She needs to persuade her partner to come with her to a counsellor so that he can dig out and explore and so dispose of his unhappy feelings or resentment.

Q *'I love my fiance but however hard I try I can't enjoy sex with him. It isn't his fault, I've always been the same — I've had a lot of boyfriends in the past — and now he is thinking of leaving me because he is afraid he is no good to me. He says we must be incompatible though we both love each other a lot. I'm afraid I'm just abnormal and can never be a real woman'.*

To blame a man for a woman's failure to enjoy sex is not just. It takes two people to make successful love, and it takes the same number to share unsuccessful sex. So a man who says he must leave a woman because she has sexual difficulties is helping no one, least of all himself. His penis is no sort of magic wand that is meant to make a woman react; to think so is to be both absurdly arrogant and self-damaging.

It is also rather foolish to talk of 'incompatibility'. To assume that there are people who match each other sexually, the way pieces of jigsaw fit, is to put a colossal strain on the workings of chance. To match people successfully, if they actually had to pair up precisely, would be impossible.

The basic fact is that any man and any woman can share successful sex if they want to. There is no magic about it. But, because we are a thinking and imaginative species, we do often, as individuals, put barriers in the way of a normal response. An adult female body that is capable of reacting like any other female adult body is prevented from doing so by the actions of the mind. A block is set up between the organs' ability to respond and the stimuli which could make them do so.

There can be a great many different reasons for a woman putting up a mental barrier against sexuality, and preventing herself from becoming aroused and ultimately reaching orgasm.

She may be ignorant. Ignorance breeds fear and fear breeds tension and anxiety. They all prevent normal sexual arousal.

She may be frightened. However complete her knowledge of her own body, she may have been exposed in childhood to alarming experiences involving sexuality. The child who was sexually abused may grow up into the girl who can't respond to sex — and it is estimated that one child in ten is so abused, with a large proportion of those being incestuously abused by their fathers.

Or she may have been frightened in adult life; an experience of assault or rape can prevent arousal and orgasm even with a much loved partner.

She may have been conditioned to hate sex. The 'teachings' of the Dr Actons of the Victorian period remain with many of us to this day. We are all the daughters of our mothers and they are the daughters of their mothers; we don't have to go back many generations to be slap in the middle of Actonian ideas about female sexuality. Even modern women may unwittingly be rearing their daughters to fear and despise that which should give them satisfaction.

In this list of barriers it will be clear that there is no physical reason given. That is because there are no physical reasons for continuing failure to arouse, excite and experience orgasm. There are, of course, times in every women's life when she will be uninterested in sex, and so will be unresponsive; a woman who is ill, or in pain, or deeply unhappy or suffering from an illness such as depression, or who is abusing drugs or alcohol, may lose her sexual appetite, just as she can lose her appetite for food. When the temporary circumstances causing the disease are removed, so will her lack of interest in sex.

However, in some women, a period of such illness may lead to a sexual arousal problem, even when the illness is over, because of lack of understanding of the way the sex drive, like any other human function, can be temporarily spoiled. A woman may be conditioned by one illness-inspired period of sexual uninterest, to expect it always to be so. And there is nothing like thinking that to make it so.

Sensate focus

The following steps should be gone through, ideally every night, when you have plenty of time and no fear of interruption. Choose a place where you can be quiet and which is pleasant to be in. Dismal surroundings make it difficult for anyone to feel sexy.

Do take lots of time. This isn't time-wasting, but a way of greatly improving your sex life.

Don't rush into complete intercourse before both partners are equally eager. Being in too much of a hurry can increase the problem.

Do take your self-help plan seriously. You may feel a little foolish at first, but in time, you'll learn just how helpful and worth while these exercises are.

Don't set any goals. All you are trying to do with sensate focus is recover your natural feelings. Then you can leave it to those feelings to do the rest.

Enjoy what you are doing, one second at a time, and give no thought to the outcome.

1 You need a large bath towel and a bottle of baby oil or lotion. Spread the towel on your bed (or on the floor as long as it is warm and clean) and then both undress completely. Keep the light on.

2 Lie on your front on the towel and go through a series of relaxation exercises, alternatively tightening and then relaxing your muscles, from your face down to your feet, and then tightening your whole body and relaxing by imagining you are floating. (See Section ten.)

3 Now, using the oil, your partner should start to massage you gently. On no account should he or she touch any sexual areas — breasts or genitals — but simply caress you gently. You on your part should concentrate entirely on the sensations you receive from this touching. Think of nothing, certainly not about whether you will go on to intercourse; only 'listen' to those gentle fingers, fixing your mind on the sensations you get. You will be a little tense at first, may even feel a bit silly — but concentrate on what you are feeling and keep your muscles relaxed. The tension and embarrassment will soon melt away.

4 Now turn over so that the stroking massage can be repeated on the rest of your body. And throughout, talk — actually describe what gives you pleasure. This is a vital part of the new communication system you are creating. Don't criticize movements you enjoy less; just say quietly, 'no', and be very positive with appreciation of those you enjoy more. Don't go on to intercourse until you really want to. If your partner wants to enjoy a climax and can't hold back, you can help by caressing his or her body with your hands. If you both agree that you won't have intercourse until you really want it, this will remove any sense of 'trying to succeed' or 'fearing to fail' and in itself makes it more likely you will want sex again.

5 Change places, and give the same gentle oil-based massage and caresses to your partner.

These few steps are the only ones. As time goes on, and you find your responses strengthening, you will want to go on and share more caressing, and eventually intercourse. Listen to your feelings. They will tell you all you need to know.

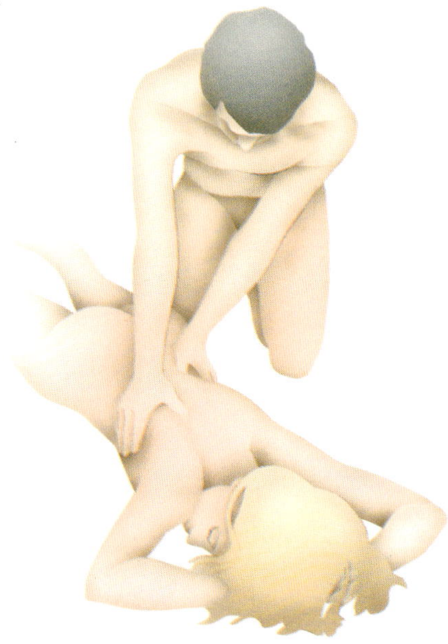

The remedy for this problem is sex therapy, if this is possible, or a self-help system can be tried to start with. It can do no harm to attempt a self-cure, and may well have the desired effect. But if it doesn't, then the sooner help is sought the better. The longer a woman goes on with a problem like this, the longer it is likely to last.

Sexual self-help

Firstly it is important to realise that a sex problem is nothing to be ashamed of. If you had a sore throat, or an aching joint that was making you miserable and spoiling your life you'd seek help for it. A sexual problem, if it makes you miserable and spoils your life, should be approached in the same way — as worthy of attention. Give yourself full permission to be sexy — you have the right.

Secondly learn more about sex and how the body works. That is the purpose of this whole book, of course, but also read others. Several others. Some will annoy you, some will amuse you, and some will anger you, but all will educate you. Read them together with your partner. There is no such thing as a solitary sex problem. It always involves both partners, so both of you need to do the reading. And sharing reading is the first step to sharing honest talking — which many couples have never yet managed when it comes to sex.

Thirdly don't blame sex if the trouble is deep in your relationship. Some people have sex problems because they have partnership problems. Being on bad terms over money, each other's relations, working women, the way the children are brought up, the amount of help a man gives in the home — all this can damage a love life profoundly. So make sure you aren't using sex as a way to cover up what is really the problem. If you may be doing that, then talk to a marriage guidance counsellor.

Fourthly seek expert help as soon as you feel you just can't cope any more. Struggling on, hoping a sex problem will right itself in time, never works. All that does is make the problem harder to solve. Use the 'sensate focus' exercises (shown opposite) devised by Masters and Johnson to help people get in touch with their own ability to be excited (this is as effective for men as for women, incidentally).

Q *'I read a lot about sex and I'm still not sure what happens when a woman has an orgasm. What is the difference between the vaginal and the clitoral one? I'm not sure what I have. It feels different sometimes?'*

This is an argument that has raged for a long time. Do women have orgasms because of sensations in the vagina, or is it solely stimulation of the clitoris that has the effect? In the past, some thinkers (Freud was a leader amongst them) said that the vaginal orgasm — that is, one that happened as a result of the penis stimulating the vagina — was the truly mature kind. The clitoral one, the sort a woman could give herself by masturbating, was described as 'immature'.

This sounds to many women remarkably like penis pride. The idea behind this definition of the 'vaginal' orgasm is that the powerful penis is all a woman really needs, if she is a real live mature woman.

Later research, notably the work of Masters and Johnson, showed that the clitoris is the source of the orgasm (a book on midwifery, published in 1855, labels the structure as 'the organ of voluptuousness'; not all Victorians were as purblind as Dr Acton.) Masters and Johnson made the point, however, that a vigorously thrusting penis in a comparatively short vagina — there are considerable individual variations — may pull on the clitoris in such a way that it is stimulated and also rubbed against the man's pubic bone. The result is stimulation of the clitoris, leading to reactions in the vaginal muscles — orgasm.

However, many women do maintain that they have different sexual responses with some orgasms that seem to arise deep inside the vagina as well as from the clitoris.

It is true that the vagina does show some response to sensation, but by no means all along its length. The opening and the outer third are the most sensitive, and so are the deeper areas. Deep pressure can indeed be very agreeable, as can the sensation of the rhythmic entry and exit and re-entry of the penis. But there is little felt elsewhere inside the vagina; most women do not feel the sensation of the semen being pumped out of the penis, for example. The fluid is of the same temperature as the vaginal walls and so there is no real awareness (though to go by some pornography, there are men who think women ought to experience it as though a hosepipe were spurting in them under pressure. More penis pride!).

The probability is that both vagina and clitoris contribute in their own ways to the total experience of orgasm, with the clitoris probably being the most significant, since stimulation of it, whether direct or indirect (and many women find it too exquisitely sensitive to tolerate direct touch) will virtually always lead to orgasm, even if it takes a very long time — and it is recorded that some women need to use a vibrator on the clitoris for up to half an hour or longer to obtain adequate stimulation.

Vaginal thrusting, on the other hand, does not always create orgasm. That this is so is shown by the discovery in research that the vast majority of women masturbate by direct attention to the clitoris, rarely with a dildo (a false penis).

It is normal to find that orgasm on each occasion feels different; there will be some extremely exciting ones, some that are little more than 'sneezes', some that seem almost to hurt, some that only tickle.

The state of mind and the erotic thoughts a woman has will be at least as important to the experience as what is happening to her genitals — and it is important to remember that some women with powerful imaginations can have orgasms just by thinking of sex or love. (Look some time at the famous statue of St Teresa by Michaelangelo. It is thought by many to depict a woman experiencing a physical orgiastic response to religious ecstasy.)

Whatever sort of orgasm a woman has, she needs to enjoy it for what it is, rather than to try to compare it with others, either her own or her friends'. Sometimes she will not have one, nor want one, and that is normal too. Variation is what we're all about.

Q *'Sometimes it hurts me to have intercourse. I get a deep ache inside and burning sensations.'*

Dyspareunia is the name given to painful intercourse. If it is persistent, it may be labelled vaginismus (see page 70).

Physical causes include local infections such as thrush, trichomonas, or 'cystitis' (see Section seven), post-birth injury, for example after stitching for a tear or an episiotomy (see Section six), disorders of the ovary (pain on deep penetration is usually linked with this) or disorders of other pelvic structures.

Psychological causes include fear of intercourse, fear of rejection by a partner, fear of pregnancy, all leading to a degree of muscular spasm and failure to lubricate. Also, disorders of the vaginal lining so that there is limited lubrication may contribute, and this is a common cause in older women. (See Section nine.)

The obvious answer is always to seek medical advice to exclude any physical cause — and then, if necessary, to seek the help of a marriage guidance counseller or sex therapist for any emotional one. This is not really an area suitable for self diagnosis or self treatment.

Q *'I've been told that women can ejaculate just like men if the right part of the vagina is stimulated. Where is that part?'*

This is another of the controversies about women's sexuality that have been aired over the years. Some writers have suggested that there is a 'G spot' (named after a German doctor called Gräfenberg) which is similar to a male structure — the prostate gland — and which, when pressed, produces a liquid that is like male semen without the sperm.

The spot has been said to lie in the front wall of the vagina near the place where the bladder meets the urethra, being about 1 or 2 cm deep and measuring between .75 to 3.0 cm in diameter. There is no firm evidence that it exists, though it is common in some sex books to find descriptions of female ejaculation. Many experts think that the fluid that may escape from the vagina during intercourse and orgasm is made up of excess vaginal lubrication mixed with some of the male emission and possibly some urine, since some women do lose momentary control of the bladder at the point of orgasm.

That the front wall of the vagina is, in some places, sensitive is true. That the congestion of the spongy tissue there — part of the general congestion of the area — can be agreeable is undoubted, just as pressure on the spongy tissue on the other side of the vagina, between it and the rectum is pleasurable (see page 68) but whether this constitutes a specific structure that can create a female ejaculation is unknown. There is simply no proof.

However, in support of the G spot enthusiast, it must be said that it is possible that those women who do prefer to use a dildo in masturbation have a somewhat different response to the majority.

It would be a fool who would dismiss the possibility out of hand, but it must be said that the claim has been made by a few over the years, and refuted by many. Either way, it doesn't seem really to matter very much.

Q *'Is it all right to use sex aids?'*

There are all sorts of aids to sex, ranging from soft lights and sweet music to scents and silks and satins, and there are some cynical people who say diamonds and minks are sex aids, too. And it has to be said that anything that helps a woman to feel relaxed and receptive and more ready to be aroused must also be regarded as useful and enjoyable.

However, the term 'sex aids' is generally used to label mechanical or chemical items thought to be sexually arousing. The search for 'love potions' has been going on for centuries. People have used potentially dangerous drugs such as cantharades ('Spanish Fly') which, when it is excreted in the urine, sets up an intense irritation in the vulva which may lead to a willingness for intercourse to scratch the itch. This has killed some women.

People have also used 'magical' ideas, seeking out things which look like sex organs and which are thought to make the sex organs behave in the desired way if they are swallowed. For example, men have fed on rhino horn, celery or asparagus and many other phallic shaped foods in the belief that the hard erectness of the food would somehow be transferred to the penis. Similarly, women have been fed on oysters and other bivalves and on certain nuts and fruits because they look rather vulval. Smooth slippery foods have also been thought to help, by making the vulva smooth and slippery — i.e. lubricated — so jellies and syrups and emulsions of many kinds have been fed to women in the hope of making them feel excited.

All the evidence that has been collected about such aphrodisiacs comes to the same conclusion; that the mind is the only true aphrodisiac, so anything the mind believes to be sexually arousing is. If oysters make a woman feel sexy it is because she expects them to.

Mechanical aids, including vibrators to stimulate the clitoris and 'geisha balls' which the woman holds inside her vagina to encourage her to contract her muscles, and various penile sheaths with attachments that give added stimulation to the clitoris during intercourse, have been used by many women and seem useful for some.

There is no harm in such things at all, apart from the possibility that the woman could possibly come to attach more importance to the mechanical aid than to the person using it when making love to her, or when she used it for herself. That would tend to depersonalize both the partner and herself — and that surely would be a little sad. But for women who want to use them, why on earth not?

Q *'Some people say women can only enjoy sex if they are in love, while men don't have to be. Others say that women can be as casual as men, and that is why prostitutes exist. Why are there prostitutes if women really do need to be in love to enjoy sex?'*

The assumption here is that all prostitutes are the same, and that they all enjoy sex and engage in the sexual liaisons they have for this reason. The evidence seems to point more to financial and social needs than to erotic ones. Most prostitutes do the job because that is what they need — a job that will earn them a living. There are for some women in many parts of the world, and for many in a few parts of the world, few opportunities to earn a living in any other way. As long as men are willing to pay for sexual favours, especially those which involve 'unusual' needs (such as being beaten or tied up, a taste many men seem to have, probably because of having been reared by 'spare-the-rod-and-spoil-the-child' zealots who teach them to equate pain with sexual arousal) women will take their money. And of course there are male prostitutes, though they mostly serve male customers too.

It is not possible to say whether women 'need to love' to enjoy sex. Some do, some don't. There can't be a simple answer for all women. We are, as women, more than our sexuality, after all. We are all minds and intellects as well as bodies; and that means that for all of us, our sexuality is extremely idiosyncratic. It is ours and no one else's, and what suits one of us may not suit another. There is no need to make standards, anyway, and it is depressing that so many people seem to need them.

Q *'I have never been particularly interested in sex. I loathe it when people talk about it so much and when there are sexy scenes on TV. I have a good absorbing job, my own home and a top income. I look good and I like that, but I just don't like sex. Am I abnormal?'*

There are plenty of women who feel this way, and they have as much right to do so as any woman has the right to be very eager for sex. Any woman who can say calmly and comfortably that sex is not a major matter in her life is certainly normal.

However, women who maintain that they 'hate' sex and find it embarrassing or distressing to hear talk about it, or see representations of it, are almost certainly blocking out of their minds, for whatever reason, a normally average interest in sex. It is possible to use sexual energy for other purposes — in work, in involvement with others' needs and in religion (think of nuns) — and that is a perfectly valid choice. But if there is anxiety about sexuality and anger, and especially fear about being normal, then it is reasonable to suggest that there may be some underlying psychological or emotional disorder that may need digging out and dealing with. Of course, if an individual prefers to hold on to her anger and doubts rather than experience the painful self-revelation that is part of psychotherapy, that too is a valid choice.

Q *'What is a lesbian exactly? What do they do? I'm not sure what I am. I have sex with men sometimes and enjoy it, but I also get great crushes on women. It frightens me.'*

The theories about why some people happen to find themselves falling in love with members of their own sex rather than, or as well as, the opposite one, have been as thick as leaves in Vallombrosa. It's hormonal, some say. It's due to uneven parental care, others announce. It's all down to pre-natal influence, or it's really the way all humans are supposed to be, only they are brainwashed into being heterosexual (that does seem a little far fetched, actually, if you consider the biological imperative to reproduce the species), it's an expression of the depravity and disorder of our times, and so on and so on.

The end result remains ignorance. No one knows why some people make this choice. But they always have; homosexuality has been part of the human experience for as far back as we have historical records. It is discussed in the Bible (disapprovingly) in Greek and Roman writings (with grudging approval) and in many others ever since.

As for what women homosexuals do (they are called lesbians, by the way, after the Isle of Lesbos where the great Greek woman poet Sappho lived with her women lovers) that is easily explained. They fall in love, just as heterosexual people do. They make love by kissing and caressing just as heterosexual people do. The only thing they don't do is use a penis.

Some women are able to enjoy sex with both men and women. This is labelled bisexuality, and is very common.

Whatever they do, with so many people in the world it seems a pity that some can't be allowed freely to select non-reproductive sexuality without the rest getting angry or critical or controlling or punitive, but there it is; it was ever thus. So many people seem to have a desperate need to make everyone behave in the same way, despite the rich human diversity that makes such a task impossible. Those who try to enforce a sexual conformity to one norm are particularly foolish. As long as humanity lives on this planet it will be what it seems always to have been; sexually curious and sexually adventurous.

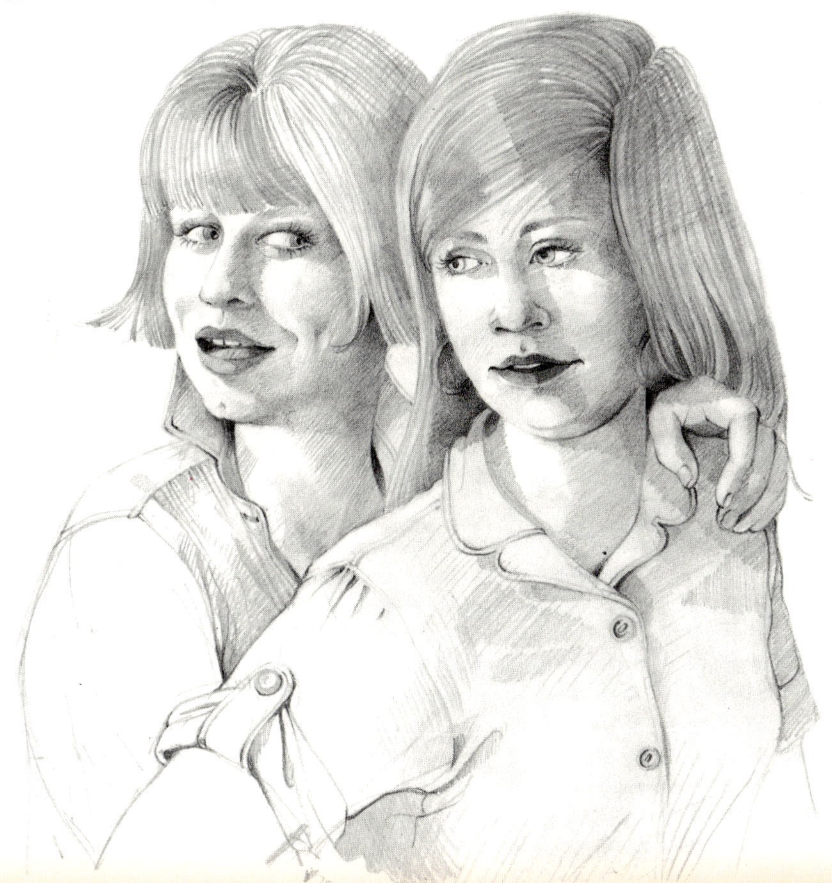

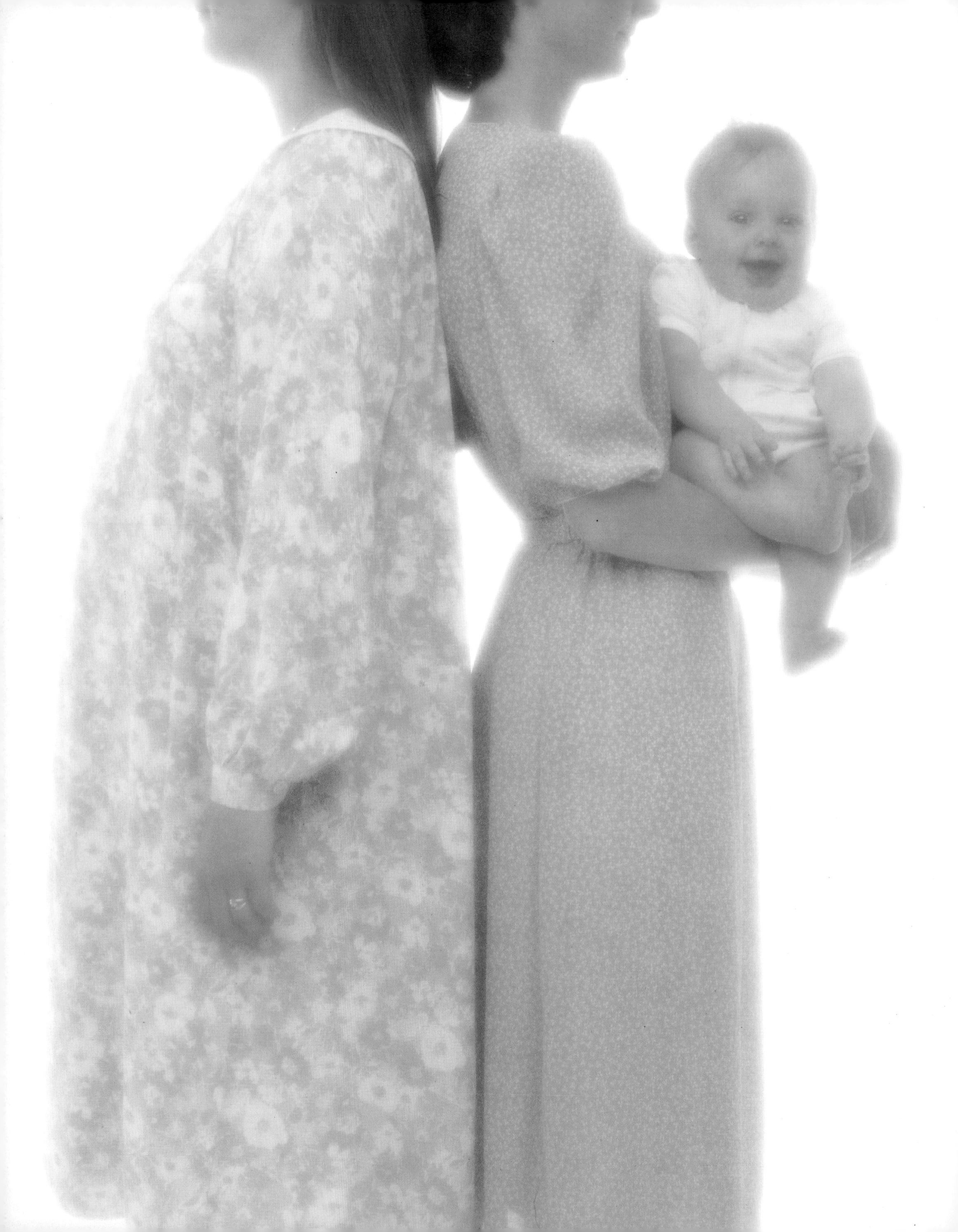

6

WOMAN'S FERTILITY

There is only one biological reason for woman's sexuality; the creation of new people. That woman should find pleasure — and sometimes distress — in her sexual activity is a by-product. The principle was built in as an inducement to engage in the making of new people, but it is by no means an end in itself.

That being so, it is really rather odd that women are as sexy as they are. Unlike a great many other animals, including several of the higher ones which are our close cousins, we seem willing and able to engage in sexual intercourse at any time. Other female animals generally only do so when they are fertile — that is, have (or shortly will have) a ripe egg in their reproductive system which is capable of merging with a male sperm to start the development of a new individual. We all know that bitches and cats 'come on heat' and behave in a very randy fashion as they seek out a mate for their ripe eggs; but women, by and large, do not do so, although some have reported that their tide of desire seems to be at its highest roughly half-way between periods, when they are most likely to be fertile. Others, however, report being at their sexiest during a period (when the dead egg is being shed from the uterus) or having no specially sexy time of the month at all.

All of which shows how much our big imaginative brains interfere with the hormonal control of our reproductive systems. If we didn't think about sex (partly because sexual stimuli are thrown at us from all directions all the time and partly because we have, over the centuries of our development, come more and more to seek the pleasure principle in all aspects of life) we would be governed far more by the ebb and flow of our hormones. We would accept intercourse willingly only during the few days when a ripe egg was making its journey from ovary to uterus, via one of the fallopian tubes.

Having said that we value the sexual pleasure we get from our bodies so highly, it must also be said that some women yearn so much for pregnancy that their bodies behave as though they are pregnant even when they are not. The phenomenon of 'phantom pregnancy' was first described by Hippocrates and it has happened to many people in many parts of the world, including Queen Mary of England in the sixteenth century. Today it seems commonest in Africa, and in any society where there is a powerful social pressure on women to have children. It is marked by swelling of the belly and breasts, loss of periods, morning sickness and reports of 'feeling the baby move'. It is a similar condition to that suffered by animals prevented from mating when 'on heat'.

Fertilization

Let us assume that an ovulating or about to ovulate woman has had intercourse with a man who has been able to reach his orgasm and deposit his semen in a pool at the top end of the vagina, where the cervix dips down to meet it. Although it is not vital for the purposes of fertility, if she has an orgasm after he has left his semen there, so that her muscles go into rhythmic spasm and her cervix gapes a little, the semen will actually be sucked up to enter the cervical canal. But by no means all of it.

A normal healthy man when he ejaculates leaves some 400 million sperm behind him, suspended in a comparatively small amount of semen; the average emission is about three millilitres — that is, less than a teaspoonful. Not all of the sperm will be fully formed and healthy; some will be lame or abnormal or damaged in some way and could, if they reached an ovum and managed to penetrate it, create a damaged infant. If this does happen there is a high likelihood that the ovum will fail to implant itself into the wall of the uterus successfully, there to grow into an infant. And even if it does, the chances are high that the woman's body will in some way recognize the fact that it is nurturing a 'blighted ovum' and throw it out — Nature's own quality control mechanism. There is a high rate of loss of early pregnancies; it has been estimated that one pregnancy in four fails in the first few weeks, sometimes so early that the woman doesn't even realise she has conceived; many of these are 'blighted ova'.

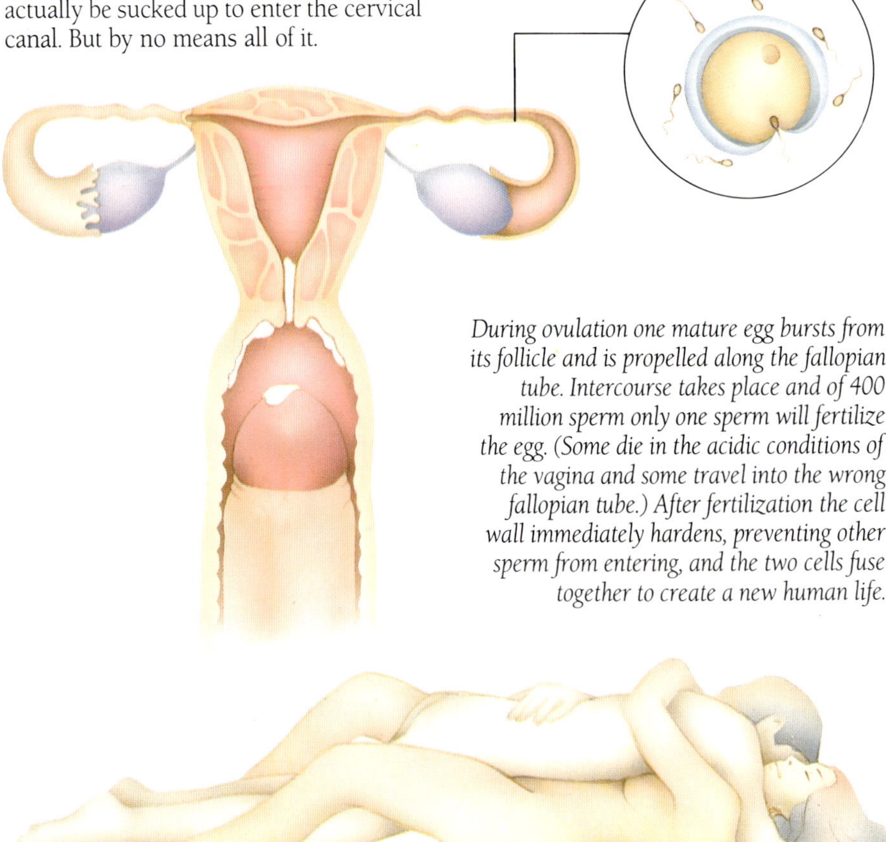

During ovulation one mature egg bursts from its follicle and is propelled along the fallopian tube. Intercourse takes place and of 400 million sperm only one sperm will fertilize the egg. (Some die in the acidic conditions of the vagina and some travel into the wrong fallopian tube.) After fertilization the cell wall immediately hardens, preventing other sperm from entering, and the two cells fuse together to create a new human life.

This protection against the creation of damaged infants is exerted quite early in the process. The semen that carries the sperm is, when it is newly produced, almost jelly like, but after about fifteen to twenty minutes it liquifies. This frees the sperm so that they can swim on their way more easily — but it also frees them to be attacked by the normal acidity of the vaginal secretions. Any that remain free in the vagina, having failed to enter the cervical canal, will be killed by this acidity. And the ones most likely to have failed to reach the opening are the sick, the lame and the halt.

Those sperm that do manage to enter the cervical canal find a much more hospitable environment than the unfriendly vagina. There the secretions are alkaline — which sperm enjoy — and rich in foods which nourish them. Also, if there is a ripe egg awaiting them at the end of their journey, the mucus becomes even more hospitable. Usually thick and sticky, at the time of a woman's fertility it becomes thinner and almost transparent, and actually pushes the sperm on their way.

Of the army of sperm that start on their hazardous journey, some ten per cent will make it to the comparative safety of the cervical canal. That is still a great many of them – around 40 million. They now have to travel a long way, considering their size (they are about a five hundredth of an inch long and made up of a head, which contains half of the genetic material needed to make a new person, and a long whippy tail) and they travel by means of lashing their tails. They are also assisted upwards by the contractions of the uterus, which are generally not felt at all by the woman, and by the movements of the tiny hairs – cilia – inside the fallopian tubes. The sperm have to get from the cervix up the uterus to the far end of the the fallopian tubes, a journey of around nine inches, and it takes them only forty-five minutes or so to do it.

But by no means all of them achieve the journey. Of the 400 million sperm which set out only one to two thousand reach the outer portion of the tubes. (Incidentally these figures are collated from a number of sources; there have been many estimates made by any number of physiologists and they vary wildly; but these numbers here seem to be those given by the majority of the most assiduous sperm counters.)

Here, in the outer third of the fallopian tubes, the sperm lie in wait for their target. There is a rich supply of food for them, in the sugary mucus which is secreted by the tubes, and they can survive for between forty-eight and seventy-two hours, while above and beyond them a ripening follicle gets ready to shed its egg. If the egg has already been shed, and is on its way down the tube, then there is no need to wait. The sperm converge on it in whichever tube it happens to be, while those that took the wrong tube perish for their misjudgement.

The cluster of sperm round the ovum — which compared to them is huge, since the ovum is the largest single cell the human body produces — now behave in a remarkably altruistic fashion. They work together to make it possible for one of their number — and only one — to enter the egg.

They all have a tightly fitting cap (it's called an acrosomal cap) which they all shed at the same time. No one yet knows precisely why they do this, or what triggers the reaction; it could be a signal from the egg that doffs their caps for them. The acrosome is thought to contain a substance which partially dissolves the outer membrane of the egg, so that one of the sperm can push its head through and enter.

So brotherhood leads to fatherhood — for one. For as soon as that one sperm has entered, the others seem to know (or perhaps the egg does in some way) and no more are able to get in. They fall away and are either swept out of the tubes and into the uterus and on out of the body in the normal secretions, or are scavenged by the body's army of cleaners, the white cells.

But for one sperm the journey is over. The egg has been fertilized.

Implantation

Conception has not yet taken place, however. The fertilized egg has still some hazards to overcome before it can be said to be on its way successfully to becoming a new individual.

Almost as soon as the sperm enters the egg, growth begins. The sperm contains twenty-three chromosomes which are the genetic material which carry messages on what we are and how we are to grow from generation to generation; they govern our colouring, our height, our gender — to an extent probably even our personalities; and the egg cell contains the same number. Every other human cell contains forty-six chromosomes, so by merging two sets of these remarkable structures, one set from each parent, a totally new human being is made. Even identical twins, which develop as two individuals from one set of egg and sperm, vary in some way, even if they are chromosomally the same. (Fraternal twins are different; they occur when two separate eggs are fertilized by two separate sperm and are no more alike than ordinary brothers and sisters even though they occupy their mother's uterus at the same time rather than in succession.)

The incidence of twins in the UK is around one in eighty pregnancies, with people of African origin more likely to have them, and the Chinese less often. Twinning is unusual in women under twenty or over forty, and most likely in mothers in their thirties. The bigger the family a woman has the more likely she is to have twins — it's a statistical effect. It is also an inherited characteristic which tends to skip generations. Having a grandparent who was a twin means you may have them too. (Triplets and more are even less common and these days are more likely to be the result of over-enthusiastic treatment with fertility drugs rather than Nature's generosity.)

Once the two cells have merged to make a complete new one, the new person's gender is decided. It all depends on what sort of sperm entered the egg. There are some which contain a special sex chromosome called an X chromosome, and some which contain one called a Y. Y makes males, X makes females. The egg also contains a sex chromosome — always an X. So if an X sperm meets an ovum the result is an XX individual, a girl. If it is a Y sperm, the result is an XY individual, a boy. Which is sad for the many women of the past who used to sit around during their pregnancies thinking 'masculine' or 'feminine' type thoughts in order to influence the development of

Foetal development

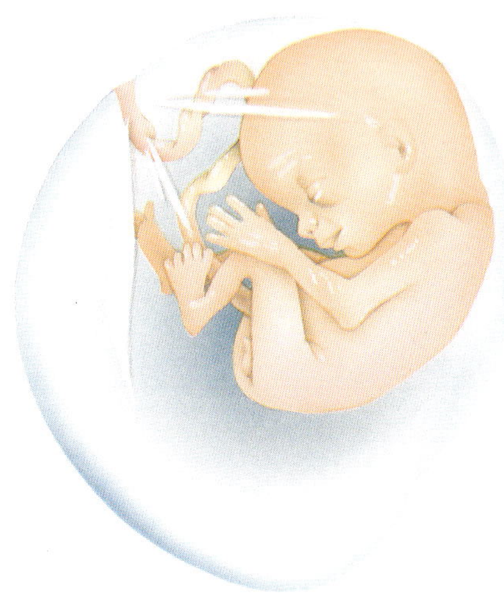

The key stages in a baby's development occur before the 32nd week.

Week 12

By this stage all the essential organs have been formed. The external genitalia are developing rapidly; there is frequent movement of the limbs and spine. The baby is now about as long as the mother's little finger.

Week 20

The baby is now at the 'quickening' stage and is moving and rotating within the amniotic fluid. Hair has begun to appear on the body, head, eyebrows and eyelashes. It is about 25 cms (10 inches) long and weighs about 350 grams (12 ounces).

Week 32

The baby is now perfectly formed with its head in normal proportion to its body. It can open its eyes and moves freely and vigorously. The average length is about 40 cms (16 inches) and the weight $1\frac{1}{2}$ kgs ($3\frac{1}{2}$ pounds).

Sex selection

The desire to select the sex of a child is a widespread one; in societies where women are subservient and males overvalued (for example in some Asian and African communities as well as Mediterranean countries) the birth of sons is a joy and of daughters a disappointment. More reasonable is to want to select a child's sex because of a family history of sex-linked disorders — for example, haemophilia, which generally affects males, though carried by females. Much research into the possibility has been done, and a US doctor, Landrum Shettles, has come up with the following 'rules' based on his observations of the behaviour and responses of X sperm and Y sperm.

For what it is worth here is this information, but many people feel that since a couple have a fifty-fifty chance of getting what they want anyway, it's not much better than some of the old fashioned witchcraft methods.

First, find out when you ovulate; this means taking your temperature every morning for several months and keeping a record on a chart (see page 56). There is a small but observable dip followed by a rise when ovulation takes place. Once you know when ovulation is likely to occur you can then plan your sexual activity.

Making girls

To produce a girl you should have intercourse two or three days before ovulation and then desist.

X sperm survive the acid environment best so you should use a douche made up of two tablespoons of white vinegar to a quart of water.

You should also have intercourse face to face to allow shallower penetration and ensure that the X sperm have a better chance of survival.

Making boys

If you want to have a boy, you should avoid intercourse from the beginning of the period until the day of ovulation and then have intercourse as frequently as you like, after that date.

Y sperm live longer in an alkaline environment, so you should use a douche containing two tablespoons of sodium bicarbonate to a quart of water.

You should have intercourse using the rear approach to encourage the survival of the Y sperm.

(A douche is a vaginal wash-out. You need a special nozzle to put up into the vagina, and a jug and a tube with which to pour it in. Quite a complicated and messy procedure.)

As you will see, the 'rules' for this chancy method are rather complex, and that may put some people off trying them. And it has also been said that douching may actually reduce fertility.

But there is something else parents should think about. Too much concern about sex selection could damage a mother's feeling for her child. If she uses one of these methods to have the sex of her choice and it doesn't work, isn't it possible that she will take a dislike to her child because it's the 'wrong' one?

Also, people who make judgements about a child on the basis of gender may suffer a great deal of distress if the little girl they longed for and visualized as a frill-bedecked little darling turns out to be a tough little tomboy with a taste for blue jeans and scorn for dolls. Similarly, a parent who wants a son because he will be butch and tough, may be very disturbed to find that he is a tender, gentle and rather frail chap. If the only way a couple is prepared to enter pregnancy is if they can be sure of a particular sort of child, then perhaps they would be better off not having a baby at all. Each child surely ought to be loved and wanted for itself. It could be a dreadful thing for a child to be less loved or rejected because it happened to be the 'wrong' sex.

Stages of pregnancy

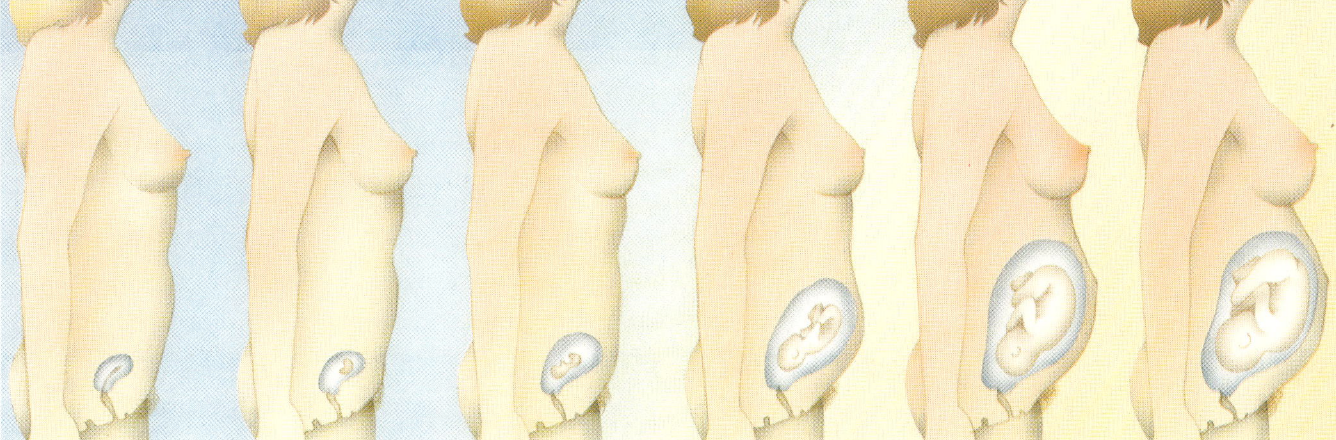

Week 4 — the pregnancy is just visible to the naked eye.

Week 8 — all the important inner organs are now present.

Week 16 — hair starts to appear on the body, head, eyebrows and eyelashes.

Week 24 — the vital organs are now mature enough to allow the baby to survive for a short while.

Week 32 — the baby is now perfectly formed, it can open its eyes and move freely.

Week 40 — usually the last week of pregnancy when the baby is ready to lead a separate life.

their baby into the desired sex. It couldn't matter less what a woman does — as soon as her egg is fertilized the sex die is cast. It is also grossly unjust that some women have been spurned by their husbands for 'failing to give them a son', when the real reason is the man has failed to create one.

Immediately the new cell of forty-six chromosomes is formed, it starts to multiply by dividing, the familiar process that governs all life on this planet. The cells divide and divide again, regularly doubling their number as the whole bundle travels slowly along the fallopian tube, driven along by the tube's actions and its waving cilia, and about a week after fertilization, it arrives at the uterus. It now contains thirty-two or maybe sixty-four cells.

In a few cases, if there is a narrowing of the tube, the egg cell may be trapped there, and try to implant, growing quite large. The result of this is an ectopic pregnancy, which mimics a normal pregnancy at first, but soon leads to abdominal pain and illness. Surgery is the only answer. Fortunately, even a woman who has lost one tube this way can still have a successful pregnancy; she still has a second tube.

Even more rarely, a fertilized egg escapes the tube from the top end and tries to imbed elsewhere in the mother's belly. There have been a few — very few — successful caesarian deliveries of such babies.

All the time, while the egg cell has been travelling down the tube, the uterus has been busily preparing its surface, under the influence of progesterone (see Section three) and it is now thick, richly supplied with blood and waiting for its guest.

The ball of cells attaches itself to the wall of the uterus, usually in the upper third or so, and special cells on its surface burrow into the lining, sending out little fingerlike projections to hold it on to the lining. They also eat into maternal blood vessels, thus releasing blood to bathe the embryo and so feed it. At the same time, the cells which are burrowing into the mother's uterine wall are growing their own delicate blood vessels, so fine and so many that by the time of birth they would, if they were stretched out, cover a distance of fully thirty miles.

The number of things that are happening at this stage is really breath-taking. The woman has as yet no idea she is pregnant, since she hasn't even missed a period, but the cells that will become the baby are dividing at a rapid rate. The placenta (the organ that will attach the baby to the wall of the uterus and act as go-between for blood, oxygen and essential substances as well as remover of the baby's waste products) is not yet formed, though its preliminary cells are there and the whole structure is sending out essential hormones needed to maintain the process of baby-making. Although the woman does not yet know she is pregnant, tests could show the presence of these special pregnancy hormones and actually give her a diagnosis.

All this early multiplying-by-dividing will continue for around 266 days from the moment of conception, and will result in a baby weighing on average about 3½ kg (7½ pounds) and measuring some 45 to 50 cm (18 to 20 inches). It is a remarkable process and incredibly speedy, when you consider just how much happens. Bones and muscles, nerves and blood, skin and internal organs, all are derived from these two small single cells, the sperm and the ovum, in just 266 days. Incredible, but commonplace — a mundane miracle.

Once the fertilized egg is safely implanted, conception is said to have happened. And it is still only three weeks since the woman had her last period.

Week 4

The pregnancy is growing rapidly. By the 28th day — the end of the week — it is just visible to the naked eye. Because growth is so rapid from now to the end of the 12th or 13th week, the developing infant is particularly vulnerable. If the mother uses certain drugs at this stage she may profoundly affect the way the baby develops; similarly, an attack of rubella (German measles) may damage the infant, causing in some cases blindness and deafness and some heart defects.

An infection in the mother, accompanied by a very raised temperature for a very long period of time (a week or so) could also damage the infant. This is why in the early stages of any pregnancy prompt care for infections so that fevers are kept under control is a good idea.

Week 5

The developing baby is now about 2 mm long and lying in a transparent membranous bag called the amniotic sac in which it will float in shock absorbing fluid as it grows. The spine can be seen and the beginnings of the nervous system is just recognizable. The spine ends in a 'tail' which is clearly visible.

Week 6

The head now forms very rapidly and then the chest and the abdominal cavities are established. The young brain is completed — considerable growth is still needed of course — and the spinal column as well as the spinal cord is properly formed. The tail begins to disappear and the limb buds are more visible. The umbilical cord is more clearly seen now; this is the thick, twisted lifeline which connects the infant to the mother via the placenta. One set of blood vessels in it carries blood rich in oxygen, food, and the mother's own body chemicals to the baby, and the other carries back the infant's waste materials.

The face is not actually looking like a face yet but little depressions are beginning to appear where the eyes will be situated. By now the baby is about 6 mm long.

Week 7

By the end of this week, the limb buds have grown so rapidly that they are clearly visible as arms and legs, and at the ends of them little clefts are appearing which will eventually separate into fingers and toes. The baby now has its own blood cells inside its own circulation, blood vessels which reach right into the head and throughout the body, and the heart, although it is a very simple pump, is beating with just enough force to send those cells through the blood vessels. The lungs are there now but they are tiny and solid. There is a liver and kidneys which are, of course, not functioning yet. The head is growing at great speed and is beginning to be quite clearly a head. It is bent forward on the chest and there seem to be odd lumps and bumps at the back, but the ears are beginning to form and the eyes are developing. There is a skin over them which is completely intact. Later this skin will separate and become the eyelids. There is no nose yet, but apertures for the nostrils are beginning to show. The baby is now 1.3 cm long.

Week 8

All the important inner organs are now present and they continue to grow towards their final shape and position. The heart beats strongly now and the lungs have grown a great deal but are still solid, of course. It is during this week that the eyes and ears do most of their growing. The head of the baby is still extremely large in proportion to the rest of the body, but it is a recognizable human creature. Its genitals can be seen and the eyes are beginning to show their pigmentation beneath the overlaying skin. There are nostrils and the upper and lower jaws have grown together so that there is a mouth, and the growing limbs have developed shoulders, elbows, hips and knees. Now, the spine begins to move, although the baby is now only 2.2 cm long.

Week 9

The head is still bent forward on the chest, but the baby looks much more like a baby. The eyelids are still intact over the eyes although they have completely grown. There is now a nose and the mouth is developing rapidly. Hands and feet are now obvious and the fingers and toes can be seen. There are more definite movements although the mother won't be able to feel them for some time yet. The baby is now about 3 cm long and weighs about 2 grams.

Week 10

Although the mother is not yet obviously pregnant – she has no bump to speak of – the baby is now $4\frac{1}{2}$ cm long and weighs about 5 grams. It looks far more human than even a couple of weeks ago. The ankles and wrists have formed and the fingers and toes are clearly distinguishable although they are still joined together by webbing. The umbilical cord is now complete and blood is circulating along it. The placenta – the afterbirth – is not yet completely formed, but it is developing rapidly.

Week 11

The baby is now about as long as its mother's little finger – $5\frac{1}{2}$ cm – and it weighs about 10 grams. Now all the essential organs have been formed and the majority of them are beginning to do the work they are going to do for the next seventy odd years. The external genitalia are developing rapidly; the face is more clearly a human face; there is frequent movement of the limbs and spine. The period of danger for the infant is now almost at an end. The organs are almost completely grown and any outside factor operating after this week will have at the most a very minor effect upon the development of any particular part of the body.

Week 13

Now the mother is said to be three months pregnant. The risks of miscarriage – spontaneous abortion – are diminishing. During the first few months when the organs are forming, it is possible for development to fail and the foetus to be thrown out. (There can be other causes for miscarriage – see later). The uterus has now grown to accommodate the pregnancy and measures about 10 cm (4 inches) round, to use more familiar measurements. If the mother lies on her back and relaxes it is possible for the uterus to be felt as a soft round swelling just rising out of the pelvis.

Inside the uterus the amniotic sac which is holding the baby contains 100 millilitres of fluid within which the baby has plenty of room to move. The head is now quite round and the neck is formed so that the head can move easily on it. The mouth, nose, and eyes are properly developed, as is the outer ear, and the infant can move fairly easily. It is not yet fidgety enough for the mother to be aware of it, or so the doctors always say. Some mothers, however, especially those having a second or third pregnancy and who are therefore experienced in the sensations of pregnancy, say they are able to feel movements of their infants at about this stage. However, they won't be very vigorous because the baby is just $7\frac{1}{2}$ cm long and only weighs around 30 grams. (In imperial measurements it is 3 inches long and weighs just over an ounce.) By the end of this thirteenth week, the baby is fully formed. It could not possibly survive, of course, if delivered, because the organs, although they are present and complete, are not mature enough to do their job. But for all practical purposes this is a completely new human being almost ready for a separate life. The job the mother now has to do is not so much to grow a baby as to accommodate one that is developing the maturity of its organs, which need time not only to get bigger but to learn how to do their jobs. Much of a human body's activity is incredibly complex, after all.

Week 16

This is when hair starts to appear, first showing itself over the whole body in a downy layer called lanugo, and also on the head, the eyebrows and the eyelashes. The baby by now is 15 cm (nearly 6 inches) long and weighs 135 grams (nearly 5 ounces).

Week 20

Growth is now considerable. The baby's length is about 25 cm (10 inches) and it weighs about 350 grams (12 ounces). There is a great deal of fluid around the baby in which it can move and rotate with ease, and it does. Some babies are much more vigorous than others and cavort freely, and usually the mother is well aware of this athleticism. (The father can be aware too, if she is thin; he can put a hand on her belly, and feel the infant's movements.)

Interestingly, the umbilical cord, although it is long and sinuous, seems not to become too kinked to do its job. This is the stage called 'quickening'. The ancients believed that this was the time when life and the soul entered the new person. The baby is now said to be 'viable' in Australian law.

Week 24

The vital organs are now sufficiently mature for the baby actually to survive for a short time if it were born at this stage. It is unlikely however, for a baby born after only 24 weeks gestation to survive normally.

Week 28

The baby is now said to be 'viable' in English law, and that means it is capable of a separate and independent existence. If it is born at this stage it must be registered as a live birth. (A baby born before this stage would be regarded as a miscarriage and would not be registered.) In Australia a baby is considered viable at 20 weeks.

The question of viability is important because of the matter of legal abortion. In the UK under the present provisions of the Abortion Act of 1967, a mother may have a pregnancy terminated before the 28th week under certain circumstances (if two doctors agree that this is necessary for her health and in certain circumstances). Any interference with the pregnancy after the 28th week is regarded as the induction of a premature labour and it is not illegal to induce this in any circumstances, even if it is clear that doing so means that the baby's chances of survival are virtually nil.

Week 32

The baby is now perfectly formed with its head in normal proportion to its body (although in fact the fully developed baby's head is much bigger in proportion to its body than an adult's). The skin is covered with a thick greasy wax-like material called vernix which protects it from becoming waterlogged because it is continually immersed in the amniotic fluid. The baby can now open its eyes and moves freely and vigorously, often kicking quite hard. If it is delivered at this stage, its chances of survival are approximately thirty per cent.

The baby is comparatively thin, since there is not a great deal of fat on its body; this will be laid down in the succeeding weeks of the pregnancy. At this stage, the average baby is about 40 cm (16 inches) long and weighs $1\frac{1}{2}$ kg ($3\frac{1}{2}$ pounds). It usually lies with its head downwards, towards its mother's pelvis, although it is still moving freely and may change its position from time to time.

Week 36

By this time the baby is almost completely grown and has a ninety per cent chance of living healthily if it is born. The only part of the body that is not fully developed yet is the lungs. It is lung function that causes the doctors the most anxiety in the prematurely delivered baby.

About half of all babies now take up their permanent position. They lie with their heads pointing well downwards — this is the best way for the infant to be delivered, because the head is the largest part and needs to push its way out to make room for the rest of the body. There is now less room for the baby to move and when it does it causes its mother considerable discomfort as it kicks upwards and hits her stomach or lower ribs.

In about half of all pregnancies, the baby's head will now move down into the pelvis. It is said to be 'engaged' — a stage that used to be called 'lightening' because the mother feels as though her baby is less heavy. Once the baby's head goes down, there is less bulk above the rim of the pelvis, she feels less crowded inside, and the baby's kicks are less likely to hit her stomach and make her feel sick. He is in fact still comparatively small — 45 cm (18 inches) long and weighing about $2\frac{1}{2}$ kg ($5\frac{1}{2}$ pounds).

Week 40

This should be the last week of the pregnancy, because the average pregnancy is supposed to last for 266 days from conception. For convenience many people say a pregnancy is 280 days long, because they count from the first day of the last normal menstrual period. However, this is an average, not a rule. Some women will have perfectly normal pregnancies that will last 38 weeks, while others will have equally normal pregnancies that will last 42 weeks. Some babies will be mature and ready to live a separate life outside their mothers well in advance of the fortieth week while others will need two or three weeks more to complete their development.

The size of the baby and its maturity may have an effect on how long the pregnancy lasts. For example, a woman carrying twins will very often go into premature labour in terms of the weeks of the pregnancy because the combined weight of her babies triggers her body into starting labour.

At full term, the baby is not only fully developed but has a considerable quantity of fat which has been deposited over the last ten weeks. It is this which gives the classic rounded appearance to the newborn baby. The buttocks, however, will still be scrawny because it is the development of muscle which comes with leg action which creates the classic baby bottom shape.

The baby may be completely bald or may have hair up to 2 to 4 cm long. The eyes are blue — all babies are born with blue eyes which later change colour (sometimes within a very few minutes of delivery but mostly after some weeks) and finger and toe nails are fully developed. The vernix is extra thick in the creases of the groin and elbows and round the neck and so on, but it is comparatively easily removed.

The woman's body has now done the first part of its reproductive job; she has taken her own egg cell and one of her partner's sperm to the stage of creating a new human being. The next part of the job is to deliver it from her body to the outside world.

The pregnant body

But before seeing the mother's body through the birth process, we should look at what the process of pregnancy has done to it. The creative labours of making a new human being don't leave it entirely as it was before conception. There are considerable changes, some of which may be more obvious than others.

The most obvious is growth of the uterus. This organ is the only one in the human body that can both grow and ungrow; that is, it develops extra tissue to accommodate the developing infant — it doesn't just stretch — and after the birth that extra tissue is actually reabsorbed, so that the uterus returns almost to its pre-pregnant state. Almost, but not quite, because it will always be a little more bulky than it was before the first pregnancy.

The breasts change too. Under the stimulating influence of progesterone they enlarge considerably, putting on extra milk-making tissue and often added fat too. The nipples darken and enlarge and develop tiny white lubricating glands which look like pimples.

Some of these changes are permanent; the darkened nipple colour will never go away, and the little white pimples stay too. The enlargement is not permanent, however; once the baby is born and the mother feeds with her extra milk-making tissue the bulkiness will go down, but it can happen that while the breasts were so much larger, they become heavy enough to stretch the supportive tissue that holds them in shape. The result can be that post-pregnancy breasts are heavier and more drooping than virginal ones.

This is normal. It is totally unrealistic to expect breasts to remain always the same throughout a sexually active woman's life. In a few cases they will, but mostly they won't. But, sadly, fashion has decreed that women should always have breasts like pubescent girls, and there have been some women so brainwashed by this sort of rubbish that they have refused to feed their babies on the grounds that it might 'spoil their figures'. This has to seem, to any sensible adult woman, a form of childish vanity that is positively lunatic. To deprive yourself on such grounds of the benefits and pleasure of breast feeding (and they are considerable) and the baby of the great protection a mother's milk gives, has to be ridiculous to put it at its mildest.

It isn't only breasts that are affected by pregnancy hormone. The belly muscles too soften and stretch to allow the rising bump of the pregnancy more room. If they didn't the inner condition would be appallingly crowded. The loss of the tone in these muscles can usually be regained without too much trouble with the right sort of exercises after the birth. The cartilages of the body — the gristle like material that is involved in many joints and in the muscles which operate them — are also softened by the hormone. One area that is particularly affected is the sacro-iliac — the joints that link the sacrum at the base of the spine with the pelvic bones to complete the girdle. These joints don't normally allow much movement, but in pregnancy they loosen and so have the effect of opening the space a little — to make more room inside the pelvic girdle.

This can sometimes be seen most easily when looking at a woman walking away from you. If she has never been pregnant she may have a wiggle to her walk, as the pelvic bones fit on each side in the usual way, but if she has been pregnant the sway will be even more visible. (The same thing happens to cattle — look at the different gait of heifers and cows after they have calved and it will be very clear).

This softening can cause a good deal of backache during pregnancy, which can be made worse by the tendency pregnant woman have to change their posture to accommodate their new centre of gravity as their front 'bump' grows. They tend to curve their spines and this adds pressure to the area and causes aching. Wearing shoes of the right heel height, neither too high nor too flat, can help a good deal.

The blood vessel walls may also be softened by progesterone, and this may lead to some of them becoming less efficient at their job of pushing blood back towards the heart. This can make some veins become varicose (swollen and lumpy) and this shows most in the legs, and in the anus where they are called piles. Mostly the veins lose some of their varicosity after the birth, but there will always be some residue of the state.

Some women feel sick and giddy at times during pregnancy. This again is likely to be a hormonal effect. The change in the levels can affect the way a woman smells and tastes food and generally reacts to it. There can be a psychological element in the sickness of pregnancy, some doctors say, though others dispute that. In general only about fifty per cent of pregnant women suffer from sickness in pregnancy (and by no means only in the mornings — it happens at any time of the day).

Fainting may be due to the fact that the woman needs a larger quantity of blood to feed her baby. The volume she has must travel not only her body but the baby's and that puts great demands on it. In the early stages of pregnancy her blood volume increases by about twenty per cent, but the number of red cells she has does not increase by so much. So, the blood is less able to carry oxygen than it usually is, this is why there may be dizziness as the brain gets less oxygen than it needs. The blood slowly gets better at doing its job and the tendency to fainting then lessens. (It is sometimes necessary to give pregnant women iron and folic acid supplements to improve their level of haemoglobin and so reduce anaemia.)

The skin and hair may change too. In many pregnant women these are particularly well lubricated, and look healthy and gleaming and glossy. Not all skin changes are as welcome as this, however. Some brunettes may find that they develop patches of darker skin, especially in exposed areas such as the face, hands and arms. This is called chloasma. There is a phenomenon called the 'mask of pregnancy' in which the patches appear on cheeks, brows and chin. The darkening is more likely if the woman sits in the sun for long periods. (It is similar to the skin darkening that affects some Pill users.) There may also be a tendency to develop new moles and freckles, and for existing ones to darken and/or enlarge. Particularly striking enlargement should always be checked of course, in case it is unhealthy, but generally the moles are harmless and normal accompaniments to pregnancy. They never fade, incidentally. Once they appear they are there for always.

Another place where this permanent darkening may appear is on the *linea alba*, the line that runs down the belly from the navel to the pubis. Its appearance led to the odd belief that this is 'where the belly splits to let the baby out'. The experience of labour and birth usually puts paid to such notions.

The layer of fat immediately under the skin often thickens as more fat is laid down all over the body. This is part of the normal store a woman will need to make breast milk for her baby. (The total weight increase in a normal pregnancy, made up of baby, placenta, fat and fluid is around 9 kg [18 to 20 pounds].)

Whether or not a woman will have an agreeable and comfortable pregnancy depends on so many factors that it is not possible honestly to guide anyone into rules of behaviour and activity that will ensure enjoyment of these forty or so weeks. There are plenty of books of advice available, many of them wise and useful, but ultimately a woman's own basic health, both physical and psychological, the amount of support and love she gets from her partner and/or from the other people in her life, and of course the healthy development of the baby, will affect her experience more than anything she does herself. But her own behaviour can affect her and the outcome of her pregnancy; the woman who smokes cigarettes and drinks alcohol is obviously putting herself and her infant at risk. The woman who fails to take adequate rest, food and exercise may also put herself at risk. But having said all that it must also be remembered that women can go through the most appalling privations during pregnancy and yet produce healthy normal infants. Babies were born alive and well in concentration camps; Nature's drive to people the world with succeeding generations is a very powerful and effective one.

What can go wrong?

The commonest anxiety pregnant women face in the early weeks is fear of miscarriage. Threat of loss of pregnancies is high (estimated at being one in four) and even if a miscarriage can in fact protect women from the much greater distress of having a sick baby who would never be healthy and normal, it can still be a deeply unhappy experience. Women who miscarry can and do grieve as deeply as those who lose live full term babies.

Why does it go wrong?

One common cause of miscarriage at around the tenth to twelfth week is the 'blighted ovum' already discussed on page 78, but the next commonest is hormonal disorder. If the hormone control is not established as it should be, the pregnancy cannot survive. One of the most vulnerable times is between actual fertilization and implantation in the wall of the uterus, but the next few weeks of pregnancy are also vulnerable because there are stages at which the developing placenta — the afterbirth — has to take over some of the hormone production from the mother's ovaries. These times tend to coincide with what would have been a period time, which is why some doctors advise extra rest over these few days, until the fourth period has been missed. There is now some evidence that some miscarriages are due to the actions of the woman's own immune system. Instead of tolerating the 'foreign body' that is the baby, the system treats it as a potentially dangerous invader and destroys it. Research into treatment for this is currently being carried out.

Sometimes miscarriage is due to a mechanical failure. Women who consistently lose their pregnancies between the twelfth and the twenty-eighth weeks of pregnancy may have an inefficient cervix; instead of remaining firmly closed to protect the developing baby, it gapes a little, and allows the pregnancy to fail. The cause of this incompetence may be a natural fault, or damage due to previous childbirths, or operations of various kinds (including instrumental or suction abortions, if they are clumsily performed).

The problem can usually be treated by inserting a 'purse-string' suture round the cervix (it is called Shirodkar's stitch) at about the thirteenth or fourteenth week, and then removing it when the baby is ready to be born. This is successful in about three quarters of all cases of cervical incompetence.

General illness in the mother can lead to miscarriage, though by no means always. Remember the women in concentration camps who had normal babies. But it can happen, just as it can occasionally happen that the old wives' tale that severe shock or upset can lead to miscarriage is shown to be true. If a woman's hormones are thrown out of balance by emotional response then her pregnancy may suffer. But it is rare.

There are also tales told about stretching, reaching and lifting causing miscarriage. There is little evidence that this is so, although excess or violent exercise at times when a pregnancy is vulnerable may precipitate the loss. However, it could be that the loss would have happened anyway, and the exercise only speeded things up. Generally speaking in a normal healthy woman it is not necessary to treat pregnancy as a time to be excessively passive, or to avoid exercise. Pregnancy is not an illness.

Sexual intercourse has also been blamed by some people for miscarriage, but here again unless a doctor specifically forbids it for a special reason there is no need to be alarmed. Sex is only likely to be forbidden if the woman has miscarried before, is suffering from pain, or is bleeding.

With so many causes of miscarriage, including disorders of the uterus itself, no one can ever foretell in a particular woman what the outcome of her pregnancy will be. But the majority of women who have suffered miscarriage go on to have perfectly normal pregnancies and babies.

Sometimes — depending on the cause — the loss is inevitable (if there is a 'blighted ovum' or, an occasional occurrence, if the developing baby has died). But often the problem is simply that the pregnancy is a little fragile and needs time to settle down and become more stable. So, when there is any sign of threatened miscarriage — notably bleeding — bed rest is advised. Just resting and being still and quiet can enable the hormone control to establish itself as it should. If there is rhythmic pain as well as bleeding, then the likelihood is that the miscarriage is inevitable.

Sometimes doctors may use hormones in careful doses to protect a fragile pregnancy, but they are used very carefully, because it was found in the past that over-enthusiastic use of some hormones led to damage to the baby. Modern methods of dosage estimation are very precise so mothers generally need not fear hormones if they are advised to take them — though mistakes in dosage can happen.

Pregnancy cancer

A rare but important disorder of pregnancy is hydatidiform mole. The fertilized egg, instead of growing normally into a baby, develops a cluster of little blisters — it looks rather like a bunch of grapes — which destroy the embryonic baby. In a few cases, the mole may undergo malignant changes and become a very malignant form of cancer. If this happens, very careful treatment is needed to save the patient's life — but today this once inevitably fatal complication of pregnancy is successfully treated.

Infertility

Most couples think they will be able to have babies as and when they are ready. They think they will only have to stop any contraception, continue to enjoy intercourse and then expect the birth of a baby forty or so weeks later. In fact it has been estimated that fifty per cent of people in the UK are involuntarily childless — that's around $2\frac{1}{2}$ million people. And there can be a great many different causes.

A general illness can have a considerable effect on fertility. This does not mean that an ill woman cannot conceive; far from it. There have been many women with severe tuberculosis or a malignant disease from which they were dying, who still conceived. So it must never be thought that a general illness can be regarded as a contraceptive. An obvious example is hormonal disease, which has the effect of disturbing the ovaries. Thyrotoxicosis, due to an overactive thyroid gland, is one. The various forms of anaemia may also lead to temporary sub-fertility. In these cases, treatment of the general illness will usually lead to conception.

There may be local problems in the sex organs. For example, an infection in the vagina or cervix, causing offensive and heavy discharge may prevent sperm from making the journey to the uterus (see Section four).

Lack of cervical mucus can also affect conception. At the time of maximum fertility, there is usually an increase in the mucus which helps sperm to swim on their way to meet an egg. Some women don't make the extra mucus needed.

Treatment and cure of any local infection (see Section seven) may lead to conception, but treatment of inadequate cervical mucus is not so easy. It may be due to disorder in the ovaries (which produce the hormone which encourages the cervix to produce the mucus), and treatment of this will therefore be needed. And that can be more complicated, involving a course of hormone therapy.

There may be a blockage of the fallopian tubes. These tubes have such very fine channels that it takes very little to close them, thus preventing the egg from reaching the uterus. Chlamydia infections are a sadly common cause of scar tissue which blocks the tubes (see page 101).

Doctors checking for this problem inject an opaque dye into the uterus and then take an X-ray. This will show whether the dye can travel from the uterus and along the tubes. It is also possible to measure the resistance it meets. If there is a blockage, it is sometimes possible to restore the clearway by an operation. There are now some surgeons who specialize in this sort of care, using microsurgery. (They can also sometimes restore a fallopian tube tied or cut for sterilization purposes.)

In some cases the ovary does not produce ripe eggs. This may be obvious in some women; they will not have periods. Absence of periods usually means absence of ovulation. However, the reverse is not necessarily true. It is possible for a woman to have periods even though her ovaries are not producing ripe eggs. This is because of the effects of other body hormones.

Treatment of failure to ovulate can be difficult. Much research has been done in recent years with various hormone treatments but there were problems with them. There have been cases of women who have undergone these treatments, producing several ripe eggs at a time, all of which have become fertilized. This has led to multiple births. Some of these unlucky women produced six or seven babies at once, none of whom lived. But doctors using these 'fertility drugs' (they include clomiphene, gonadotrophin, tamoxifen and monotrophin among others) are getting more and more skilful with them, and multiple births do not happen often now. Any woman offered the treatment today should not be afraid of it; it has helped many childless women to become mothers, and is widely and successfully used in many of our fertility clinics.

In some cases, the hormonal problem is not based in the ovaries, but in the pituitary, the controller of the endocrine system (see Section one). If it produces too much of a hormone called prolactin, this can damp down normal ovarian function. Prolactin — its name means 'milk maker' — is the hormone that stimulates the breasts when a baby is being fed, and because it has the side effect of preventing ovulation, it exerts a contraceptive action. It is because of prolactin that breast-feeding women generally do not conceive. In some women, for unknown reasons, the hormone is produced when there is no pregnancy or breast-feeding baby to account for it. Then treatment is needed to reduce its levels and so allow the ovary to function normally. (The drug used is bromocriptine; it can also be used to stop milk-making in women who would normally lactate, after they have given birth.)

Other causes of sub-fertility

Although the popular belief is that childlessness is always a feminine problem, in fact as many men as women suffer from reduced fertility.

They are perfectly potent. That is, they are able to enjoy intercourse and orgasm and eject semen, but the sperm they produce are somehow inadequate. It may be that the man is producing a large number of sperm but they are not fully developed or he may not be producing enough. Although only one sperm is needed to make a baby, many millions must be produced to make it possible for one to complete the long journey to meet the egg.

An examination of a woman within a few hours of intercourse will reveal whether or not a man is producing healthy sperm. Some will still be living within her body and can be seen under a microscope. This is a post-coital test.

If sperm are not seen, or appear to be of poor development, there may be several causes, all of which will need investigating and treatment.

In some cases there are couples who are perfectly fit and apparently capable of conceiving, yet are not able to start a pregnancy. The commonest cause is that the couple are just not having intercourse during the time of the woman's fertility. As this time is such a short one this is quite possible, even in a sexually active pair.

An even more common problem, especially in very young couples, is that they lack understanding of the mechanism of sexual intercourse. There have been quite a few reported cases of people seeking medical help who were found not to have fully consummated their relationship. For such a couple, clear explanation of the mechanism of intercourse may be enough to help the consummation and therefore conception. (See Section five.)

Yet another cause may be an exaggerated attention to hygiene by a woman. Some, while actively wanting babies, are distressed by the presence of semen on their bodies and immediately after intercourse get up and wash. While this is not exactly a contraceptive practice it can certainly spoil the chances of starting a pregnancy in a couple of low fertility.

In a few cases there may be a form of allergy problem operating. Some women react to their partner's sperm as though it were a dangerous invader. Their bodies make antibodies which kill the sperm. Treatment of this problem may be complex, but some doctors are using modified AIH — artificial insemination by the husband — to overcome the difficulty.

It has been noted that a woman who is very tense and distressed by her apparent infertility is very unlikely to conceive until she is able to relax and turn her energies and thoughts to other things. The classic example of this is the woman who gives up her job immediately after marriage, confident she will start a family at once, yet does not. When she takes a job again and stops thinking about babies at all, pregnancy often follows almost immediately.

This can happen to a childless woman who adopts or fosters a child. As soon as she is caring for a baby she becomes pregnant.

Sometimes the psychological problem is that a woman has unconscious fears of sex or pregnancy and childbirth strong enough to prevent conception, even though she is not aware of them. A woman who is helped to recognize such fears and their causes may be able to lose them. Once she has real insight into her problem, often a pregnancy will result.

The process of birth

No one knows precisely why labour starts when it does. There is now a good deal of evidence to suggest that it is the baby itself acting through the placenta — which it controls — which sends out a special hormone that starts the process going. And it could well be that it is not until the baby's body reaches a critical weight, in relation to the mother's body and the food supply she is able to give, that this stage is reached.

But whatever triggers it, the process follows much the same pattern.

All through pregnancy the woman will be aware of the fact that from time to time her uterus goes into contraction. Her belly will go hard and if she puts her hand on it, it will feel quite board-like. These contractions are painless and are called Braxton-Hicks after the doctor who first described them. Although women tend not to notice them every time they happen, they are probably occurring throughout pregnancy at irregular intervals of every fifteen, twenty or thirty minutes and lasting about twenty-five seconds.

As the pregnancy nears its end, these contractions become more powerful and they occasionally can be quite uncomfortable, though still not painful. Once labour commences then they become regular (almost to the second) more powerful and more forceful and begin to be more painful. This is the point at which the doctors will say that labour has started, but in fact it will have started long before. The cervix will have begun to get a little softer under the influence of hormones, and the bag of waters in which the baby is floating will be pushed against the cervix by the baby's head. This will have the effect of opening the cervix a little and the plug of mucus which has been keeping it closed as the pregnancy progressed — it is called the operculum because it is pearly white, the meaning of the word in Latin — comes away. It might be slightly bloodstained and is often referred to as a 'show' when it appears at the surface of the body.

As the pressure of the baby's head increases and the contractions push it more and more against the slightly open cervix, a small pouch of the amniotic sac — the bag of waters — may be pressed against the cervix or even through it and under the continued downwards pressure the pouch will burst open. The result will be a flood of fluid known as 'the breaking of the waters'.

Once this has happened labour is likely to go on fairly briskly. The contractions will come every fifteen to twenty minutes and may be uncomfortable though not necessarily painful. The hardening of the uterus now lasts for rather longer. The Braxton-Hicks contractions usually lasted for no more than thirty seconds, but those that are true labour contractions will last for forty seconds or even longer.

If for any reason it is decided to hurry labour along — perhaps because the mother is distressed or there is anxiety about the baby's welfare or for any one of a number of other reasons — deliberately breaking the waters can set labour going, as can giving drugs and hormones that have a directly contracting effect on the uterus.

Whether a labour is artifically started or starts by itself, the progress will continue to be the same. (One word of warning; there may in some women be a false labour — the normal Braxton-Hicks contractions, which do become stronger towards the end of pregnancy, impinge themselves more on the woman's mind and she may become apprehensive and interpret these as labour pains. If she goes then into hospital or calls her midwife or doctor she may well be told that 'it will be some time yet' and be sent home to wait. There is no shame in making this mistake; even women having second, third or fourth babies have been known to misinterpret signs of labour.)

Labour has been well named. It takes a great deal of effort on a mother's part to expel this large baby, and the by-products of its growth, from her uterus.

Generally labour is described as being in three stages.

The first stage of labour

This stage lasts from the beginning of true labour to full dilation of the cervix. The contractions of the powerful muscles of the uterus not only push the baby down towards the vagina and the way out, but also eliminate the cervix without actually damaging its muscle. The whole system seems to 'remember' that it may be needed again, so the emphasis is not just on delivering the new infant but leaving the mother fit and able to go through the whole process again.

The contractions of the upper part of the uterus pull on the lower part which in turn pulls on the upper part of the cervix, thus smoothing it out. It is a very complicated mechanical process and eventually the cervix is obliterated so that the way through to the vagina is completely clear.

Once the cervix has disappeared all the uterine contractions now work at opening the space left behind more widely. At first the process is slow and part of the work of the midwife or obstetrician is to measure that progress. Various descriptions of the degrees of dilation of the cervix have been used; some older midwives will talk of a cervix that is 'one finger', 'two fingers', 'three fingers', dilated. That means that it will admit that many fingers. Nowadays it is more usual to measure it in centimetres; when the cervix is opened five to six centimetres, it is said to be half-dilated; when it is seven centimetres open it is three-quarters dilated, and when it is fully dilated it is eight to ten centimetres across.

This first stage of labour is generally the longest. It can take up to thirteen or fourteen hours for a first baby (though this can be much longer) and as little as seven or less in later pregnancies (in a few cases women have been known to have a labour that has lasted one hour or less, but this is extremely unusual).

However long it lasts it should never be thought that the whole period is of agonizing pain. It is not. Yes, the contractions can be powerful and frequently uncomfortable, but during the early part of this stage they are coming at fifteen to ten minute intervals so there is ample time to rest in between or wander about or watch TV. (Some women get very energetic at this point, and get a great urge to wash the curtains or bake bread or polish the kitchen floor. It's almost like the animal 'nesting' instinct.) And even at the end, when the contractions may come every two or three minutes apart and last for as much as a minute or more, many women find them at least tolerable.

But if it does become painful, there are safe drugs that can be used. Safe in the sense that they relieve a mother's discomfort, but do not damage the baby. It must be remembered that any drug given to the mother will reach the baby via the placenta and the umbilical cord. In some cases, if it is considered necessary, it is possible to give an injection into the mother's spine that will remove all sensation in the birth area without removing her ability to push and use her own muscles, which is very necessary for the second stage.

The second stage of labour

Stage two lasts from full dilation of the cervix to delivery of the baby. It is often ushered in by the mother feeling and sometimes being sick. This could be a protective mechanism; the mother with a completely empty stomach probably does a better job of pushing the baby out of her uterus.

Hitherto the contractions have been of a particular type, powerful waves of sensation that arise often from the back and, travelling right across the belly, sometimes send tension down the legs. Now they begin to change their nature. Instead of making the mother want to lie still and wait for the contraction to rise to a peak and then die away, she will find that she has an urgent need to push downwards. In fact she won't be able to prevent herself doing so. It is an incredibly imperative feeling as any woman who has ever had it will report, and once the need is there, no power on earth will stop a woman from pushing, apart from a complete general anaesthetic. Which is not to be recommended unless it is really essential (remembering the possible effect on the baby).

Positions for childbirth

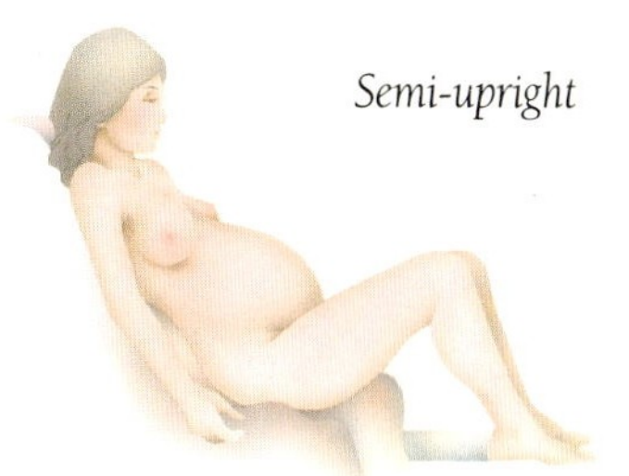

Semi-upright

Left lateral

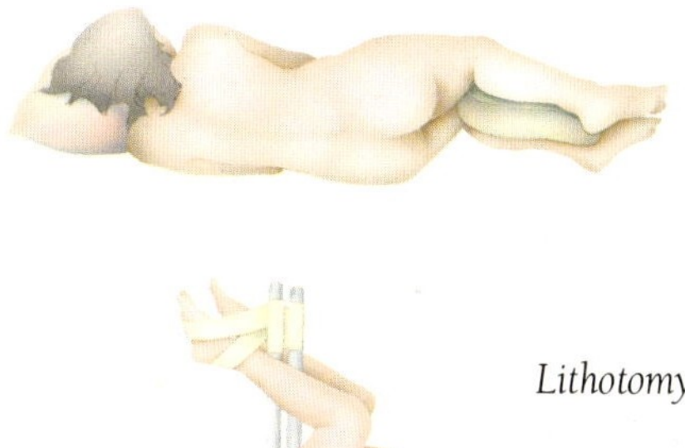

Lithotomy

Dorsal

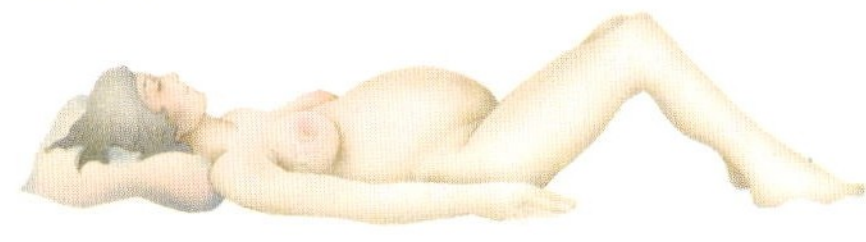

At this stage many women will automatically bend their knees and lift their heads forward and tighten their shoulders – so creating a posture which helps to make pushing more effective. In the recent past most women were delivered of their babies while lying on their backs, which is not the easiest way in which to push effectively.

It has been said that this fashion derived from the desire of King Louis XIVth to watch his mistresses give birth; a woman on her back provides a better view to others of what she is doing. Before this time, women were allowed to sit up to give birth, if they wanted to.

Now more and more women find that it is much more agreeable to behave as their ancestors did, and to deliver their babies while they are kneeling or squatting or sitting in a birthing chair. Thus gravity aids their pushing efforts.

The three stages of labour

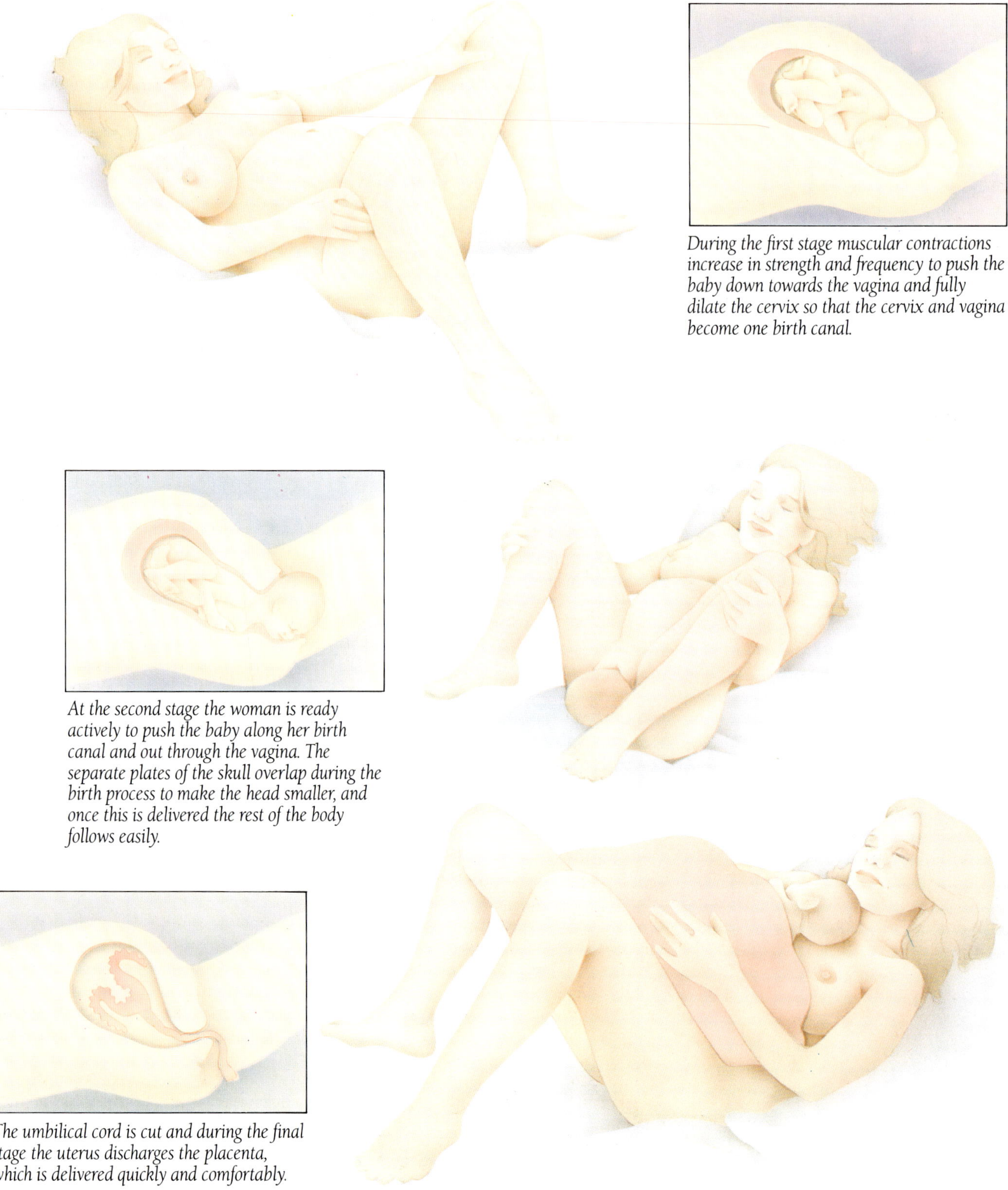

During the first stage muscular contractions increase in strength and frequency to push the baby down towards the vagina and fully dilate the cervix so that the cervix and vagina become one birth canal.

At the second stage the woman is ready actively to push the baby along her birth canal and out through the vagina. The separate plates of the skull overlap during the birth process to make the head smaller, and once this is delivered the rest of the body follows easily.

The umbilical cord is cut and during the final stage the uterus discharges the placenta, which is delivered quickly and comfortably.

With each contraction and desire to push, the mother will be forcing the baby a little further along her birth canal. It is probable that the baby also makes efforts, possibly moving its legs against the down-pushing muscle of the uterine wall in which it has lived all its life so far, so that it is pushed even further along the birth canal.

The vagina stretches easily as the baby's head moves down it. Its ridged elastic walls allow that. Only when the head reaches the opening may there be any difficulty. The muscular wedge of tissue (the perineum) between the opening of the vagina and the anus needs to be well relaxed so that the baby's head can pass across it and through the ring of mucous membrane that edges the opening. If the mother is not sufficiently relaxed or the head is pushing too hard and too fast, a tear may appear through the side of the opening of the vagina and run into the perineum behind. If this happens it can be very difficult for an obstetrician to stitch it as well as it should be stitched, so very often a cut is made deliberately to widen the opening. This is called an episiotomy and is to be preferred to a tear because it is so much easier to stitch neatly and successfully, giving a good cosmetic as well as comfortable result.

Once the head reaches the opening and comes through, the contractions stop for a while and then start again as the baby's head rotates and first one shoulder and then the other is born.

After that the rest of the body follows easily, for the widest parts have led the way. The head is really quite massive compared to the rest of the baby's body (even though it is made smaller for the purposes of birth by the gaps in the infant skull; the plates move together and over-ride each other a little — thus reducing the overall diameter).

This marks the end of the second stage and is often greeted by the mother with intense emotional exitement. Some burst into floods of excited tears; others laugh while some just lie staring at their infant in amazement. The delight a mother feels at this stage can be extremely infectious and often the whole staff of a labour ward will become involved. It's as though everyone was flying on an enormous 'high' — and why not? If this has been a normal birth and has resulted in a healthy baby who is loud and lusty (probably crying by now), a great thing has been achieved. A very good reason for excitement.

The second stage usually lasts about half an hour to an hour for a first labour, though it can be much longer, and maybe only twenty minutes or even less for subsequent labours. Every midwife and obstetrician will tell tales of an experienced mother who produced her second or subsequent baby with just a couple of good pushes in the second stage.

The third stage of labour

Stage three lasts from the delivery of the baby to the delivery of the placenta — the afterbirth — and this is the easiest and most comfortable stage for the mother. Often she is hardly aware it is happening at all.

In a well run maternity ward, or in her own home under the care of a well-trained obstetrician or midwife, she will have been given her baby to hold as soon as it was delivered and possibly will be able to put it to the breast immediately. If this can be done while she and the baby are naked, a very rapid bonding can occur. The baby will obtain food from the breast as he suckles — and he has a powerful ability to suck from the moment he is born, because he has been sucking his own fingers for many weeks while inside his mother's uterus — from a substance called colostrum. This is thick and yellowish and very, very rich in many protective substances. The mother will have been able to produce some of this by squeezing her nipples any time during the last few months of pregnancy.

When the newly delivered baby suckles in this way he not only helps himself and his mother to bond together; he also sends a rush of hormone from her breasts to her pituitary which sends more hormone on down to her uterus, which causes it to contract down hard. This contraction separates the placenta from the wall of the uterus and closes down any open blood vessels that may release too much blood, and pushes the placenta out through the birth canal.

By this time the umbilical cord, which has been attached to the baby, will almost certainly have been tied and severed, leaving a stump on the baby's belly and the remainder on the placenta. The cord and placenta can now be examined by the mother's attendants to make sure it is complete. If any fragments are left behind, by any chance, they can set up inflammation and infection and cause a good deal of bleeding and disease. So careful examination of the placenta is vital.

An interesting detail; the placenta is very richly supplied with important hormones and food substances and in many societies women used to eat their own placentae after birth in order to give themselves back these vital substances. It had a mystical value rather than a nutritional one. In other societies it was the men who were given the placentae to eat, again for mystical reasons. Occasionally there are people today who like to do this, but it is not a common practice and by no means necessary for successful childbirth, or recovering from it. In modern hospitals and maternity units it is very common to collect the placentae and deliver them to factories where vital hormones and other substances can be extracted and turned into very useful drugs to treat various illnesses.

As the infant goes on suckling the uterus clamps down even harder and the flow of blood from the naked area on the wall of the uterus where the placenta was attached is heavily reduced. However, there will continue to be a flow for some time — even up to six weeks — as the raw area heals.

Lactation

The stages of birth ideally end with the first experiences of suckling the infant. It cannot be said too often that the sooner this first experience is shared by the mother and baby the better, because breast feeding is a skill like any other which both in the feeding partnership have to learn. True milk does not appear in a mother's breasts until the third day after delivery (for the first three days her breasts remain comparatively soft and produce only colostrum) and in the past some doctors and midwives did not attempt to put a baby to the breast until the third day. Now, fortunately, it is known that the more vigorous suckling there is in the first three days the more comfortable will be the established breast feeding.

Breast feeding is often a deeply enjoyable physical experience for a mother. It's meant to be. It encourages the uterus to contract, as we've already seen, and these contractions are needed for a long time after birth to help the uterus to lose the excess tissue that it has put on during the pregnancy. Sometimes the contractions following breast feeding can be uncomfortable and are referred to as 'after pains'. Sometimes they are so uncomfortable that the mother needs pain killers to give her relief. But they are useful contractions and worth tolerating for that reason.

The pleasure a woman gets from breast feeding is partly psychological and partly physical. Psychologically there is the awareness that she is giving her baby something that no one else can; she is giving it protection as well as food, love and warmth as well as calories. Physically she will gain sensuous feelings from her breast feeding. Just as having her nipples kissed and played with by her sexual partner as a preliminary to intercourse gives her pleasure and arousal, so does she get the same feelings when she feeds her infants — even if she has problems establishing a comfortable feeding routine at first. Some women have been so embarrassed by this and thought it in some way so 'shameful' that they abandoned breast feeding, but that really is a tragedy. There is no shame in finding sexual pleasure in suckling an infant and some women have been fortunate enough to experience an orgasm as a result of it. All of which helps to bind the mother even more closely to her infant and to improve the quality of care she can give him, and the satisfaction he can give her. When a mother/baby relationship is based on this sort of closeness in the very early weeks it bodes very well indeed for a peaceful and happy childhood, a successful adolescence and the final emergence of a complete, happy and well-adjusted adult. Which is, after all, the whole purpose of women's fertility.

The baby learns to latch on to the mother's breast and take part of the areola as well as the nipple into his mouth. This stimulates milk production and prevents the nipples becoming sore.

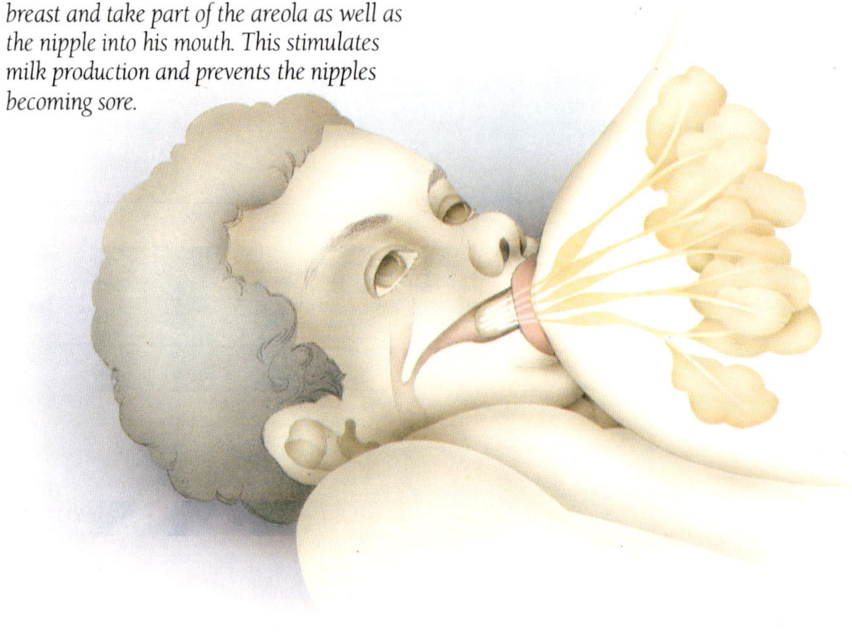

What can go wrong?

Sometimes a birth is complicated because a baby is not in the ideal position. The vast majority of babies are delivered with their head pointing downwards and with the crown presenting at the opening of the cervix and then at the opening of the vagina. If the head is misplaced, being tilted backwards so that the face presents, this can cause considerable difficulties because that diameter of the head is much greater in that position, and it needs more space to get through. Also, if the child is upside down — that is head upwards, presenting his bottom to the birth canal — this can cause difficulties because, it will be remembered, it is the sizeable head that opens the way for the smaller body. This is called a breech presentation and happens in about two per cent of all births. However, with careful control on the part of the obstetrician and/or midwife, a breech delivery can be made without too much difficulty. In a few cases it has been found possible to turn a breech baby before labour begins by manipulating him from the outside of the mother's body through her belly. However, this is not always possible and a breech delivery is then inevitable.

Sometimes the head does not come down sufficiently and it is necessary to give it some assistance, and for this purpose forceps can be used. These were first designed by the Chamberlen brothers more than two hundred years ago and they have indeed saved many, many mothers' and babies' lives over the centuries. Beautifully shaped and curved, they can be inserted into the mother's vagina to hold the baby's head safely without pressure and encourage its movement down the birth canal. If a forceps delivery has to be done, then it is necessary to perform an episiotomy.

In some cases it is not possible for the baby to be born through the vaginal route at all. It may be that the position the baby is in means that a safe delivery is impossible; it may be that the mother has too small a pelvis or some distortion of the pelvis, which means a big baby cannot be delivered vaginally. Or it may be that there are signs of stress in the baby or in the mother that make a rapid birth essential. Many of the monitoring techniques now used in hospitals are designed to ensure that no baby is left too long inside the uterus when a rapid birth is needed to save its life.

In recent years there have been many passionate articles and books written, and television and radio programmes made, decrying the 'takeover of childbirth' by technologically minded doctors. It has been suggested that more harm than good has been done to mothers and babies by the proliferation of equipment that makes it possible to measure the child's welfare while in the uterus; to perform operations and blood transfusions on the baby while it is still unborn, and to monitor its progress and wellbeing throughout labour. Those who object to these techniques maintain that Nature, left to herself, can safely deliver babies with the minimum of trauma for the mother. They fear that mothers are intimidated by the presence of equipment that depersonalizes them and makes them merely into objects out of which babies are delivered rather than living, breathing, human beings. And it has to be admitted that the rate of Caesarian births is rising. In 1963 the rate in the UK was 3.1 per cent of all births (in the USA it was 5.5 per cent)

Caesarian section

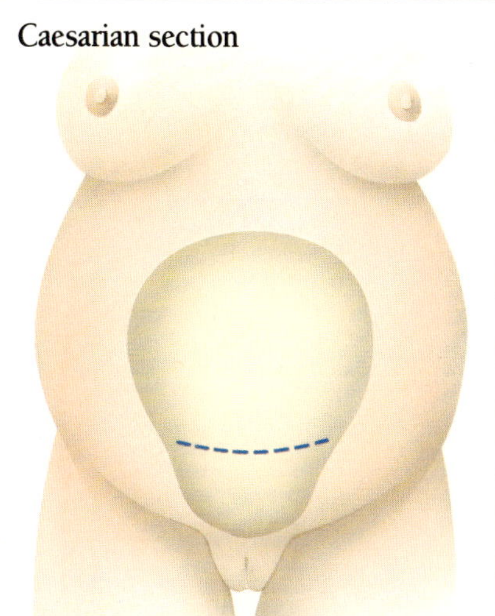

A Caesarian section in which an incision is made into the mother's belly and uterus, so that the infant can be extracted, these days is a safe and successful operation and has saved many babies' and mothers' lives.

It may be needed because of a disproportion between the size of the baby and the mother's pelvis (damage to the pelvis because of rickets used to lead to many Caesarian operations) or because of distress in either the mother or the baby, making a normal vaginal delivery risky.

Complications in childbirth

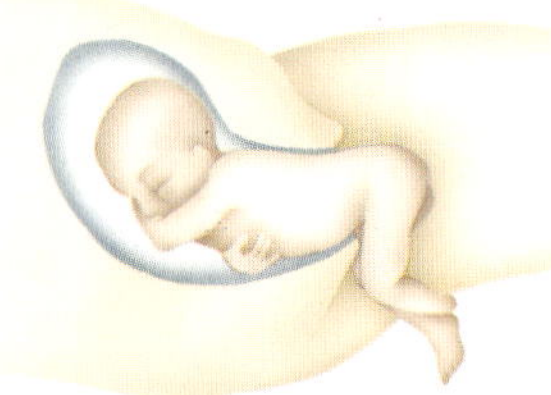

In the extended breech position the baby lies with the buttocks and the head uppermost and will need skilful delivery.

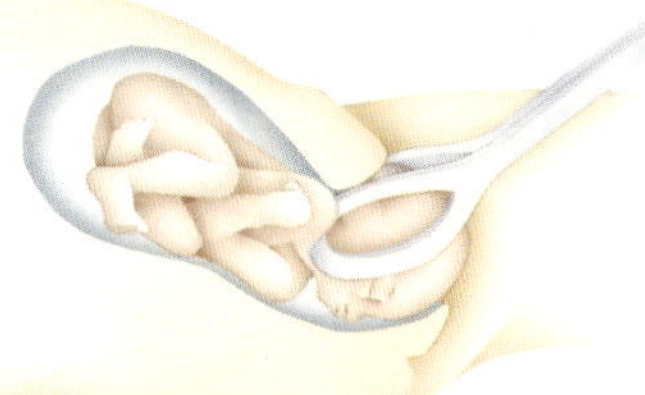

Sometimes the head needs to be encouraged to move down by inserting forceps. These are specially designed to hold the baby's head safely without pressure.

and by 1978 it had risen to 7.5 per cent (in the USA even higher — 15.2 per cent). In Australia the rate lies somewhere between the UK and USA figures. In some places it is still rising, though many modern obstetricians agree with those women who resist the use of high technology aids to birth and say that some Caesars are unnecessary.

So there has been a great deal of sympathy for this stance and understanding of the feelings of many women who quite deliberately 'fly from science' and insist on giving birth to their babies at home with the minimum of care, apart from that of a qualified midwife. And, for the vast majority of them, this may indeed be successful and safe. Many babies have been born alive and well in this way to relaxed, happy and comfortable mothers who are content to be in the bosom of their families. But — and this is the important point — there are babies who have been lost because of refusal of technical aids. Childbirth, while being perfectly normal and natural, is still a potentially hazardous experience for both mother and baby. If we left it to Nature we would probably lose the majority of our babies, just as animals living in the natural wild still do. Technology can be a superb aid for a modern woman and protect both her and her baby. The great reduction in the very high rate of prolapse that used to bedevil many women who had had babies is ample evidence of this. (See page 120, Section eight.)

Contraception

Despite the fact that we are fertile for only three days or so in each month of our reproductive years, and despite the fact that our reproductive life only lasts for about half of our total life span — thirty-five years or so — we are still capable of producing vast numbers of offspring. If each of us produced the number of children we were capable of producing, we would be overrunning this planet even more than we are. As it is we are the most numerous of all the higher animals (only outnumbered by some species of insects) and are doing ourselves and our planet a great deal of harm because of our sheer weight of numbers.

It is therefore essential that as well as understanding what happens when we give birth, we should have a deep understanding of how not to give birth.

The methods of contraception that are available today would have amazed our great great grandparents. One hundred years ago it was a choice between abstention or 'coitus interruptus' (also known as 'being careful', which involves a man withdrawing his penis from the vagina just before he ejaculates and therefore releasing his sperm outside her body) and thick and clumsy condoms (sheaths for the penis, a gadget said to have been invented by Don Juan who made his out of sheep's bladders, tied them in place with pink ribbons and wore them to protect himself from venereal disease rather than to protect his partners from pregnancy). Today we have many more methods, some good, some not.

Even with the information offered in the chart overleaf at your fingers' ends, it can be difficult to make the ideal choice of contraceptive; each woman has different needs at different times in her life.

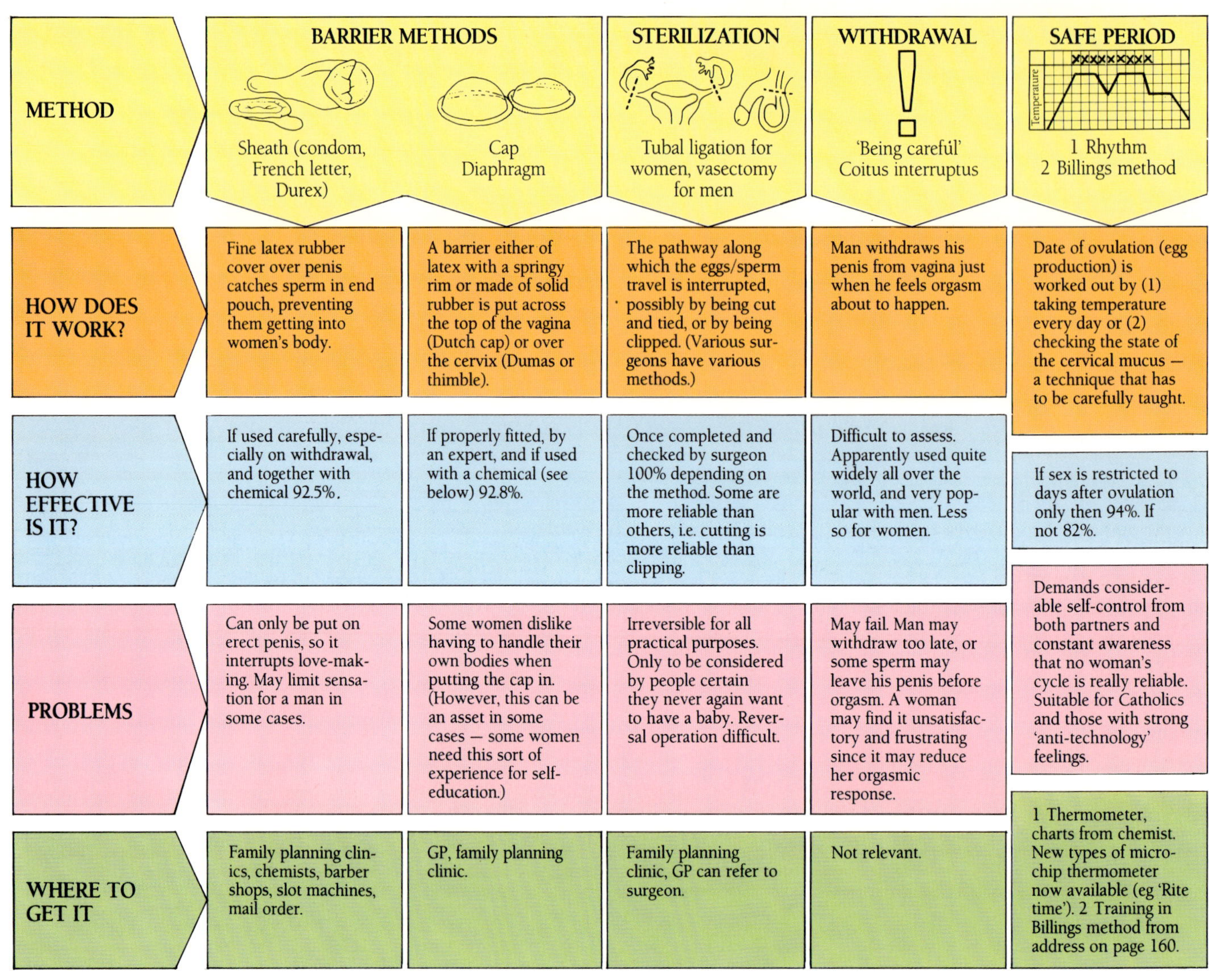

	BARRIER METHODS		STERILIZATION	WITHDRAWAL	SAFE PERIOD
METHOD	Sheath (condom, French letter, Durex)	Cap Diaphragm	Tubal ligation for women, vasectomy for men	'Being careful' Coitus interruptus	1 Rhythm 2 Billings method
HOW DOES IT WORK?	Fine latex rubber cover over penis catches sperm in end pouch, preventing them getting into women's body.	A barrier either of latex with a springy rim or made of solid rubber is put across the top of the vagina (Dutch cap) or over the cervix (Dumas or thimble).	The pathway along which the eggs/sperm travel is interrupted, possibly by being cut and tied, or by being clipped. (Various surgeons have various methods.)	Man withdraws his penis from vagina just when he feels orgasm about to happen.	Date of ovulation (egg production) is worked out by (1) taking temperature every day or (2) checking the state of the cervical mucus — a technique that has to be carefully taught.
HOW EFFECTIVE IS IT?	If used carefully, especially on withdrawal, and together with chemical 92.5%.	If properly fitted, by an expert, and if used with a chemical (see below) 92.8%.	Once completed and checked by surgeon 100% depending on the method. Some are more reliable than others, i.e. cutting is more reliable than clipping.	Difficult to assess. Apparently used quite widely all over the world, and very popular with men. Less so for women.	If sex is restricted to days after ovulation only then 94%. If not 82%.
PROBLEMS	Can only be put on erect penis, so it interrupts love-making. May limit sensation for a man in some cases.	Some women dislike having to handle their own bodies when putting the cap in. (However, this can be an asset in some cases — some women need this sort of experience for self-education.)	Irreversible for all practical purposes. Only to be considered by people certain they never again want to have a baby. Reversal operation difficult.	May fail. Man may withdraw too late, or some sperm may leave his penis before orgasm. A woman may find it unsatisfactory and frustrating since it may reduce her orgasmic response.	Demands considerable self-control from both partners and constant awareness that no woman's cycle is really reliable. Suitable for Catholics and those with strong 'anti-technology' feelings.
WHERE TO GET IT	Family planning clinics, chemists, barber shops, slot machines, mail order.	GP, family planning clinic.	Family planning clinic, GP can refer to surgeon.	Not relevant.	1 Thermometer, charts from chemist. New types of microchip thermometer now available (eg 'Rite time'). 2 Training in Billings method from address on page 160.

A young woman, not in a committed relationship, and having intercourse only occasionally, would not need the Pill method; that would be like keeping the central heating on all the time when you're never in; what you need is just to light the fire when you're going to be at home — in other words, an occasional method like a cap or sheath plus a chemical.

A new mother who wants to space her family may prefer to use the POP mini-pill rather than the combined one. The woman who suffers from recurrent thrush may need to avoid the Pill altogether and use a barrier method. The woman who is sure she has completed her family may feel ready for sterilization. All any woman can do is discuss her special needs with her own trusted doctor or family planning clinic, as well as her partner, and make her choice accordingly. But it could be useful to know that an estimated ninety million women round the world have been sterilized, making this the most popular form of birth control, selected by a third of the 270 million who use contraceptives at all; that about twenty per cent use the pill; fifteen per cent the coil, ten per cent the sheath and the remaining twenty per cent use other methods such as rhythm and/or withdrawal.

Abortion

For most people this is the least acceptable form of birth control, though it has long been used for this purpose. The laws governing its use that exist in various countries around the world reflect the deep distaste many feel for the concept of killing a developing infant. They can countenance with equanimity the prevention of conception, but balk at the destruction of it afterwards.

Many women feel the same way and have their fears exacerbated by knowing that of those women who have abortions many suffer great distress afterwards. This can be partly due to moral or intellectual concerns, but also to hormonal effects; once a pregnancy is established a woman does feel 'different'. It is hard to describe, but it is very real for all that, and even the most determinedly commonsensical woman may find herself surprisingly bereaved if

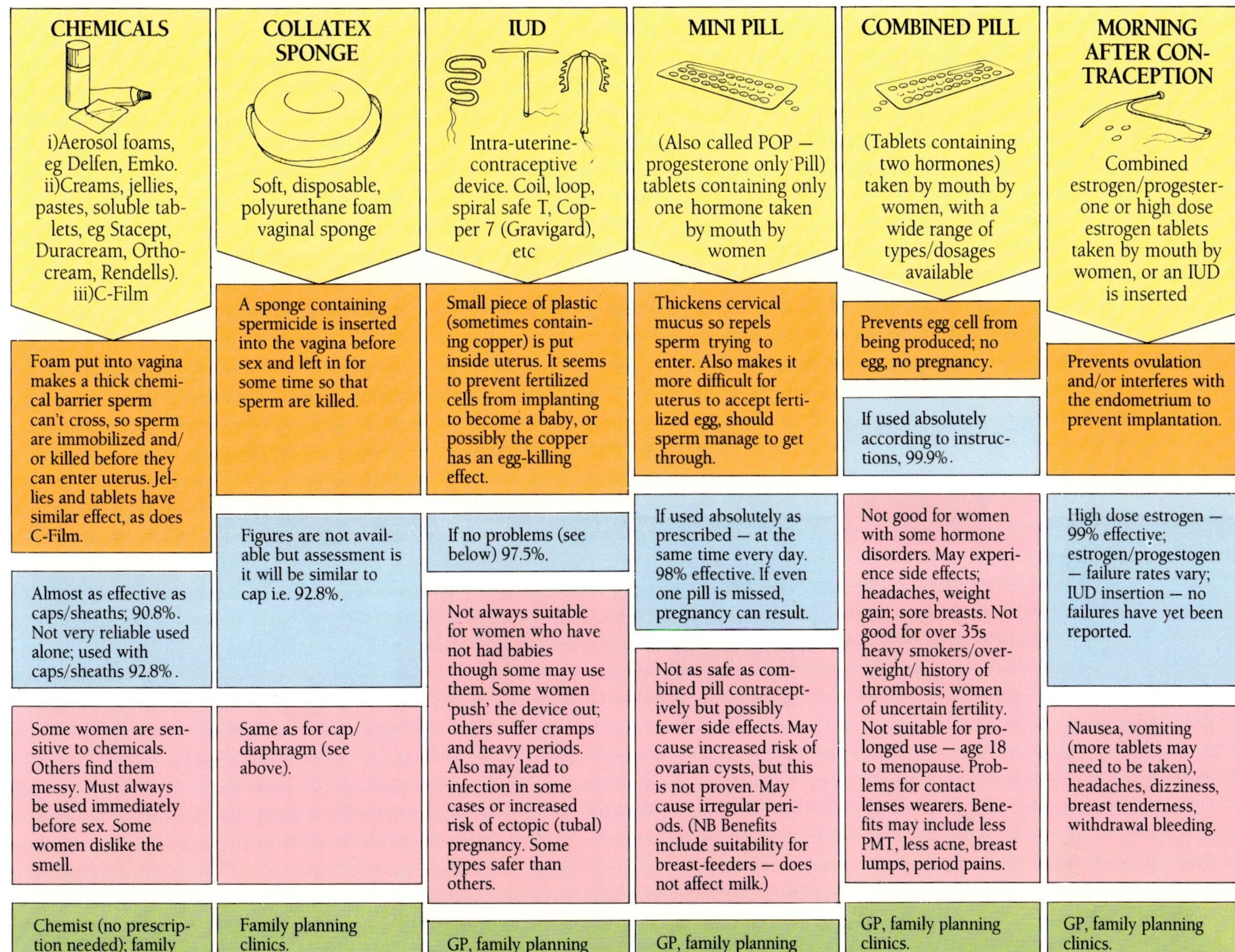

CHEMICALS	COLLATEX SPONGE	IUD	MINI PILL	COMBINED PILL	MORNING AFTER CONTRACEPTION
i)Aerosol foams, eg Delfen, Emko. ii)Creams, jellies, pastes, soluble tablets, eg Stacept, Duracream, Orthocream, Rendells). iii)C-Film	Soft, disposable, polyurethane foam vaginal sponge	Intra-uterine-contraceptive device. Coil, loop, spiral safe T, Copper 7 (Gravigard), etc	(Also called POP — progesterone only Pill) tablets containing only one hormone taken by mouth by women	(Tablets containing two hormones) taken by mouth by women, with a wide range of types/dosages available	Combined estrogen/progesterone or high dose estrogen tablets taken by mouth by women, or an IUD is inserted
Foam put into vagina makes a thick chemical barrier sperm can't cross, so sperm are immobilized and/or killed before they can enter uterus. Jellies and tablets have similar effect, as does C-Film.	A sponge containing spermicide is inserted into the vagina before sex and left in for some time so that sperm are killed.	Small piece of plastic (sometimes containing copper) is put inside uterus. It seems to prevent fertilized cells from implanting to become a baby, or possibly the copper has an egg-killing effect.	Thickens cervical mucus so repels sperm trying to enter. Also makes it more difficult for uterus to accept fertilized egg, should sperm manage to get through.	Prevents egg cell from being produced; no egg, no pregnancy.	Prevents ovulation and/or interferes with the endometrium to prevent implantation.
Almost as effective as caps/sheaths; 90.8%. Not very reliable used alone; used with caps/sheaths 92.8%.	Figures are not available but assessment is it will be similar to cap i.e. 92.8%.	If no problems (see below) 97.5%.	If used absolutely as prescribed — at the same time every day. 98% effective. If even one pill is missed, pregnancy can result.	If used absolutely according to instructions, 99.9%.	High dose estrogen — 99% effective; estrogen/progestogen — failure rates vary; IUD insertion — no failures have yet been reported.
Some women are sensitive to chemicals. Others find them messy. Must always be used immediately before sex. Some women dislike the smell.	Same as for cap/diaphragm (see above).	Not always suitable for women who have not had babies though some may use them. Some women 'push' the device out; others suffer cramps and heavy periods. Also may lead to infection in some cases or increased risk of ectopic (tubal) pregnancy. Some types safer than others.	Not as safe as combined pill contraceptively but possibly fewer side effects. May cause increased risk of ovarian cysts, but this is not proven. May cause irregular periods. (NB Benefits include suitability for breast-feeders — does not affect milk.)	Not good for women with some hormone disorders. May experience side effects; headaches, weight gain; sore breasts. Not good for over 35s heavy smokers/overweight/ history of thrombosis; women of uncertain fertility. Not suitable for prolonged use — age 18 to menopause. Problems for contact lenses wearers. Benefits may include less PMT, less acne, breast lumps, period pains.	Nausea, vomiting (more tablets may need to be taken), headaches, dizziness, breast tenderness, withdrawal bleeding.
Chemist (no prescription needed); family planning clinics.	Family planning clinics.	GP, family planning clinics.	GP, family planning clinics.	GP, family planning clinics.	GP, family planning clinics.

she has an abortion. It is not a decision to be made lightly, therefore.

If a woman has been raped, or is carrying a child known to be defective then she may be able to face an abortion with equanimity and recover rapidly and gratefully afterwards, though even in these cases there may be some deep grief. Talking about all the feelings and problems involved before the operation is therefore vital.

It can be performed by doing a D and C operation (see Section eight) or by using a suction apparatus that removes the contents of the uterus via a fine tube. Alternatively it can be triggered by giving prostaglandins, the chemicals that are similar to hormones, and which govern the way the uterus contracts and relaxes, so expelling its contents.

Abortions performed before the twelfth to fourteenth week are much simpler and less traumatic in physical terms than those performed later. In later pregnancy it may be necessary to open the uterus to extract the infant. This (it's called hysterotomy) is rarely performed and then only under special circumstances (in the case of a sick mother, for example).

End word

Our fertility remains still, in many ways, a major burden as well as the source of much of our joy as women. We are capable of gaining far more from our sexuality and our reproductive abilities than are men — because our reproductive role is so much more complex — but we have to pay a high price for that benefit.

Fortunately, most of us seem to think it is worth it. It will be even more so when men learn to be much more involved with childcare than they are now (childbearers don't have to be sole childcarers) and when the somewhat dilatory search for an effective and reliable male method of contraception is successful and willingly used by men. At present both childbirth and contraception are seen mainly as women's concerns and it's high time that they became truly the concern and responsibility of both partners.

7

WOMAN'S INVADERS

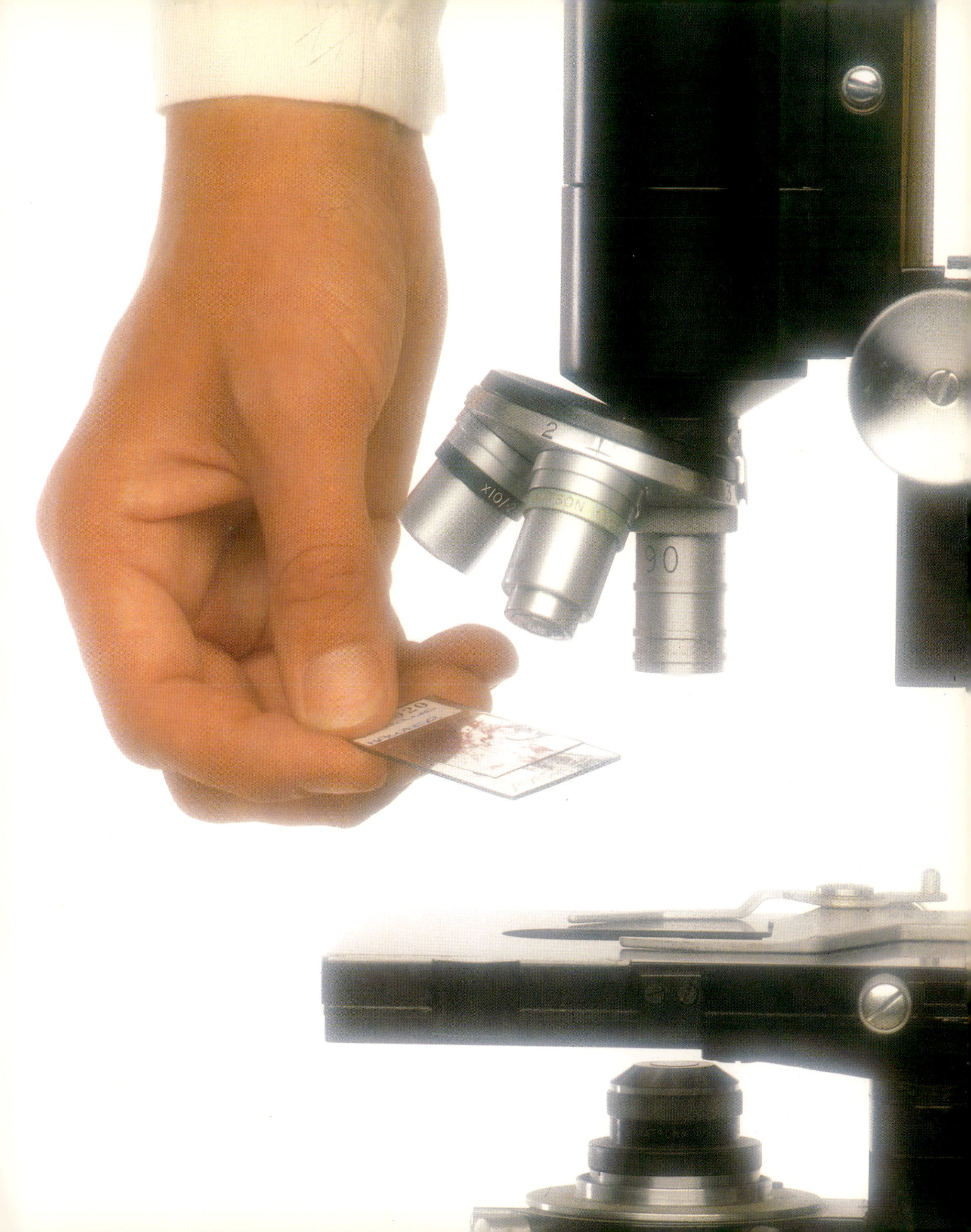

It is difficult for creatures as egotistical as we are to see ourselves as merely part of the life chain of the planet, but that is what we are. We are predators on certain animals (every time we eat a chicken sandwich we're behaving like animals of prey) and certain animals are predators on us. Notably bacteria, viruses and other minute organisms that we can't see, but which play a very large part in our daily lives.

Some are useful; those that clean up dead materials which would otherwise litter our world very disagreeably; those that work in our own bodies to keep us healthy (it is the presence of friendly bacteria inside our digestive systems that keep unfriendly ones — they're called pathogens — under control) and those that work on organic material to make it more useful and interesting to us by turning it into wine, yoghurt, cheese and so on. But there are others that are less benevolent, and which may cause all sorts of disagreeable symptoms and unpleasant disorders.

They are the micro-organisms which have led to a great deal of human misery, illness and death over the centuries. Diseases caused by them, ranging from smallpox to bubonic plague, tuberculosis to cholera, have decimated whole populations, and in spite of considerable scientific progress that makes it possible to control the effects of some infections (smallpox, for example, has been officially declared as eradicated) we still labour under attacks from a great many more.

Organisms are not, by and large, choosy about gender. They will get into any human body any way they can; but their effects can be altered by the gender of their host. A woman's body will react differently from a man's when attacked, say, by an organism called *candida albicans* (a chaming name for a far from charming attacker) because not only is her body made differently — her hormone status creates a different environment for the organism to live in.

So let us look in some detail at the sort of infections that a woman may suffer because she is a woman. We won't look at coughs and colds or measles or mumps since they affect men too, and in this context we aren't interested in them.

Vaginal discharge

Most vaginal infections will cause vaginal discharge — but not all vaginal discharges are due to infection. All adult women have a natural flow of healthy vaginal secretions, which may in one woman be scanty, in another copious. Most women will know what is normal for them, and will also know that there will be times when this flow increases; before a period, say (when the increased blood supply to the area increases mucus production) but they may be puzzled when it happens at other times.

A girl who is just embarking on an active sex life may be startled by the quantity of flow that accompanies sexual arousal. A girl having sexual intercourse for the first time may not realise that her partner's semen could later reappear as a vaginal discharge, and a girl who is pregnant for the first time may not realise that a fairly heavy flow is a common experience (again, it is due to the increased blood supply to the area during pregnancy).

It is when there are variations in this normal-for-me discharge that there may be cause for concern, because of the possibility of infection, but it's important to check there are no other possible reasons.

Foreign bodies

The presence of a foreign body in the vagina can lead to a heavy, smelly sometimes discoloured discharge. There are women who manage to forget the last tampon of a period, and fail to realise it is in place because it settles up behind the cervix in the pouch that is made there by the shape of the vagina.

Sometimes there can be other foreign bodies; all doctors and nurses know of women, often suffering from some form of emotional illness, who tuck items into their vaginae. I once nursed a woman who had folded a five pound note very small, wrapped it in fine latex and hidden it in her vagina, and then forgot it till she got a nasty discharge. The fiver emerged unscathed under our care and she was delighted to be given it back since she'd put it there and forgotten it fully two years earlier.

Trauma

Trauma is another cause of vaginal discharge; over-rubbing of the mucous membrance may make it produce extra mucus, but often this is bloodstained; any trauma severe enough to make excess mucus will often cause some bleeding too. But not always; an example is the damage done by sexual intercourse when in an unaroused state. For enjoyable, comfortable sex, the vagina needs to be well lubricated — and arousal ensures it is. A woman who accepts the penis before she is really eager for it may find she experiences damage to the vaginal wall, and allows organisms to enter the body's defences and so cause a discharge.

Chemicals

Another common sort of injury is that done by the excessive use of perfumes, deodorants, scented soaps and talcs. These can damage the vagina's natural ability to keep itself clean and healthy, and lead to a form of inflammation of the vaginal walls — vaginitis — that causes a bloodstained discharge. No one needs more than simple clean water — without the addition of disinfectants of any kind — to wash the area. And no one, but no one, needs douches (internal vaginal washes) unless they are medically prescribed for a precise reason. So if you see advertisements for such 'feminine hygiene products' ignore them; they are a snare and a delusion.

Erosion

Some women suffer discharge, see a doctor who examines them and are then told they have 'cervical erosion'. That sounds horrendous, as though part of the cervix has actually been rubbed away, but this is not what has happened. There are cells in the mucous membrane that line the channel in the cervix — the os — which make extra mucus (the reasons for variations in cervical mucus are explained on page 79, Section six on Fertility). These cells are usually inside the os, but in some women they protrude into the vagina and there produce quantities of mucus, felt by the woman as a discharge. If there is also an infection present, the discharge can be most unpleasant. The remedy is to get rid of the extra mucus-producing cells and the simplest way to do this is to use a cautery (either electric, chemical or laser) to 'burn' them off (see page 117) although most cervical erosions are symptomless and best left alone.

Also, polyps (little fleshy outgrowths of mucous membrane) can cause vaginal discharge as they too sometimes produce extra mucus; and so can our increasing age. Women past the menopause develop a thinning of the mucous membrane (see page 128, Section nine) and this can lead to a form of vaginitis that causes bleeding and discharge.

Vaginal infections

All discharges can occur on their own, but often they have the problems of infection added on. And some women can get these infections when everything else in the vagina is fine — no lost objects, no injury, no erosions; just a healthy vagina into which organisms have moved. Before looking at some of the particular organisms that can do this, it's worth knowing why some women suffer from them. If you are in good general condition and you have a healthy vagina which, remember, has a built in self-defence system, how is it that organisms can flourish enough to cause symptoms?

There are times when a woman may find her defences are low. Women who are pregnant are more likely to be attacked by some organisms; so are women who are using the Pill (remembering that the Pill mimics pregnancy — see Section six) and women who are taking antibiotics for some minor infection elsewhere in the body, such as toothache or sinusitis. In this situation the antibiotic kills not only pathogens but friendly bacteria as well — including those that help resist invasion by hostile bacteria, which explains the paradox that the use of antibiotics can actually cause infection. Women suffering from uncontrolled diabetes may also find they get more attacks of thrush, because the higher sugar levels in their bodies make them extra attractive to the invaders. They need food just as do all other life forms.

And some women without realising it create an environment which is irresistible to organisms. They wear tight non-porous underwear so that the vulva is entirely enclosed and air excluded. This keeps the temperature of the area at a higher level than it should be. They wash the vulva too often, using over-hot water, and so not only keep the temperature high but alter the vaginal pH (acid level — remember that this is one of the vagina's defences). There is nothing the organisms like better than a hostess who sits in hot baths every day. Also, some women may eat a high carbohydrate/refined sugary diet, which will produce extra sugar in the urine, again making the area sweetly attractive.

So, the best basic advice to anyone who tends to get vaginal infections easily is:

Wear loose cotton panties rather than tight man-made fibre ones (cotton allows you to sweat and dry comfortably) and either stockings or open crotch tights.

Avoid tight jeans.

Shower rather than bath so that you don't sit in hot water.

Don't use soaps or talcs around the vulva.

Aim for a sensible low sugar diet rather than a sweet one.

There is of course one other vaginal infection; exposure to the sort of organism that will always set up an infection if it can just get into the body, and which gets there only via sexual intercourse. These used to be called venereal diseases, the word deriving from the name of Venus, goddess of love. Modern science, however, prefers less romantic labels and calls them sexually transmitted diseases.

When they were called VD the only ones listed under that heading were those then known to be transmitted solely by sex; the new label includes those that are not necessarily spread by sex, but which may be. For example, thrush, the very common condition caused by candida albicans, can affect babies, nuns and the most faithful and virtuous of wives married to totally faithful men — yet it is regularly treated at STD clinics. So never think that because a GP sends you to such a clinic he is suggesting you or your partner are sexually promiscuous. He is simply sending you to a hospital department where such conditions are best understood and treated; and indeed in some British hospitals even the label STD clinics has been abandoned, partly because of patients' resistance to it. They are called 'Departments of Genito-Urinary Medicine'. But whatever they are called, the care they give is good and is aimed at a number of common conditions, including the following infections:

Non specific genital infections

This is the most common diagnosis made in STD clinics. It means a woman has symptoms — discomfort, extra discharge, some pain on peeing, together with frequency and possibly chronic, dull, low belly pain — but no actual organism can be identified as causing the trouble. Recent research suggests the cause may in fact be an organism called chlamydia (see page 101) but by no means all are due to this. The treatment is usually antibiotics, given in the hope that whatever the organism is, it will succumb to it. Or, treatments usually given for specific infections may be tried to see if they have the desired effect. They often do, fortunately.

Candida albicans: 'thrush'

This one, already mentioned, causes a great many women a great deal of misery. It is a fungus — a statement which has made some startled women imagine they are growing mushrooms in their interiors — and you may hear it described as a yeast infection because the organisms which cause the infection are very similar to those which make bread and beer, and in the vagina can be very active indeed. There are actually hundreds of such organisms and labelling all these as 'thrush' due to candida is inaccurate. However, that is how most doctors describe the problem, so we might as well do the same.

The symptoms are a thick creamy yellowish discharge that may form a 'cottage cheese' like appearance.

The discharge may stain fabric, and on underwear dries to a powdery substance that can be brushed off. It can smell somewhat like cheese too, though that can be very variable. Most people find it a disagreeable odour.

The worst thing about the discharge is not simply that it is there — tiresome though that is — but that it causes a sometimes severe itching and soreness. There may be swelling of the mucous membrane and it will look red (check in a mirror — it's the easiest way to see your own vulva).

The treatment of thrush is first to make sure that the environment is made as inhospitable as possible (see page 99) and to prevent further damage to the vulva. The best way to cleanse the area is not to wash, but to use pure olive oil BP (get it at the chemist) on clean cotton swabs to remove the discharge. Use each swab once only — that is, wipe in one direction with it, discard it, and then take a fresh one. This is better than washing with water and gives considerable relief from itching.

Then, the use of a specific anti-fungal remedy may be provided by a doctor. This can be used either as a local cream, or as a pessary. It's essential that the whole course of the prescribed remedy is used; too often women find they get relief of symptoms fairly soon after starting with a cream or pessary, and stop using it thinking they're cured. They are not, because there are still organisms there. They flourish once the treatment stops, and so become resistant to the treatment in future. So always use all of what is prescribed, just as you do with antibiotics and for the same reason.

In some cases a doctor will prescribe tablets taken by mouth to kill off the organisms, and these too must be taken as a full course. They work by killing off the organisms that may be lingering in the gut (most of us probably have some candida there most of the time) and prevent any from escaping via the anus and getting into the vagina.

A popular self-help non-medical way of dealing with thrush is to use a substance that deters the growth of thrush organisms by putting in another one — the one that turns milk into yoghurt. Insert plain, live yoghurt (is it necessary to say that using a strawberry or pineapple flavoured one would defeat the object of the exercise?) into the vagina — it can be put in with curved fingers, or by using a simple applicator you can get from the chemist, or by dipping a tampon into it — and it will (in theory) defeat the yeast. A great many women use this method very successfully — preferring it, despite its undoubted messiness and dairyish smell, to doctors' prescriptions. It's certainly worth trying. It also may bring relief actually to eat a pot of live plain yoghurt which will attack the organisms in the gut that might cause re-infection of the vulva.

But it has to be said here and now that some women will have recurrent attacks of thrush all their lives. Whatever they do they just can't seem to eradicate it, in which case all that can be done is to be as cheerful as you can about your unwanted guest and make yourself as unwelcoming to it as possible. The regime on the previous page won't cure the condition — but it could go a long way to controlling it.

Trichomonas vaginalis — TV

This one is also pretty common. It causes an even more intense itching and soreness than thrush and the redness associated with it can be more extensive, stretching over the inner thighs, between the buttocks and part of the way up the belly. The discharge it creates is usually said to be watery, copious, bubbly, greenish and very smelly, but again this can vary.

The treatment of TV is comparatively straightforward — a drug called metronidazole. It is marketed in the UK under various names, of which the best known is Flagyl. This can make people who take alcohol at the same time feel dreadfully ill, so people using it should never drink anything alcoholic as long as treatment lasts (and it must be maintained, as with anti-fungals, for the whole prescribed course. That usually is for five days).

Because there may be a teratogenic (baby-damaging) risk, this drug is not usually offered to women who may be in the first three months of a pregnancy. There are other drugs that can be used which, though less effective, still deal with the infection. The same alternatives may be needed for a breast-feeding mother as the drug metronidazole can pass through her body into her breast milk.

Because this infection is one that is so often sexually transmitted, it is common for doctors to want to treat a woman's sexual partner too, with the same drug. Generally doctors won't give this treatment by proxy, however. The man has to be seen himself, because there is always a possibility that there is more than one infection present (TV can co-exist with other infections) so he'll need as careful a medical check-up as his partner.

Gardnerella

This is a comparatively new label for a well known infection. It used to be called *haemophylis vaginalis* and not every expert is convinced that this new label is accurate. Whatever the academic medical arguments, it can be said that women showing soreness and itching — as usual — together with a rather greyish discharge may have gardnerella.

The treatment for it is the same as that for TV — metronidazole.

Anaerobic infections

There are some organisms that are killed by the presence of oxygen, and which get into the body during surgical operations, say, and then thrive in places where there is no air (incidentallythe prefix 'an-' to a word means absent, so anaerobic means absent air). So, any infection which arises immediately after such an operation as dilation and curetage perhaps, or cone biopsy, (see page 117, Section eight) and which is accompanied by a discharge that is very offensive to smell, with a fishy odour about it — the colour is immaterial — should be checked by a doctor.

Treatment is yet again by metronidazole. This drug is indeed widely used, and very effective in most cases.

Chlamydia

This has been described as a 'new' infection, which of course it is not. It is just newly identified — the likelihood is that it's been amongst us for a very long time indeed. It is usually sexually transmitted and is a particularly difficult one to deal with because it can cause severe infections of the fallopian tubes (salpingitis) which can lead to sterility as the tubes become blocked by scarring and won't let the eggs through. It therefore contributes to the problem of ectopic gestation — when a fertilized egg, instead of moving through the tube to embed itself in the uterus becomes stuck inside the tube (See Section six — Fertility). If infection and its subsequent scarring has narrowed the tube, it's harder for the egg to escape from it.

Recent research reports that there has been a marked increase in the incidence of tubal pregnancies of this sort, an increase which matches the rise in the reported incidence of chlamydia infections in the last few years. Many British gynaecologists fear that there are a number of women who have symptomless chlamydia infections, calling it 'a quiet epidemic'. They would urge all women, who are sexually active and who can't be sure their partners are free from any risk of giving them an infection, to seek check-ups at STD clinics. Other gynaecologists feel that suggesting this is to spread unnecessary alarm and despondency.

Perhaps the best answer is to suggest to women that they should use STD clinics not as a place of last resort, to visit after symptoms appear, but as a first-aid post to consult as soon as there has been exposure to risk — that is, sex with a partner they can't be sure they can trust in health terms.

Chlamydia can be transmitted to unborn babies, being a well-known cause of eye infections in the newborn and in some circumstances leading to blindness.

The major trouble with chlamydia infection is that it is often symptom free. Some women may get a messy discoloured discharge (greyish white and frothy) and some may have a sore vulva and suffer pain when they pass water or deep in the pelvis (the condition called Pelvic Inflammatory Disease — PID — is often due to persistent infection with chlamydia) but a great many have no symptoms at all. It is only when they arrive at clinics and are carefully tested that the diagnosis is made. And it is made with depressing frequency. There are 17,000 new cases a year in the UK alone. It's important that it should be carefully diagnosed not only for the woman's sake, but for any baby she may be carrying. As well as a risk to the eyes of newborn babies from this organism there is also a possibility that babies born of mothers with chlamydia may develop breathing disorders.

The treatment for chlamydia is the ever resourceful metronidazole, but also antibiotics may be used, notably tetracycline though this cannot be used in pregnancy, because it may cause permanent yellowish stains on the unborn baby's teeth. So, for a pregnant woman with chlamydia infections, another antibiotic (erythromycin) can be used. This is another infection in which treatment of a woman's sexual partner is essential, both to ensure that her treatment is successful and that she doesn't suffer re-infection, and to prevent problems occurring in him.

Gonorrhoea

All that has been said about chlamydia applies to gonorrhoea. It tends to infect somewhat different areas of the reproductive system — notably the opening of the urethra (causing pain on peeing) the Bartholin's glands (those which lubricate the vagina) and the cervix, so it can spread to the inside of the uterus — but the effects and the risks are much the same as chlamydia. And in fact it is often the case that there are mixed infections; people who have chlamydia may well have gonorrhoea too.

Treatment depends on the strain of gonorrhoea organism that is present. There are a number of them and they need different care, and it is best given not by family doctors, but by specialist clinics. Gonorrhoea, like chlamydia, is always sexually transmitted and care must be taken to identify and treat every patient's sexual partners. Antibiotics are once again the method of treatment, though many patients will also be given metronidazole, because of the presence of mixed infections.

Syphilis

This was once the sexually transmitted disease people found most alarming. It was a killer before penicillin arrived and it destroyed not only the people who caught it but the unborn as well. Syphilis used to be a major disease, with very large numbers indeed infected.

Today the numbers seen are less than a fifth of those seen in clinics just after the Second World War, in the middle and later nineteen forties. Also, although it once affected men and women equally, now it is much commoner in men because in the UK most cases now occur among homosexuals.

But it still exists, and must not be ignored, because untreated it is a potentially very severe illness. Syphilis goes through three distinct stages:

Primary syphilis shows itself sometime between nine and ninety days after infection — the average length of time before symptoms show is twenty-one to twenty-eight days. The first sign is a painless sore at the point of infection, which in a woman can be the vulva, or the mouth or the anus. There is associated swelling of nearby lymph glands. If a woman is pregnant, the infection can pass from her to her unborn baby. There may be miscarriage or stillbirth, or if the child is born alive, both physical and mental handicap. The child may develop notched teeth, damage to bones, affecting notably the nose (the bridge disappears completely) and the shins, which become very sharp and curved. Fortunately a test can be done on a pregnant woman's blood to check whether she is infected (it's called a Wasserman) and this ensures that any disease is treated and the infant protected.

At this primary stage syphilis is very simply treated. A blood test and other checks to confirm the diagnosis are followed by a course of penicillin. There is no evidence at present that the organism that causes syphilis (it is called *treponema pallidum* or the spirochaete — because it is shaped like a corkscrew) is resistant to penicillin and adequate treatment given in these early stages can produce a complete cure in virtually all patients.

But if it isn't treated — and it is all too easy to ignore the primary sore because it is painless, or because it is so high inside the vagina that a woman doesn't know it is there — the sore will heal (within three to ten weeks) and the condition enters the next stage.

Secondary syphilis shows a great many more symptoms than the primary form, and sometimes these can appear while the painless primary ulcer is still present. They include non-itching skin rashes which are a dusky red in colour, sore throat and hoarseness, swollen glands and a general flu-like illness. Indeed syphilis can be misdiagnosed because the symptoms are so like so many other feverish illnesses. At this stage the patient is very infectious to his or her sexual partner.

In addition to the skin rashes there may be large lesions that appear in areas where two skin surfaces touch — say between the buttocks, or beneath heavy pendulous breasts — and there may be ulcers which appear on mucous membrane — in the mouth, on the tongue or on the vulva — and these are called 'snailtrack' ulcers because of their glistening greyish white colour.

All these signs and symptoms will eventually fade and disappear; it may take several weeks or months, but they will go and the patient may think she is quite well again. But she isn't.

Tertiary syphilis may show itself many years after the first infection with a distressing range of symptoms, affecting the brain and nervous system (resulting in forms of paralysis and insanity) heart and blood vessels (causing severe heart disease) and quite dreadful permanent sores affecting skin and bones. Fortunately late stage syphilis is very rare nowadays.

Herpes

The virus infection known as herpes is one that has lived in and around humanity for many centuries. Shakespeare mentioned it in *Romeo and Juliet* — 'o'er ladies' lips, who straight on kisses dream, which oft the angry Mab with blisters plague...' He was talking about cold sores, the painful blisters which appear on lips or chin when you're run down — as you are when you have a cold — and which turn into painful scabs and take their time about healing. And the virus which causes them — herpes simplex — can attack other parts of the body too.

In recent years the number of people suffering from attacks of painful herpes affecting the sex organs has increased hugely. It has been estimated that in the USA there are some twenty million people and that the numbers are increasing at the rate of half a million a year, while in the UK there has been a 168 per cent increase in the past ten years.

It is now regarded as one of the commoner sexually transmitted diseases, and it causes a great deal of distress — not only because it is painful, but because the condition tends to recur. One attack may herald several more, because the organism is difficult to eradicate. So people with herpes tend to become withdrawn and anxious, feeling themselves to be sexual outcasts. They need not be, of course — but that is how too many of them feel.

The herpes organism comes in different guises. There is Herpes Simplex Virus 1 (HSV1) and this is most commonly the cause of cold sores on the face and eyes. There is also Herpes Simplex Virus 2 (HSV2) and this one shows a marked preference for the genital area. However, either can affect either site, and it is generally believed by experts that the reason for the huge upsurge in cases is the growing popularity of oro-genital sex; once it was considered totally wrong to kiss your partner's sex organs; now it is regarded as normal sex play by a great many. Also, it is possible for an individual to infect her own genitals with herpes from cold sores on her lips if she touches them in succession and carries the virus that way.

The virus probably actually enters the body via tiny abrasions that the person doesn't even realise she has. Since about half of all people who are exposed to infection don't actually get it, this seems the most likely reason — that they have no abrasion through which the virus can enter. But once it has entered, then it can exert its effects.

The illness tends to follow a predictable pattern, though the severity of it can vary greatly; first, within a few days of infection, there is severe itching, tingling or aching in the affected area. Then some red spots may appear very briefly, almost immediately becoming small blisters. Sometimes the blisters are so tiny they can't be seen.

These fluid-filled blisters, which are swarming with the viruses, eventually break, leaving a small ulcerated area. This can be very painful and tender — in some cases the whole area of the skin nearby becomes swollen and sore too. It may be painful and there may be swollen glands in the groins or difficulty in peeing. As well as these local symptoms there will be a sense of general illness, with shivering and perhaps headache and nausea.

Gradually the symptoms subside, the fever goes, the swelling flattens and the ulcers dry up and after a couple of weeks heal completely.

If this were the end of it, it wouldn't be so bad, disagreeable though an attack of herpes clearly is, but unfortunately the virus tends to lie dormant in the area, and that means that there can be recurrent attacks of blistering in precisely the same place as before. Some people never have any further problems after the first attack; they are the fortunate ones and happily they are in the majority.

Others have only mild and rare repeat attacks, but there are some people who have many recurrences and who become very miserable as a result. In fact the body does gradually build its own defences against the virus, and in due course, for the majority, the problem diminishes and finally disappears, as long as there is no reinfection.

The risk of transmission of the virus is when there are blisters present. If there are no blisters, nor signs of threatening blisters — the tingling or aching or tenderness — then the likelihood is that there is no risk of infecting your partner. It is even safer if the man always uses a sheath, and if the couple uses a lubricant such as KY Jelly to make sure there is no undue roughening of the mucous membrane.

Treatment at present is, frankly, limited. Patients need care of symptoms during attacks (aspirin for the pain and any feverishness) but there is nothing that can be done to cure the condition. There is no drug that gets rid of the virus, in the way that penicillin gets rid of the spirochaete that causes syphilis. Research is under way to find a vaccine to prevent infection, but until one is developed, symptomatic treatment is all that can be offered.

This includes saline washes; local applications of pain-killing drugs such as Lignocain or Locan and oral painkillers such as aspirin or paracetomol. Some doctors will also give antibiotics, not because they can affect the virus — they can't — but because that will prevent any secondary bacterial infection. Some also use spiritous substances to dab on the sores to dry them out, but this takes a spartan patient. It hurts a good deal to apply spirit to an open sore. Other doctors use coloured applications such as gentian violet, copper sulphate or potassium permangate which are thought to speed healing.

In addition to this, there are some anti-viral treatments that can be given but their value is doubted by some experts. The problem with killing viruses is that they live inside cells, so if a drug kills the virus, it kills the cell too. And that can be damaging to the cell's owner. That is why really effective anti-viral drugs can have unpleasant side effects. But work is being done on genital herpes using acyclovir (Zovirax is its trade name in the UK) idoxuridine (Herpid in the UK) and one or two others.

The answer at present has to be, for those not infected, to be very careful about their choice of sexual partner, and for those who are infected, to refuse to become obsessively unhappy about it. It can be distressing to have an infection that is liable to recur, but with commonsense and care it is possible to live happily and to avoid infecting people you care about. That is, you don't have sex when you suspect you have an attack, you always explain to a new partner what your problem is, and you use, if in doubt, a sheath.

It is also unnecessary to worry unduly about the risk of herpes in pregnancy. If by any chance a woman approaching labour has an attack of herpes, and there are fears her baby may be infected by the virus as he passes through her blistered vagina, then she can give birth via Caesarian section. Not ideal, but it does ensure a healthy infant. (See also Section six.)

One last important point; there has been much publicity in recent years about the possibility of a link between genital herpes and cancer of the cervix; does the first cause the second?

There is no hard evidence that it does. There is a suggestion that cancer of the cervix is triggered by some sort of agent introduced to it and that the younger the cervix is when active unprotected sex starts, the more vulnerable it is. It also seems more likely there will be potentially cancerous changes in the cervix in later life if a girl not only starts her sexual activity young (in her early to mid-teens) but also has several partners, though no one has yet worked out precisely why this should be so, though there is increasing evidence that a girl who has sex with a man who has previously had sex with a number of partners is at higher risk.

His promiscuity affects her dangerously — especially if he has penile warts (see below). But it must never be forgotten that by no means all the women who develop signs of cervical cancer have a history of early promiscuous sex and by no means all their husbands have either. At present all that can be said is that any woman, whatever her history of infections and sexuality, who does not seek out regular checks on the health of her cervix is being wilfully uncaring of her own health (see also page 115, Section eight).

Genital warts

These too are caused by a virus, just as are warts anywhere else in the body. The virus is called HPV (human papillomavirus) and when sexually transmitted causes little fleshy lumps to appear around the genitals, especially in the moist places. These may vary from small pimply objects to large fleshy masses which cause considerable discomfort because of their bulk. There may be several months between infection and the actual appearance of the warts, which means that people who lead particularly free and easy sex lives may have some difficulty in identifying the donor of the infection — which makes life difficult for those clinics which treat sexual infection. Tracing contacts and treating them is an important part of their work.

As with the other major viral infection — herpes — treatment has to be symptomatic only; there is no known way to prevent recurrences. So, the warts can be 'burned off' with electricity or chemicals or lasers (not as painful as it sounds — local anaesthesia can be used, and the warts are not in themselves sensitive to pain).

But merely burning off the warts doesn't end the story. There is considerable medical anxiety about the possible link between genital warts and cancer of the cervix. Often doctors will insist that a girl who has picked up such an infection has frequent and regular smear tests of her cervix (some doctors repeat them every three months). It is wise to accept these frequent tests; one survey showed that of a group of young women attending a sexually transmitted disease clinic for treatment of simple vulval warts almost a third had a pre-malignant lesion of the cervix after six months of observation. In other words, they had a condition that could, if left untreated, lead to cancer.

That's the bad news. The good news is that with regular smears and early identification of any suspicious changes in the cells of the cervix, vigorous treatment given promptly can and will cure the condition. The girl need not have cancer.

Parasites

All organisms that invade the human body and live there are parasitic of course, but this label is generally used for infestation by larger creatures than bacteria or viruses.

There are two particular ones that are sexually transmitted — the pubic louse (its Latin name is much prettier — *pedicular pubis*) and scabies (another stylish name here — *sarcoptes scabiei*).

The former is a small round insect, between 1mm and 2mm in length with three sets of legs. It can hang on to pubic hairs and feeds by sucking blood from its host, leaving itchy spots where it made the punctures. It lays its eggs — nits — on the base of these hairs where they hatch within a week or so, to crawl about, bite and suck and lay more eggs. They cause severe itching or sometimes no discomfort at all — only the shock of finding one wandering about on one's person.

The scabies mite is much smaller — the female is twice the size of her mate and she is only 0.3mm long — and they burrow into the skin and lay their eggs there. Unlike the louse, which is really only transmitted by close bodily contact (it is unlikely to be picked up from clothes, bedding or public loos, since the louse never leaves its host except to jump directly onto another very nearby one) the scabies mite can reach the genitals by non-sexual routes. It's a common visitor to school children and can travel through a family very quickly, causing itching and scaly little skin eruptions.

Treatment for both louse and mite is specific. The louse succumbs to one per cent gamma benzene hexachloride powder, cream or lotion applied to the body hair. In the UK the application is marketed as Lorexamene and Quellada. It is not suitable for pregnant or breast-feeding women, incidentally, because it can enter body fat and appear in the breast milk. They need an alternative remedy such as 0.5 per cent Malathion. The scabies mite can be vanquished by painting the body (all of it) with twenty-five per cent benzyl benzoate — a tedious operation since it has to be total, and has to be repeated twenty-four hours later, but it usually works very well. The most important thing about these two unpleasant parasites is that they all too often occur in tandem with other sexually transmitted diseases. This is why it is always wisest to get a complete check-up from the expert clinics.

AIDS

There has been more panic about this condition than any other disease since syphilis terrified the people of the Middle Ages.

So much research work is being done at present that no book can hope to be up-to-date in its reporting. All that can be said at the time of writing is:

That the full name of the condition is Acquired Immune Deficiency Syndrome;

That it means that a person who suffers from it loses the ability to fight off dangerous invading organisms, and therefore become very ill and eventually dies.

That it appears to be carried by blood and semen and is therefore spread by, among among other things, sexual practices that cause some tissue damage and loss of blood, such as very vigorous intercourse.

That other than those infected sexually it is most likely to afflict people who require blood transfusions or treatment with blood products, such as haemophiliacs, or those who share unsterilized needles for injections, such as drug addicts, or those who work with blood, like doctors or laboratory technicians.

That at present those most likely to suffer it as a sexually transmitted disease are homosexual men, but that cases are rapidly appearing among heterosexual men and therefore among women.

That it is probably caused by a virus which has been labelled in different ways, but which seems to be either a 'new' one (a mutation from an old one), or one that has reached man from animals or which has suddenly started to behave in a different way and which appears to have originated in the Africa continent and reached the rest of the world via Haiti.

That not all the people who pick up the virus suffer the full blown disease; the majority are symptom free, but may be carriers — i.e. capable of infecting others.

And that is all we know at present. Very vigorous research is going on around the world looking for both a cure for the afflicted and a vaccine to protect those not yet afflicted but thought to be at risk. We must hope that by the time you read these words those researches will have been more successful.

Cystitis

Many women who suffer from vaginal infections and disorders also find they have symptoms affecting the bladder and the way they pee. They complain of burning pain, of frequency, of damage to their sexuality because lovemaking brings on attacks of what is usually labelled 'cystitis'. But not all of them have associated infections to cause their symptoms.

The bladder is a muscular, elastic, hollow organ which collects the urine produced by the kidneys. It is connected to the kidneys by a pair of fine tubes through which the urine travels. At its bottom end the bladder has another tube — the outlet. In women this is shorter than it is in man, as the male urethra has to reach the end of the penis, and a woman's need reach only the surface of her body, at the vulva. So his is up to eight inches long, hers a mere $1\frac{1}{2}$ inches.

The usual cause of any inflammation anywhere in the body is invasion by germs and, for many years, doctors have said that this was the cause of the symptoms that are present in cystitis. Often they were right; a sufferer's urine, when tested, was shown to contain pus, a sure sign of infection, and sometimes there was blood as well. But not every patient showed this result. Some had sterile — germ-free — urine, and in recent years, much more study has been made of this tiresome condition, not least because women themselves have become more vociferous in complaining about it.

The dispiriting fact is that although ninety per cent of women who have an attack of cystitis can be treated by antibiotics and given permanent relief, about ten per cent suffer recurrent attacks which resist all attempts at treatment with antibiotics. Further studies of the problem suggest that not all attacks are linked with infection. In fact, cystitis is not an accurate label for these patients' condition. Instead it should be called the 'urethral syndrome' meaning a cluster of symptoms which affect the way urine is passed out of the bladder.

Sometimes it is caused by trauma, direct injury to the soft tissues surrounding the urethra, and the urethra itself. And one of the most likely ways for such trauma to be caused is by sexual intercourse. The woman may not feel any pain when love-making; none the less, there can be friction and tension which result in local swelling. This is likely to be most marked in the early days of a girl's sex life, when the combination of unfamiliarity with the experience and frequent repetition results in what has been called 'honeymoon cystitis'.

But it is not only youngsters starting out on a sex life who have this problem. It can also afflict more experienced women of any age. And again, the cause is trauma. One of the necessary factors for successful and comfortable intercourse for a woman is full sexual arousal. When she is ready for sex, then her vagina produces a clear, slippery liquid which allows the penis to move comfortably inside it. When this is not produced, there is an increase in friction, which can result in attack after attack of urethral syndrome (see Section five).

There are a great many women who say that their marriages have been ruined by cystitis, and blame their doctors for being unable to resolve the 'inflammation' when the real problem has nothing to do with the bladder at all. It is the woman's own sexual responses which need understanding and perhaps treating.

This fact has been borne out by studies made into the background of women who report frequent attacks of cystitis. Researchers say that a picture has developed of a typical recurrent cystitis patient: 'She is likely to be a thin, tense woman, who frequently discusses her symptoms, is usually in her reproductive years, habitually takes tranquillizers and is still emotionally attached to her mother.' All of which sounds a little male chauvinistic but, it has to be said, is a judgement based on accurate observation.

But, obviously, not all women suffering from frequent attacks of cystitis fall into this category. There can be physical as well as emotional causes. For example, women who suffer from vaginal discharge due to infection may get local itching. The organism which causes the vaginal discharge does not get into the bladder, but the local irritation and swelling can affect the urethra and surrounding tissues.

Also, some women suffer local damage to muscles and ligaments after pregnancy and childbirth. A prolapse — misplaced uterus — can put strain on the area and result, once again, in attacks of frequency, urgency and painful urination.

Finally, there is a group who may not have sexual problems or local discharges or itching but who still have attacks — and in this case we have to look again at the effect of the mind on the body. Most of us know perfectly well that anxiety can lead to a need to pee more often. When there is an obvious cause for the stress there is no real problem. The sufferer understands why it happens and as soon as the stress is gone the need to pee more often fades.

But there are some people who are always anxious, always worried, always expecting trouble. For them, anxiety becomes a way of life — and with it comes frequency. The anxiety that this causes adds to the burden of the wretchedly unhappy worried person, and begins to be registered as pain as well as frequency. And then, there may be a fear of 'accidents' — loss of bladder control and wet clothes — which makes the stress worse and may add urgency to the rest of it. It's easy to see how such people may be labelled as suffering from cystitis, when they are really suffering from aggravated worry (see Section ten).

What should a woman do if she is attacked by this cluster of symptoms? First of all, she needs to think about what is happening. Is this the first time it has every occurred? Is it associated with fever, headaches, general illness? In this case the likelihood is that she is one of the eighty per cent with an attack of true urinary infection. She needs her doctor's diagnosis and treatment.

If it is the second or third time it has happened and the fever, illness and so on are part of it, again, see the doctor. It may be a resistant infection which needs vigorous treatment, perhaps hospital investigation. Or, she may cope without such help if she uses a regime of self-care to abort attacks.

If you are newly embarked on a sexual relationship, this might be a cause, but you should still check with your doctor if there is the possibility of an infection. Don't assume, by the way, that a man who gives his partner such an infection is promiscuous. That may be a part of the problem, admittedly, but by no means always. We all have our own germs — bacteria that are on our bodies and which don't affect us badly in the least, but which cause a reaction when passed onto someone else who does not have a resistance to them.

If the attacks are frequent and linked with sexual intercourse to which you are not a newcomer, and the doctor has taken urine specimens and found no infection there, be honest with yourself and consider the possiblity that the real problem is not in your bladder, but in your attitude to sex.

I have no doubt that many people reading this will bristle with rage at the suggestion that their very physical symptoms of pain and frequency could have anything to do with their emotions or their sexual response, but that in itself is an argument for investigating these possibilities in women who have no bacteria in their urine, and no other signs of general infection. And what is worse? Going on with the discomfort or seeking more deeply for the cause?

Self-help for cystitis

Once symptoms start, drink half a litre (a pint) of water, and keep on drinking water, fruit drinks, weak tea etc at half-hour intervals until the attack is past.

Do not exceed 285 mls (half a pint) an hour.

Take a weak dose of bicarbonate of soda (a teaspoon to 285 mls (half a pint) of water). This make the urine less acid and less stinging to pass.

Take a mild painkiller such as paracetomol or aspirin.

Pee as often as you want to — keeping the bladder as empty as possible.

Put your feet up and relax .

If you can do this for three hours and follow the rest of the regime, the chances are the attack will be aborted.

8

WOMAN'S ILLNESSES

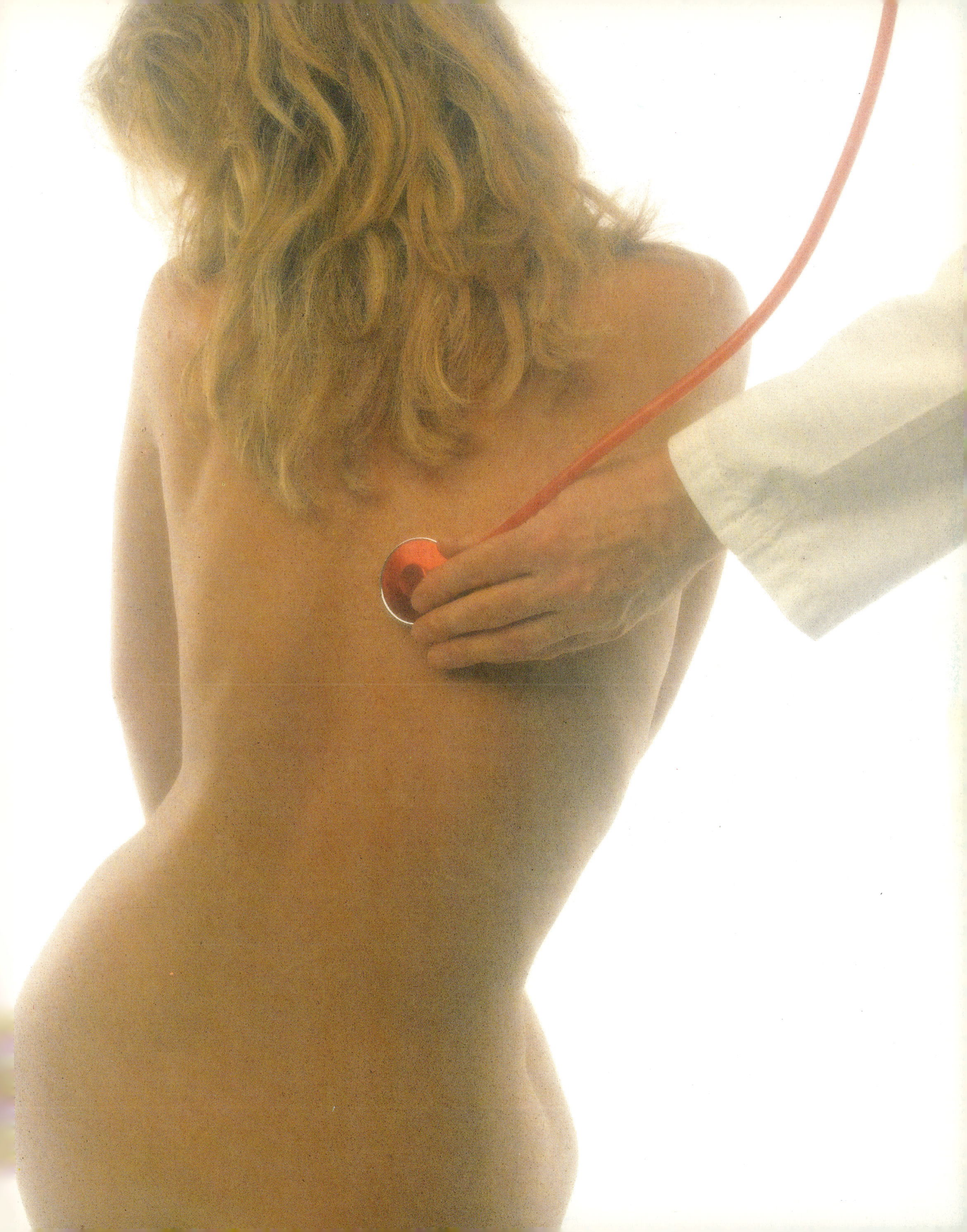

Part of the armoury of any intelligent woman is an understanding of how to deal with the inevitable ills and problems that arise in even the best kept of bodies. To know what various symptoms mean, and what weight should be given to them; to know how to relieve minor ills and when to yield to more expert knowledge — all this is as important as knowing how to read and write. Yet, amazingly, few schools make any effort to teach girls about health. Children are taught, if they are lucky, a little about how their bodies function — rarely about how they might malfunction. And even more rarely what to do if that happens.

First, then, an account of the sort of symptoms that should be taken seriously and discussed with a doctor. And that doctor should be a well trained orthodox practitioner in the first instance. I yield to none in my admiration of the many excellent therapies that are available for a wide range of human diseases. Osteopaths have done great work in easing the aches and pains of those with joint and muscle problems. Naturopaths have done a good deal to comfort the distresses of those who are ill-fed and tense. Acupuncturists and hypnotists have done much to relieve pain both emotional and physical. All have their place in the pantheon of healers — but the most important first stage of any therapy has to be accurate diagnosis. And to get that, surely you need to go to a person who has had an exhaustive and wide ranging scientific training.

I emphasize the word scientific because many of the so-called 'fringe' or 'alternative' healers seem to demand a form of faith from their patients. They make their diagnoses on the basis of limited scientific — that is, proven — data and this obviously can be risky. Maybe a naturopath or a herbalist can offer remedies for the pain in your back or your belly — but you want to be sure that the pain isn't caused by a malignant disease that could kill you if not fully treated. Even fully trained doctors of medicine can make mistakes and miss diagnoses, as we all well know, but at least their patients start with a better chance of getting accurate and therefore safe answers. And if one doctor doesn't give you a satisfactory answer, you can always ask him or her to arrange for you to have a second opinion from another doctor, of possibly wider experience (or seek such a second opinion independently). No genuine doctor ever objects to a patient seeking help elsewhere, whereas, in my experience, alternative practitioners sometimes do, and indeed some make it a condition of giving care that their clients go to no other healers.

So, with that point made, to the checklist of symptoms that should be taken seriously.

The first list here covers signs and symptoms that might indicate the presence of malignant disease. None of them are definite signs of such disease and must never be assumed to be so. There can be many different reasons for some of them, reasons which are essentially harmless. However, there is the possibility that the symptoms may indicate underlying cancers, which is why it is important to get a medical check if you notice them. But, please, don't panic.

Cancer checks

• Unusual lumps or bumps. Most likely to be found in the breast, these make women very anxious, but never forget that the majority of breast lumps are benign.

• Unusual bleeding from any orifice, in the absence of injury. Blood in the stools is very likely to be due to haemorrhoids (piles) or a fissure. Bleeding between periods or after intercourse may be due to many causes. (See Section three.) Bleeding into urine is another probably non-cancerous symptom as is unexpected bleeding from ears, and nose, but still needs attention.

• Unusual discharge. Sometimes discharge from the nipples can suggest a cancerous condition. Persistent discharges from the vagina are almost always due to non-malignant causes.

• Changes in normal functions unconnected with other illnesses. Changes in bowel habits, with severe constipation, or constant diarrhoea, or difficulty in peeing.

• Weight and girth changes in the absence of changes in appetite. A marked loss of weight, or increase in the size of the abdomen or a limb when as far as you can tell you've not changed your eating habits.

• A cough or breathlessness when you haven't got a cold. The causes of these symptoms are many, but must never be neglected, in a smoker in particular.

• Hoarseness when you haven't got a cold. Persistent changes in the voice in the absence of infections of the upper breathing tubes, particularly in smokers.

• Bruising which appears in the absence of injury. Many people, especially children, have extra delicate capillaries which break easily and result in bruises. But in a few cases (and they are very few) this may be due to a blood disease.

• Sores which do not heal. Sores appearing on skin anywhere in the body, or in the mouth or on other mucous membrane, for example, the vulva.

• Moles which enlarge or darken or bleed. Enlargement and darkening can happen normally as a result of Pill usage or pregnancy and after exposure to the sun, but must never be ignored. *Bleeding* from moles must also never be ignored.

Breasts

Most of us are, by and large, concerned about our breasts. We care about other parts of our anatomy, of course; hands, feet, noses and ears — but breasts are special. Even more than the vulva and the rest of our pelvic sex organs, the breasts seem to most of us to be Femininity writ large. If they're small, we feel less female than we should; if they're uneven in size we feel a deep embarrassment and if they're big we tend to strut a little (although some girls feel theirs are too big and grieve over that).

So, inevitably, ailments of the breasts are likely to cause a good deal of distress, and when you add on the fact that cancer of the breasts is the commonest among women (it accounts for about thirty per cent of all cancers) and that there are a considerable numbers of other sometimes uncomfortable disorders of the breasts it's quite understandable that for many women Breasts Mean Worry.

Breast cancer checks

Breast cancer is one of the most common in women (although it must never be forgotten that in fact it affects only seven per cent of women – ninety-three in every 100 of us will never get it). In the UK 24,000 women every year are diagnosed, and though nearly half of them survive and continue to lead active lives, still far too many die.

There have been a number of studies to try to discover why the rate is so high in some countries, comparatively low in others. Various factors have been suggested:

• A woman who eats a diet high in meats and animal fats is believed by some experts to be at higher risk than one who eats a high-fibre vegetable-based diet (this is also thought to help prevent other forms of cancer, notably of the gut – see Section ten).

• A woman who has her first baby later than average – in her thirties or after – is said by some to be at higher risk.

• A woman who did not breast feed her babies is considered to be a candidate.

• A woman who has a family history of breast cancer is possibly at more risk.

Fat women are considered more likely to develop tumours than thin ones (possibly such women have different estrogen levels from thin women and estrogen is considered to contribute to the disease).

Also, studies have been made of the Pill and the use of hormone replacement therapy in older women (see Section nine) to see if these may play a part. At present, there is no evidence of any link.

Finding out why breast cancer happens will of course be a major step towards stopping it; but while these studies are going on, it is important for all women to know how best to protect themselves. And there is little doubt that it is possible to identify breast cancer at an early enough stage to make a cure possible. Research suggests that regular X-ray screening of the breasts in suitable women and regular properly carried out self-examination of the breasts could cut the death rate from breast cancer in the UK for women over the age of fifty by fully one third. And that could be a considerable improvement.

Breast self-examination

This is the simplest first line test, and has a great deal to commend it. It is non-invasive, harmless and it ensures that a woman gets to know her own body well (and it really is surprising how often women shrink from touching themselves in any way that might seem to be sexual) and becomes aware of changes in what is normal for her. Every woman is different, despite the fact that we all have the same basic structure, so discovering how your own breasts are made is a vital first stage to a successful self examination programme.

1 Set aside a regular time to do the test each month. No more often than that – the last thing you need to do is become obsessive about it – but it should be done at the same stage of the menstrual cycle. The best time usually is just after the period ends. The breasts are generally at their softest then, and easiest to feel.

If you don't have periods for any reason – you're an athlete, or dancer, your weight is too low, you've had a hysterectomy, or you're past the menopause – then select a date that will be easy to remember. (The first of the month is one a great many women use) or you may prefer to select every fourth Friday, because that's the day of your committee meeting, or whatever.

2 Choose where to do your BSE. Bathrooms are popular with many women because they find it a convenient private place in which to be naked to the waist. The drawback to bathrooms is the provision of mirrors. If yours has a full length one, fine. You need to be able to get a clear view of yourself, and you can't do that in the average over-the-basin square. Bedrooms are probably better not only for mirrors, but also because you can lie flat and comfortably on your bed to do the actual feeling of your breasts. As long as you tell your family not to disturb you, or do it at a time when the children are asleep or everyone is out, you should be able to relax and do the checks in a quiet, leisurely and unanxious way.

3 Now you are ready to start your BSE. Check the appearance of your breasts in a mirror, first with your arms by your sides, and then raising them above your head. Look for changes in the texture of the skin – puckering or dimpling – and in their shape. Get to your know your breasts – they are usually slightly different from each other in their shape and in their position. Examine the nipples for any unusual discharge, including bleeding.

4 Lie down comfortably and put a folded towel or tiny pillow under your left shoulder, and put your left hand under your head and examine your left breast with your right hand, using the flat of the fingers, not the tips.

Get to know their normal texture so that you can feel anything unusual; two or three months and you'll be sure! With your left arm still behind your head, start by examining the upper, inner quarter. Work inwards towards the nipple from the ribs and chest area.

5 Keep your arm in the same position behind your head while you examine the lower inner quarter in the same way. Feel the area all round the nipple.

6 Put your arm down by your side before you examine the lower outside quarter. Work inwards towards the nipple from the ribs well outside the breast area.

7 Feel over the upper outer quarter of the breast in the same way. Check across the top of the breast to the armpit to cover the extra section of breast tissue there. Now you will have come full circle and examined the whole breast.

8 Finally, feel inside the armpit for any unusual lumps. (There will be some normal ones; we all have lymph glands there.)

Breast self-examination

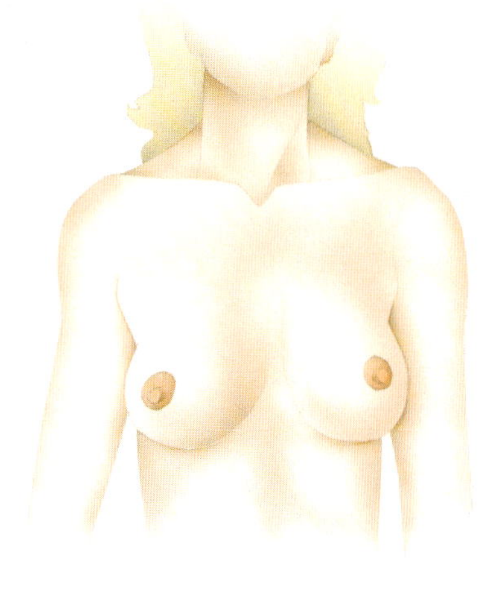

1
Become familiar with your breasts. Check them in a mirror, first with your arms by your sides and then raised above your head. Look for changes in skin texture and shape and for any unusual discharge, including bleeding, from the nipples.

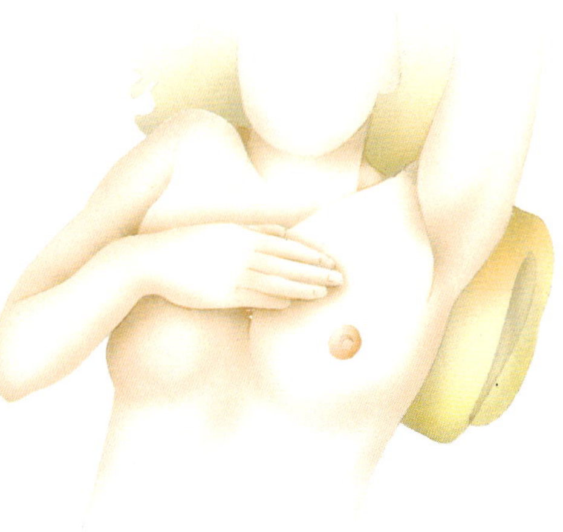

2
Lie down with a pillow under your left shoulder and put your left hand under your head. Examine your left breast with your right hand, starting with the upper, inner quarter and working towards the nipple from the ribs and chest area.

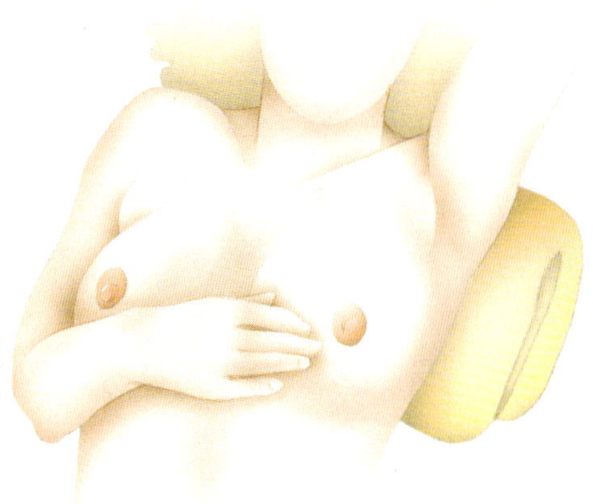

3
Keep your arm behind your head while you examine the lower inner quarter in the same way. Feel the area all round the nipple.

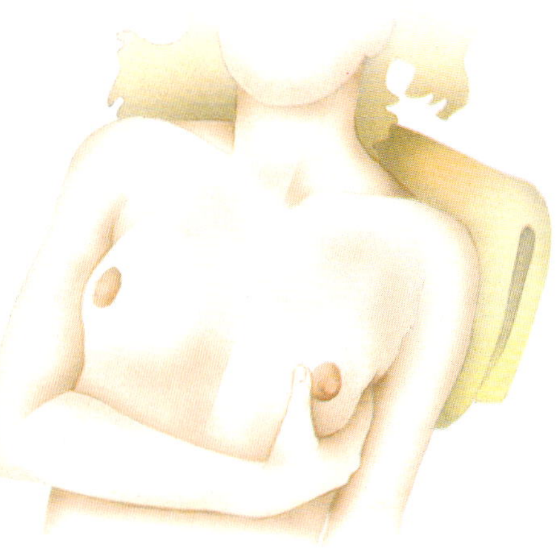

4
Put your arm down by your side and examine the lower outside quarter of the breast. Work inwards towards the nipple from well outside the breast area.

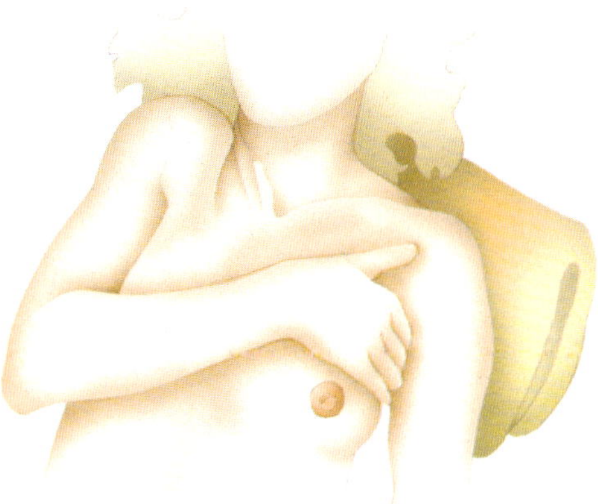

5
Examine the upper outer quarter of the breast in the same way. Check the top of the breast to the armpit where there is an extra section of tissue.

6
Feel inside the armpit for unusual lumps.

Reverse the whole procedure for the right breast, with the pillow under the right shoulder and right arm behind the head.

Reverse the procedure for the right breast — remember to change the pillow to the other shoulder — beginning again with the upper, inner quarter, with your right arm placed behind your head.

If you aren't sure you're doing it properly, or can't really work out what it is you're feeling, then get someone to go through it with you to teach you. Your own doctor, or a nurse at the doctor's surgery, or at a well woman's clinic, or at the local family planning clinic will be glad to help.

What to do if you find a lump

First, check the same area of the opposite breast; this could be something that is normal for you — or you could even be feeling a knobbly bit of rib if you are a particularly thin person. But always err on the side of being extra cautious; don't just reassure yourself, but go and check with your doctor or local clinic. There isn't a doctor anywhere who wouldn't rather examine you and put your mind — and his — at rest than take the risk of you neglecting what could be an important change in your breasts.

Make a note of any visits you make to your doctor, and why, perhaps making a little sketch to remind you what sort of change it was you felt, and where. Then if you feel it again another time, you'll know whether it's important or not.

And never forget that nine out of ten of all lumps, bumps or alterations noted by BSE turn out to be harmless and not malignant. And that even the malignant ones, if diagnosed early, can be treated successfully.

Mammography

This is an X-ray examination of the breasts. It can identify lesions too deep in the breast to be felt by BSE, and there is considerable evidence, notably from the USA and Sweden, to show that regular (two-yearly) mammographs in women over the age of fifty can give great benefit. An early study showed that there was a twenty-five per cent to thirty per cent reduction in mortality after fourteen years in women who had been X-rayed as compared with a control group who hadn't; more recent studies suggest that with the improved technology since the nineteen sixties when that first study was made, the benefit is even greater.

At present, it is strongly advised that the X-ray is done only every two years, because more frequent exposure could actually cause the malignant changes that are feared. And women under fifty are at present excluded unless there is a family history of a mother or sister developing breast cancer under the age of forty, because their breasts are thought to be more vulnerable. It is by no means true that breast cancer is an inherited disease — but there may be a family tendency (not at all the same thing) — which means that members of affected families are wise if they ensure particularly regular BSE and screening by a clinic.

Breast thermography

This test is based on the observation made thirty years ago that cancerous areas hidden inside the breasts are hotter than surrounding areas. So, machines have been developed to 'map' hot and cold areas in the breasts. The woman sits bare to the waist in a cooling draught for a period of time (up to fifteen minutes in some centres) and her breasts are then scanned for hot areas, and the result is shown as a 'map'.

The benefits of thermography are that like BSE it is non-invasive. No X-rays to cause risks, just observation. The drawback is that it is not as accurate a technique as mammography. It's a useful preliminary check, but many experts prefer to use other tests after they get a positive result from a thermogram, in order to confirm any dubious diagnosis.

Computerized tomographic mammography

Although this is a technique that, like mammography, uses X-rays, it really is a separate technique from mammography. It is not often used as a first line diagnostic tool, because it is cumbersome and costly, but it can be useful to pin-point the precise area needing treatment in a woman who has been diagnosed by a doctor as having a suspicious lump.

Transillumination

This has been called very prettily 'diaphanography' or 'diaphanoscopy' or more soberly 'light scanning'. In simple terms, a light is shone through the breast to identify any darker, and possibly doubtful, areas. The system used is generally microwave light and does no harm to the woman because the amount of power actually used is the equivalent of a single 25 watt lamp bulb. The system is said to be particularly useful for women who have breasts in which the tissue is dense and therefore difficult to examine with the hands or even by X-ray. The developers of the equipment and the doctors who use it have claimed a ninety per cent success rate in detecting cancers, and also say that the sort of cancers their system picks up are different from those that X-rays identify. The system isn't yet widely used for screening, but may be used for patients in whom there is already concern about worrying lumps.

Ultrasound

This is a system in which sound waves are bounced off body structures so that the echoes made can be collected, and shown as a picture. It's the system used to study the infant in the uterus (see Section six) and for other forms of body study, and can be useful in screening for breast disease. It is particularly valuable when used with mammography, but not quite so useful on its own. It is difficult for the sound waves and their echoes to demonstrate the difference between various breast structures and so the system can't give as accurate a picture as a doctor needs. But it's a very useful adjunct.

Digital radiography

This is a technique that it is hoped will be available in the future. It will make it possible for small areas of tissue to be examined with lower doses of X-rays. This will mean that women can be examined safely whatever their age.

Magnetic resonance imaging

Some scientists are getting very excited about this. It involves placing an individual in a strong magnetic field, and then measuring the signals sent back by body cells when their nuclei are 'pulsed' with radiofrequency radiation. The physics is exceedingly complex, but the simple message is that this, at present costly, technique could produce highly accurate 'pictures' of deep body tissues, including breasts, without inflicting any damage at all on the patient, being non-invasive and very safe.

The value of screening

Having said all this about the value of early diagnosis in the treatment of breast cancer, I have to report that there are some experts in the field who do not believe it to be of any value at all. They say that the long term results of treating breast cancer are not affected by early self-diagnosis, and that encouraging BSE amongst healthy women, far from helping them be well, actually causes them to become psychologically disturbed, leading in some cases to obsessive self-examination and constant fear of breast cancer. In a survey of family doctors in the UK about two thirds believed that there was convincing evidence of the value of BSE and screening systems, while the remainder expressed some doubts.

It is important for women to know this; any one of us could come across a doctor who, while still being deeply concerned for an individual woman's welfare, would dismiss self examination and screening as a waste of time. This can be very bewildering, if you've been told elsewhere that it can protect your health and even your life. As a woman, all I can say is that I believe awareness of what diseases might strike, and knowledge of the sensible measures I can take to deal with it, is part of my equipment for living. If the pessimistic doctors are right and screening has small effect on the long-term outcome, the fact that I have sought screening will have done me no harm and at least I will have the comfort of knowing I tried to take care of myself. I will never, certainly, blame myself if I ever do get an illness, any more than any other sensible woman would.

Other breast problems

There are other ailments of the breasts that affect some women. The statistical likelihood is that you'll have no problems, but some people will, and they need all the information they can get about what their symptoms mean and what can be done about them.

Fibrocystic disease

This has been given a bewildering variety of labels. Mastitis. Lumpy breasts. Cystic disease. Cystic mastitis. Take your choice. What it means is that pain starts in the breasts and there may be some generalized swelling. In the very young girl — and the disorder is generally commoner in younger women — there are few separate lumps to be felt, but as she gets older, and reaches her thirties, there are multiple little nodules that can be felt almost like hardish little peas under the skin. Sometimes the little nodules run together, as it were, and become fibrous — hardening tissue appears in them — and an actual lump can be felt. Later there may be cysts — little sacs which fill with fluid and feel to the touch like soft rubber balls. Sometimes a woman may have a discharge from her nipple, though by no means always.

All this is likely to feel worse in the week before a period when the hormonal balance is designed to stimulate the breasts in case a pregnancy occurs and milk-making will be needed. The areas affected will not just be the breasts themselves but often the 'tail' of the breasts which reaches up into the armpit. The whole area feels full and tender, so tender sometimes that being touched at all is exquisitely painful. Some women say their lives are dominated by their miserable breast discomfort.

Incidentally, it is because breast pain of this sort makes women so miserable that in the past many male doctors labelled women who complained of it 'neurotics'. Now it has been proven they are not. Careful studies have shown that there are many causes of breast pain (for example, gall bladder disease can be registered as pain in the right breast because of the way the nerve supply to that organ runs up the chest wall, so referring the pain) and all are entitled to be taken seriously. Doctors today do check carefully to see why breasts hurt, and do what they can to give relief, though it has to be said, in reply to the question, 'What can be done?', 'Not a lot.'

Hormones — given, say, as the Pill — have been tried and help some women. For others, diuretic drugs — to rid the body of excess fluids — have been tried especially pre-menstrually (see Section three). Male hormones have been tried to see if they can damp down the breast's reactions, but there has been small success with them. The drug Danazol is very effective but only if used in dosages so high that it stops periods — and it has to be taken indefinitely. This is a drawback to its use which makes some people prefer to tolerate the pain. Surgery to aspirate (that is to draw out with a hollow needle the fluid contents of cysts) or to remove lumps helps sometimes. But for many this discomfort has to be lived with. Wearing a firm supportive bra and using painkillers such as paracetamol or aspirin is the simplest regime.

Fibroadenoma

This is a smooth, solid, rubbery-feeling lump that may appear in the breasts, either singly or in clumps, in one or in both, commonly in women aged between fifteen and forty. Happily this does not cause pain, but can cause anxiety, especially fear of cancer. In fact a fibroadenoma is not cancerous. It is simply a collection of gland tissue and fibrous cells which coalesce to form the lumps, which are so loose inside the breast that they have been called 'breast mice' by some doctors, who have difficulty in getting them to remain in place beneath their fingers when they try to examine them. Simple removal is the answer if the lumps are very tiresome, though many women once reassured they are not dangerous happily keep them, preferring a few lumps to even the smallest scar.

Duct ectasia

This is unlikely under the age of forty, though it does appear sometimes, in younger women; it is far from common but it does alarm women to whom it happens. The ducts inside the breast become distended with cellular and glandular products, and result in a sticky discharge from the nipple which may be of different colours — reddish, green, yellowish brown.

There may be itching and pain round the nipple and the nipple itself, if touched, seems to have wormlike swelling beneath the surface. If the condition isn't treated then the ducts harden and may shorten and so pull the nipple inwards. It is not in any way a cancerous or pre-cancerous condition, but some surgeons do treat it surgically, mainly to give relief from pain and anxiety.

Fibrosis

This means simply thickening, and it is an inevitable part of getting older. In some women, however, it starts fairly young, and can cause odd lumps and bands in different areas of the breast.

There are a few other reasons for lumpiness in the breast and for pain, tenderness and nipple discharges, most of which are a nuisance — but no more than that. They certainly don't threaten life. But because there has been so much publicity about breast cancer many women become exceedingly frightened about such symptoms. So, doctors will always take seriously a woman's report of a lump, or a discharge, or inverted nipples and investigate carefully. If such a condition happens to you, try not to get too agitated while you wait to go into hospital for any treatment you need. The vast majority of women like you have no malignancy at all.

This is of course an easy thing to say and a devillishly difficult thing to do, but all the same it's worth saying it again and saying it loudly. *Most breast lumps and ailments are not dangerous.* For further reassurance about what can be done to protect yourself and how to ensure the early diagnosis that makes it very treatable, see page 109 on checks and self examination.

Gynaecological checks

These symptoms affect a woman's reproductive system. The same comment made about the cancer checks above applies here. They may mean potentially severe trouble but are just as likely not to. But they still need to be investigated, just in case.

- A marked change in period patterns. (If you've always been irregular, that is normal for you. It is *changes* that matter.)

- Unusually heavy bleeding during periods.

- Bleeding between periods.

- Vomiting, pain or headaches during periods.

- Vaginal discharges.

- Pain on intercourse.

- Bleeding after intercourse.

- Pain in belly or lower back, associated with discharges.

- Abdominal pain associated with a missed period. This may suggest an ectopic — tubal — pregnancy. (See also page 82.)

- Rashes, sores, blisters or any other new eruption in or near the vulva.

Digestive checks

The usual proviso that these signs may not be sinister goes with this list, and it is also important to note concurrent eating behaviour; pain in the belly, or sickness associated with eating or drinking too much, is more likely to be due to the dietary indiscretion rather than to any underlying disease.

- Persistent pain under the ribs.

- Heartburn.

- Difficulty in passing stools.

- Diarrhoea, chronic constipation.

- Pain in the centre of the ribs, low down, moving through to the back. (This can be due to a peptic ulcer.)

- Waterbrash — the mouth seems to fill with saliva. (This is also a possible sign of a peptic ulcer.)

- Waves of belly pain — the sort usually labelled 'colicky'. (This might suggest colon disorder.)

- Attacks of nausea, vomiting.

- Pain in the right side of the belly, sometimes radiating up to the shoulder. (This could be gall bladder disease.)

- Marked changes in colour and consistency of stools. Sticky blackish stools, for example, (could indicate bleeding high up in the colon) or greasy, highly offensive yellow stools (could be linked with jaundice).

Rheumatism checks

Many people think that stiffening and weakness of joints and muscles is an inevitable part of ageing, and are stoical about the sort of symptoms listed below even when they are still as young as forty or so. But it is not true that such problems are inevitable; a great deal can be done to prevent permanent damage to the joints and muscles if symptoms such as these are dealt with promptly.

- Early morning aches.

- Swelling of small joints, such as knuckles.

- Persistent aching of a joint or group of muscles not caused by extra use (pain after, say, heavy digging in the garden is normal).

- Persistent stiffness of a muscle or group of muscles, not associated with postural changes (for example, one night's awkward sleeping).

- Loss of sensation, or tingling, or pins and needles not associated with postural changes.

General physical symptoms

Some of these symptoms may indicate such problems as high blood pressure, heart disorders, kidney disorders and so on, though many of them will have much less important causes.

• Double vision.

• 'Haloes' round lights.

• Sudden limitation of visual fields, for example, an inability to see what is at the sides.

• 'Ringing' in the ears, not associated with wax in the ears. But never dig in your own ears to remove wax, that is more likely to impact it against the drum. Always have it removed carefully either with professional syringing, or the use of wax solvent ear drops, or both.

• Pain in and around ears (always report this immediately to a doctor; ear infections need rapid treatment).

• Unusual production .of sputum — 'catarrh' in the chest, especially if discoloured.

• Frequent headaches not associated with dietary/drinking habits.

• Dizziness on exertion — or on bending over.

• Breathlessness on mild exertion (just walking a few yards, say).

• 'Wheeziness' on mild exertion.

• Unusual pain in the chest, left arm, jaw (this could be linked with heart disease).

• Change in the amount of urine production.

• Blood in the urine (remember food such as beetroot can colour it).

• Pain on passing urine.

• Unusual thirst especially if associated with marked weight loss (may be linked with diabetes).

Psychiatric illness

The symptoms listed here are regarded as 'normal behaviour' by some people and so they may be — sometimes. But if you find you are showing them often they may indicate that you need to talk about how you are feeling and behaving with an expert who can assess whether you are in need of psychiatric support or help.

• Changes in sleeping habits with either a need to sleep all the time, or insomnia or early morning waking with some daytime sleepiness.

• Changes in eating habits, either eating a great deal more or a great deal less.

• Changes in sexual appetite, especially loss of libido (sex drive) — this is often one of the early signs of clinical depression, especially when associated with childbirth and the menopause.

• Anxiety about aches and pains and constant awareness of the body's activities (if reading lists like these worries you, and yet you feel strongly drawn to them, and constantly check yourself for the symptoms mentioned, this could be a positive sign for you).

• Frequent nausea, without actual vomiting.

• Feelings of heaviness in the belly.

• Feeling of a lump in the throat.

• Frequent breathlessness.

• Awareness of a rapid heartbeat.

• Frequent 'missed' heartbeats (uneven heart beating).

• Dizziness, tingling, pins and needles in arms and legs.

• Panic attacks in which waves of fear engulf you.

• Constant bad taste in the mouth.

• Constant awareness of your own 'bad breath'.

• Increase in alcohol consumption, especially in non-social settings, drinking alone, and because you need to, rather than just for friendly fun.

• Smoking more heavily.

• Tearfulness, for no immediate personal reason.

• Obsessive anxiety about news items such as child abduction, murders, terrorism, the arms race etc. It is reasonable and intelligent and compassionate to be concerned about such matters, but if a person becomes obsessed, anxious, and the worry about the arms race, say, prevents her from coping with ordinary day to day tasks, it may indicate a degree of depressive illness rather than sensible intellectual awareness of real problems.

• Obsessive behaviour, for example, feeling obliged to repeat pointless actions or rituals; feeling a need to keep washing either yourself or your environment.

• Marked changes in thinking patterns, such as being convinced strangers are talking about you, or staring at you, or harming you from a distance, or that people are ganging up on you.

• Inability to control your own thinking so that unpleasant or frightening ideas keep going through your mind.

• Frequent attacks of irritability, bad temper, aggressiveness, especially when driving, or when dealing with strangers, on the telephone and in shops, etc.

• Periods of high excitement and excessive energy when you spend a lot of money, get over-excited about crazy schemes, and seem to need little sleep, especially if associated with matching periods of depression.

• Feelings that life has nothing to offer now or in the future. (Careful with this one; it may be that your life is indeed in the sort of disorder that makes such feelings natural and normal — for example the recently bereaved person feels like this and is certainly not ill, though she is naturally far from happy.)

Feelings of guilt and remorse especially over events that happened long ago and which are irremediable.

When using this list, it is an accumulation of positive responses that matters rather more than individual ones.

The more of them you identify as pertaining to you, the more useful it could be to seek medical advice. Many of these symptoms are part of common anxiety states and depressive illnesses for which help can be given, either via anti-depressant drugs (which are not the same at all as the much-worried-about-tranquillizers which have caused so much emotional distress, but therapeutically effective tools that work without leading to addiction) or via psychotherapy — 'talking it out'.

Once you have read these lists, give no more thought to them.

That way lies obsessive anxiety, a disorder in itself. With just one reading you will find that the important messages will stick in your memory, so that if ever you do develop any of the signs and symptoms described you will remember you should do something about them.

Tests and screening

Awareness of symptoms and what they might mean is one blade of the weapon against illness; the other is to pre-empt illness by deliberately looking for evidence that it exists, or might appear in the future.

There are some doctors who are opposed to the idea of screening healthy people for such evidence. They say that doing so is a very costly exercise which returns much smaller benefits than the outlay of time and money warrants. They also think screening may make some people 'neurotic' — that is, over-concerned about their health, repeating the aphorism that good health is unawareness of wellbeing. And up to a point they could be right. To do as some anxious people have been known to do and put oneself through a battery of tests and checks at frequent intervals is hardly healthy behaviour. But there are some tests for women that are undoubtedly worth having at regular intervals, because all the evidence suggests that doing so does protect against two of the major cancers that afflict women — cancer of the cervix, the neck of the uterus, and cancer of the breast.

The smear test

About fifty or so years ago, a New York doctor from a Greek family — his name was George N. Papanicolaou — demonstrated that early cancer cells of the cervix are less sticky than normal cells, and so are shed more easily into the vagina. He showed that by taking a smear from the cervix and looking at it under a microscope, the presence of pre-malignant cells — that is, cells that might, if left undisturbed, become cancerous — could be detected.

This early detection means that the potentially lethal disease of cancer of the cervix can be prevented; the threatening cells can be removed without doing any permanent damage to the woman's reproductive system — she can have a baby afterwards if she wants to — and the cancer cured. This is one of those rare situations where doctors are willing to use the very definite word 'cure'. Mostly they prefer to make the more modest claims of ' treating' or 'ameliorating'. But with a Pap smear as a guide (inevitably the good doctor's name has been abbreviated) modern doctors save women's lives every day, all over the world, as a matter of ordinary daily work. (And, incidentally, versions of the Pap test are used today for diagnosing cancers elsewhere in the body, for example, the stomach and the lungs, and can be used for men as well as women. But generally speaking, the term Pap test is applied to tests for cancer of the cervix.)

It would be reasonable to assume with such a test available, and the comparative simplicity of treatment of any abnormal cells (see later for details) that no women anywhere would ever die of cancer of the cervix. All would have their tests regularly and hey presto, the disease would be eradicated, much as smallpox has been eradicated.

But that hasn't happened. Despite the wide publicity given to the test in the developed countries, there are still some women who just don't bother to present themselves for it. They may not regard it as important, lacking any understanding of the unpleasantness of dying from cancer of the cervix. They may not find it possible to pay for the test, if they live in countries where there is no State health service that provides them. And even in countries where there is such a service — as in Britain — they may not come forward because they are 'too modest' and will always shun any sort of medical care involving the sex organs, or because they are so frightened of the very word cancer that they'd rather not have a test that might reveal they are candidates for the disease — even though the test actually protects them from it.

The provision of comprehensive and truly protective Pap test services is further complicated by differing opinions on when and how often the test should be done in individual women. In the USA it is recommended that women should have a routine smear once a year from the age of sixteen or seventeen, or as soon as a girl starts to have intercourse, if that is earlier.

In Britain, the Department of Health and Social Security originally said that the test should be offered only to all women over the age of thirty-five, and those who have had three or more pregnancies, and should be repeated at five yearly intervals.

Under pressure from some women's groups and from doctors, the DHSS now says that screening 'should first take place for any woman who is or has been sexually active on her first presentation for contraceptive advice or whenever she first requests screening. Screenings should be repeated after that occasion at the ages of twenty, twenty-five, thirty and thirty-five, and not on any other occasion, except that every woman should be screened early in the course of care for each pregnancy.

Many doctors and their patients remain unsatisfied with this, and feel strongly that British women, like their American and

Scandinavian sisters, should have the protection of more frequent tests. They point out that there is at present a marked upturn in the numbers of young (under thirty-five) women suffering cancer of the cervix, and that more frequent screening could detect them and save their lives.

The point must be made, of course, that the DHSS recommendations apply only to women seeking tests on the National Health Service — without making direct personal payment. They certainly don't say that women who choose to pay should not have tests more often; they can have them as frequently as they like. And in practice many women who can afford to pay do have their tests on the American pattern; but meanwhile the campaign proceeds to provide all women in Britain with yearly tests for which they do not have to pay directly, from the age when they first become sexually active.

One of the problems, incidentally, in providing a fully comprehensive system of Pap smears for the entire relevant female population is not just the cost in money but in manpower; it takes a lot of expert time to read the tests accurately and to report on them properly so that any necessary action can be taken, and for this reason considerable research is going into seeking computerized and therefore faster and simpler methods of reading the tests.

How is the test done?

Setting aside the political and social aspects of the test, important and interesting though these are, what matters most to most women is what happens when a test is done, what it may reveal, and what treatment may be needed.

The process is simple and generally painless. The woman usually needs to lie on her back, with her knees bent and apart (though some doctors seem willing to cope while their patient lies on her side, so that they can reach the cervix from behind) as the first stage is a manual examination of the vagina. The doctor puts two or three gloved fingers inside the vagina, while pressing down on the uterus from above, with his or her other hand on the belly wall.

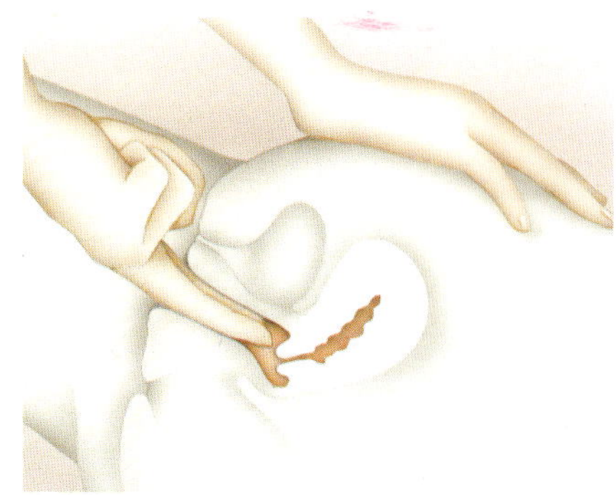

This reveals whether all the organs are in the position they should be and leads to the next stage, the actual taking of the smear.

An instrument called a speculum is passed into the vagina, which is, it will be remembered, a collapsed tube. That is, the walls are touching each other, and so hiding the

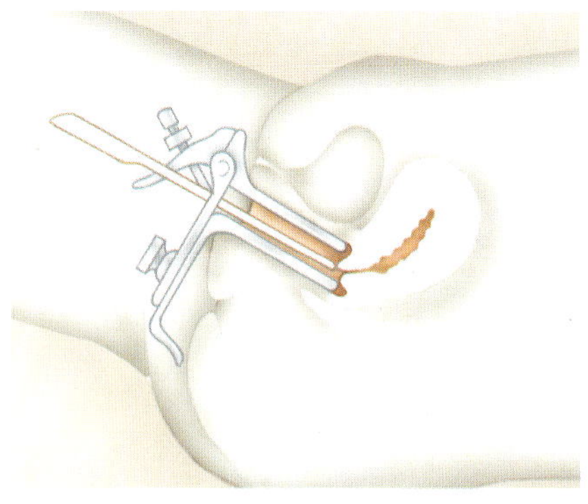

cervix at the far end. A speculum opens the vagina and allows the cervix to be seen.

A plastic spatula — similar to the tongue depressors doctors use to look at throats, but with a specially shaped end — is used to rub gently round the opening of the cervix and sometimes also the upper vaginal walls. The cells that are removed by these actions — and it must be repeated that there is no pain involved, any more than there is when shreds of skin are rubbed off our bodies every day — are put on a microscope slide, stained to make them more visible and examined under a microscope.

The only after-effect for the woman is at the most an awareness of having had the test done — not a pain, but a feeling of having had something inside for a few seconds — and a mild discharge.

What does the test show?

As well as identifying cells that might be pre-malignant, the test is now also used to look for other disorders of the vagina. Infections such as thrush, TV, herpes and warts (see Section seven) can be detected and treatment given. And it is vitally important to remember that sufferers from warts should be checked at very frequent intervals, because of the link between exposure to that virus and the later development of cancer of the cervix. It is also important to know that the test does not reveal the presence of cancer of the ovary or of the uterus of any other part of the body.

There are similar smears that can be taken to check on the levels of estrogen in the body (it is used to help menopausal women — see Section nine) but these are not the same as cervical smear tests.

What treatments are given?

If pre-malignant cells are detected, then treatment will be offered. There is no need to panic over this. These cells are not a sign of imminent cancer. In fact, it can take several years before any severe disease appears. This is a condition that has what is called a long latency period; it can lie dormant for some time before flaring into true illness. This is why the disease is commonest in women over the age of thirty-five (the DHSS in Britain isn't being unreasonable in concentrating its efforts on this age range; at the time of writing, ninety-four per cent of all deaths from cervical cancer affect this older age group).

However, it must be said that there appears to be a new development in the pattern of cancer of the cervix in younger women.

Some doctors are reporting a new and very aggressive form of the disease that progresses from pre-malignant to frankly malignant in a very short time — less than a year in a few cases — so early treatment is obviously best. An important observation is that women who smoke seem to be at higher risk from this form of the disease, though why there should be this link is far from clear.

All that is needed is to remove the cells. This can be done by taking out a cone shaped piece of tissue, in an operation usually done on an in-patient basis and under a general anaesthetic. This is called a cone biopsy. Alternatively a cautery can be used — a 'burning' technique — to destroy the cells.

At one time the ones most commonly used were chemical cauteries — powerful cell-killing substances were applied — and electrical ones, but today there is a much more popular method with both doctors and their patients. Using a procedure known as colposcopy (that means literally 'looking into the vagina'), a technique which illuminates the whole area so brightly that the operator can see precisely what has to be done, a laser is applied to doubtful cell areas, and this action shrinks them away completely.

The laser can be used not only to deal with pre-malignant cells but also warts, cervical 'erosions' (see Section seven) and a range of vaginal and vulval membrane disorders. It is a painless procedure, possibly followed by a minor discharge for a few days — which may be bloodstained — though many women don't have even that. The whole affair takes about twelve to fifteen minutes and the most uncomfortable part is lying on your back with your knees apart. But that is surely a great deal less unpleasant than having the disease.

And remember, there is no damage done to the ability to have a baby. Studies of women who have had laser colposcopy (rather than cone biopsy) to treat pre-malignancy of the cervix show they have the same rate of successful pregnancies as untreated women, with the same number of failed pregnancies (miscarriages) and premature deliveries.

So there is no reason in the world to be afraid of the condition or of its treatment. As long as you have your Pap tests at regular intervals.

Women's surgery

Some of the operations women may need have already been dealt with in these pages, as part of the accounts of the problems. But there are some operations which are widely used for a whole range of women's problems which need more detailed discussion.

Dilation and curetage

This is an operation that is exceedingly common. It is performed some 140,000 times each year in the UK alone which means now nearly half of all women have the operation at some stage in their lives. It is used:

• For diagnosis — of such problems as excessive or unusual bleeding, or failure to conceive, via shreds of tissue lining the cervix or the uterus which are removed for microscopic study.

• For cleaning — following the loss of a pregnancy (a spontaneous abortion — see Section six) or a complicated birth when any retained products of conception need to be removed, to prevent them causing inflammation and damage to the uterus.

• For deliberate ending of an unwanted pregnancy — known as a therapeutic abortion (see Section six), when the developing foetus is removed.

• For protection — post menopausal women having regular hormone replacement therapy may need checks of the uterine lining to ensure that this is doing no harm (see Section nine).

• As a general 'look-around' operation— which some surgeons use when they aren't quite sure what is causing a woman's symptoms and hope to discover something by actually looking at her reproductive organs. (This is called an EUA — examination under anaesthetic.) And it has to be said that often women do report relief of distress of various kinds after the operation even if the surgeon has not been able to identify a precise cause for the distress or did no more than the basic procedure. This is called the 'placebo effect' (from the Latin *placere* which means to please) and it is one that is often noted.

People with genuine symptoms find genuine relief merely because something has been done — a pill has been swallowed, a discussion has been undertaken, an operation has been performed. Quite why it happens no one can be sure; some experts think that the reassurance of interest and concern for one's suffering on another's part causes the release of brain chemicals (they are called endorphins, and there will be more about them in Section ten) which act as painkillers and natural tranquillizers. Whatever causes the placebo effect, certainly the operation of D and C — the familiar shortened label — can provide it.

What is done?

The patient is admitted to hospital the night before, usually, though in some cases the morning will do, if the operation is to be performed late in the day. She may be given a suppository to empty the rectum (a full one gets in the way, rather, since the structure is so close to the vagina and uterus — see Section two) and a set of routine examinations of heart and lungs, blood pressure, urine and so on will be done.

She will be weighed, so that the anaesthetist can assess how much anaesthetic her body needs (too much is unhealthy — too little is inefficient) and in some hospitals she may have her pubic hair shaved off, though these days many surgeons regard this as an unnecessary ritual.

She will have a pre-anaesthetic dose of a drug to make her sleepy and co-operative (people who are tense may become argumentative when they are anaesthetized, and that helps no-one, least of all the patient herself) and also to dry up the secretions that might cause excess fluid to enter the lungs when she is unconscious and so make her choke. This causes a rather disagreeable dryness of the mouth. (This is a routine procedure before all general anaesthetics.)

After the anaesthetic is given (usually all the patient knows is an injection into a vein — generally at the crook of the elbow —

The stages of a D and C operation

Once the anaesthetic has taken effect, the patient is placed on her back with her ankles held in high stirrups so that the vulval area is easily accessible.

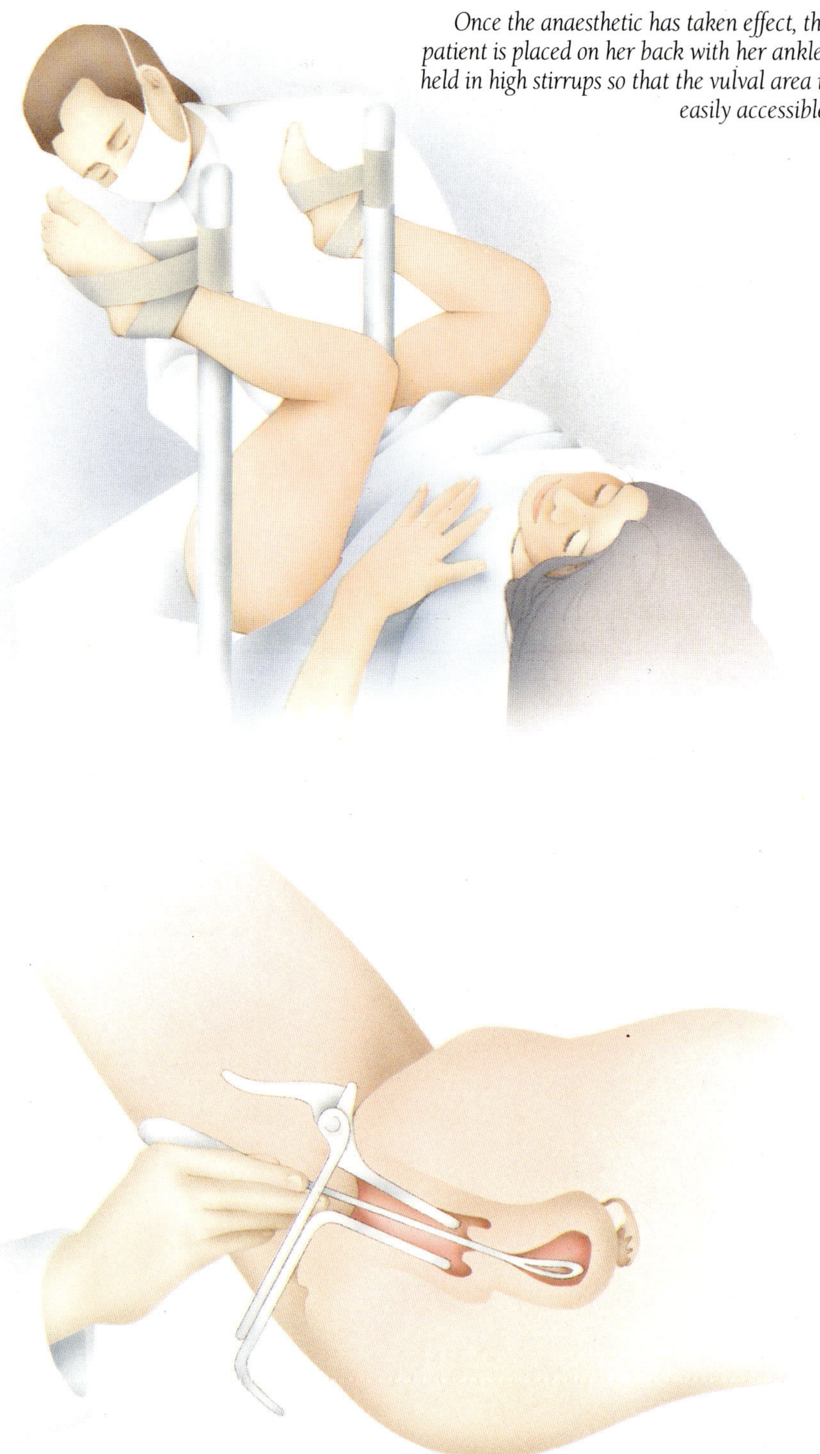

A speculum is then inserted which opens the vagina and allows access to the cervix. The surgeon can then measure the exact depth of the uterus using a sound. The cervical opening is gradually enlarged with a series of dilators and the inner walls of the uterus carefully scraped with a curette.

which knocks her out) she is put on the operating table in what is called the lithotomy position; it gets its name from the operation done in the nineteenth century to 'cut for stone' — when men commonly got painful stones in their bladders and had to have them cut out (*litho* is stone in Latin). The position involves lying on the back with the ankles held in high stirrups, so that the whole of the vulval area is revealed and is easily accessible.

The first stage of the operation is the insertion of a speculum, which opens the vagina, and allows access to the cervix, the small neck of the uterus, with its tiny central channel.

Once the surgeon can easily see the cervix he uses an instrument called a sound, which he passes through the central opening in order to measure the exact depth of the uterus, for each woman varies a little. It is important that the surgeon pushes his next instruments in only as far as they should go — and the sound tells him how far that is. Then he uses the dilators, a series of rather handsomely curved metal rods, gradually increasing in thickness. Using one after the other he carefully enlarges the cervical opening.

He then uses an instrument called a curette, slender and long and with a loop at the far end. The loop has on one side a sharp edge and on the other a blunt edge — though the sharp one isn't all that sharp. With this the surgeon carefully scrapes the surface of the inner walls of the uterus, to remove the lining there; it does no harm at all to the deeper structures.

Some of the scrapings are then sent to the laboratory to be examined to check the state of the lining of the uterus and to look for any dubious cells.

Once he has passed his curette over the whole surface to ensure it is all clear of lining, the surgeon removes his instruments, takes away the speculum which was making the way clear for him and the patient is then almost precisely as she was before he started. She has no stitches, no visible injuries, no source of any pain. She has only a slightly wider open cervix and a uterus which is free of any lining. She may bleed for a day or two, because the uterus responds to the operation by shedding some extra blood.

Most women are free to return home within four to five hours, or at most forty-eight, of the operation; some need this time to recover not from the surgery but from the anaesthetic, which is the most debilitating part of the whole procedure. Safe as anaesthetics are these days, they do involve the use of very powerful drugs and the most robust of people need time for these drugs to be excreted from the body. But the operation itself causes little more than local bleeding similar to a period for a few days. In some cases, the next period (which may appear within a week or two, or not for another month or more, as the cycle is likely to be disturbed) will be extra heavy. There is no need to panic if there is such extra bleeding, but if it is particularly profuse and prolonged of course talk to the surgeon about it. He can give a drug (it is called aminocaproic acid) to reduce the flow, by increasing the clotting of the blood.

Possible complications

There are few problems with this operation; it is a remarkably safe one. In a few cases a clumsy operator has pushed a curette too far into the uterus and caused a perforation but even then the uterine muscles heal particularly well, and in cases where excessive opening of the cervix is needed (say a late stage termination of a pregnancy) tears of the cervix may occur. But they are very rare indeed. Some people react badly to anaesthesia, but the operation can't be blamed for that. Such patients would have problems whatever operation they were having.

After-care

There is rarely any need for much. In a few cases, there is heavy bleeding afterwards, which needs to be reported to a doctor if it is prolonged, and if the patient is at all alarmed. Occasionally there may be an infection. A raised temperature, a smelly heavy discharge and pain in the belly should always be reported for any necessary treatment.

After D and C most women can resume work within a couple of days, can drive a car again after the same sort of time (you need at least twenty-four hours to recover from a general anaesthetic) and can have intercourse again within a week. Love-making up to and including orgasm is fine — it's penetration that is best avoided, because of the small risk of infection while the cervix is more open than usual.

To have or not to have

Because this operation is so common, some women accept a surgeon's offer of a D and C without question, and some surgeons forget the need to explain to their patients why they want to do it. They say with great jollity, 'We'll just do a poke and a scrape, my dear,' (if they don't mind revealing hospital slang to their patients) and wander off — or say nothing much at all. Don't ever let a surgeon off that easily. Insist on a full explanation of what is to be done to you, why it is to be done, and what the expected outcome might be. You have every right to this. It is your uterus, not the surgeon's.

Vaginal repairs

A problem that used to be more common than now is weakening of the muscles of the pelvic floor to such a degree that they no longer fully support the uterus and its appendages. There is sagging — prolapse — of the walls of the vagina, and in a few rare cases, complete descent of the uterus to the surface of the body.

The causes of this weakness include childbirth and the menopause. In the bad old days when women had a great many children, often close together in time, and suffered prolonged and painful labours to produce them, the muscles of the area were obviously weakened. Nowadays, when women tend to have fewer pregnancies and their labours are shorter because they are better managed by obstetricians (and it must be said here that despite the complaint of the lobby that demands 'natural childbirth' and which rejects the use of modern high technology care, it is safer and healthier to have a baby today than it has ever been — see Section six) there is less of the sort of muscle damage that used to be the cause of prolapse.

The main reason for prolapse today is the weakening of the muscles that may happen at the menopause. The loss of estrogen, which is involved with muscle tone and strength, can in some cases cause sagging. This can be prevented in part by the use of Hormone Replacement Therapy (HRT) (see Section nine) but even so, surgery may sometimes be necessary.

There are two main types of prolapse; that affecting the front wall of the bladder, and leading to loss of bladder control, and that affecting the rear wall, and leading to pressure on the vagina from the rectum and sometimes some constipation as the weakened rectal wall fails to push hard enough to expel its contents.

When the front wall of the vagina bulges it is called a *cystocele* (the Latin for bladder is *cyst)* and when the rear wall bulges it is called a *rectocele.*

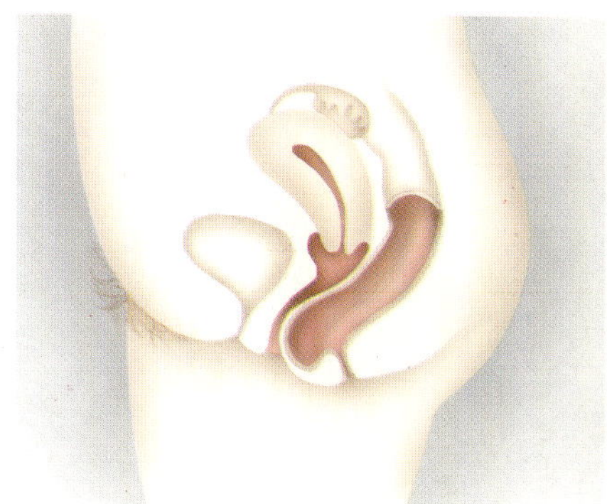

Prolapse affecting the rear wall of the vagina, leading to bulging of the rectum.

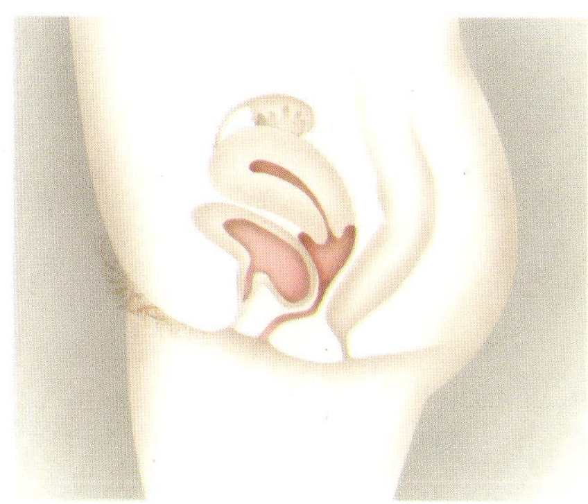

Prolapse affecting the front wall of the vagina, leading to loss of bladder control.

The symptoms these weaknesses cause vary. If there is a cystocele, trouble with urine is the commonest discomfort. There may be 'stress incontinence'; sneezing, laughing, coughing, indeed any downwards strain, causes the escape of some urine, as the muscles controlling the bladder outlet fail to hold on. There is also general frequency; when the woman needs to pee, which is often, she needs to do so desperately, and can barely hold on. There may also be some urinary infection and cystitis. With rectocele there may be, apart from constipation, a sense of dullness and dragging downwards. There is less pleasure in sexual intercourse as the vagina is unable to grasp the penis firmly enough for the woman — or her partner — to feel it.

In a few cases, in women not yet at the menopause and where the prolapse is mild, improvement can be found by exercises of the pelvic floor. These are similar to those recommended to women after giving birth. If they are performed for twenty or thirty minutes at a time twice or thrice a day, they can be very effective. Many keep fit classes offer to teach them and there is no doubt that it is easier to learn at such a class than to try and learn by yourself. But the exercises you could use are on page 152, if you prefer to be independent.

In a few very rare cases a prolapse can be treated by inserting into the vagina a ring-shaped support made of heavy rubber or plastic. These are called pessaries (the chemical ones are quite different — see Section seven) and were once very commonly prescribed. Nowadays they are used only for very elderly ladies who are used to them, having had them for many years already, or for those too frail to cope with surgery or — rarely — for newly delivered mothers who show signs of prolapse. Their muscles are likely to return to normal as their homone balance returns to the pre-pregnant state and surgery too soon is not needed. The pessary helps them to be comfortable while waiting for the muscles to take over their normal job again.

What is done?

There are a number of different operations that can be done. For some women with prolapse the simple answer is hysterectomy (see page 121), for others who want to have more children or who object to losing their uterus, a repair is possible.

A Manchester or Fothergill Repair is performed via the vagina. The cervix is removed and a large supportive stitch is put through the ligaments to sling the uterus back into position. Although the woman has no cervix it is, of course, still possible for her to have children by Caesarian section after this operation. Like so many gynaecological operations, it is performed while the patient is in the lithotomy position, as are the other repair operations.

For a cystocele, the surgeon — using a speculum to clear the way for his instruments — removes a diamond shaped piece of tissue from the front wall of the vagina. The resulting gap is then firmly stitched together so that a tuck is taken which draws in the slack, and leaves the wall taut and able again to support the uterus above.

For rectocele, the same diamond shaped incision and removal of tissue is made on the rear wall of the vagina and again closed with firm stitches.

If necessary both posterior and anterior repairs can be done at the same time to the same patient.

Possible complications

Because there are no skin stitches there is less discomfort after the operation than after other abdominal operations. There is usually an absorbent pack of gauze inside the vagina, to protect the stitches, though this is usually removed after twenty-four hours. The stitches don't need removing; they are made of organic material which means they slowly absorb into the wound and disappear, but in a few cases there may be some soreness round a stitch, and pieces of it may come away. This is normal, and nothing to worry about. The wounds usually heal with remarkable speed — more quickly than wounds in skin.

Most patients are able to be out of bed within twenty-four hours, because these days early activity after surgery is the norm. This prevents any congestion in the lungs, due to inactivity and shallow breathing, and also prevents weakness of the leg muscles and all the debility that comes from long bed rest.

The commonest discomfort after a repair operation is difficulty with urine. Some surgeons put in a tube — a catheter — which drains the urine away, and leave it in place for a few days, while others prefer their patients to try to pee unaided. If they can't then a catheter may need to be passed.

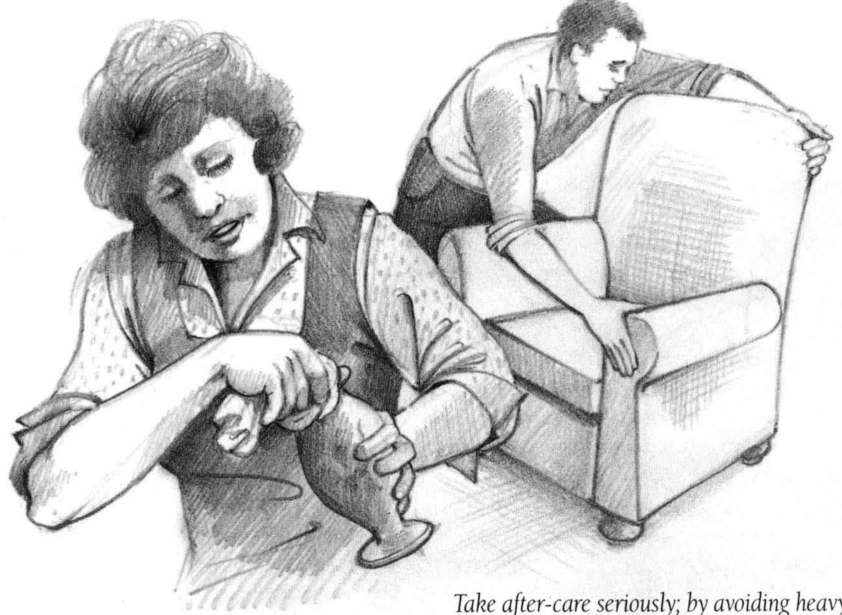

Take after-care seriously; by avoiding heavy work the wound will heal more quickly.

After-care

Most patients remain in hospital long enough for any complications such as infection to be noticed and dealt with, but if after discharge from hospital — on around the tenth day in most cases, though it may be longer or shorter — there is unusual pain, or fever, or discharge — the doctor should be told at once.

Normal activity can usually be resumed within three or four weeks — back to work, if you have a job, and back to light housework. (Get someone else to do heavy work — or leave it undone. A bit of household disorder is preferable to personal disorder because of overwork.) You can drive a car again after three weeks or so.

About six weeks after the operation the surgeon will want to examine his handiwork. Once you have had this vaginal examination and are assured that all is well and your wound has healed, you can resume intercourse. Till then nothing should be put in the vagina. Lovemaking short of penetration is again the answer. Once intercourse is resumed you need a gentle, patient and careful partner and plenty of lubricant such as KY Jelly.

To have or not to have

There is rarely any argument about the value of this operation. Most patients suffering from prolapse are anxious for help, and grateful to be offered a repair. But of course, if you're in any doubt, do ask. You may be one of those people who would prefer a pessary to an operation — though in the long term they really aren't ideal.

Hysterectomy

One British woman in five will end her life minus her uterus, having had it removed on an operating table. In the USA these figures are higher. This was because there was a time when surgeons faced with women complaining of a range of symptoms, including bleeding for various reasons, believed that the simplest way to deal with the problem was to remove the target organ. That certainly cured the bleeding, but did not necessarily cure the patient's ills.

The operation is offered to women for a number of different causes.

- For cancer of the organs. Obviously, in this case there is no question of the value of the operation.

- For large fibroids, which cause heavy and prolonged bleeding. In a younger woman of childbearing age who wants to conserve her uterus for future use, an operation called a myomectomy can be done. This 'shells out' the fibroids from the muscle wall, and leaves the uterus intact and available (though there is a possibility the fibroids may come back after the operation). In an older woman such complex surgery is not needed. Simple removal of the uterus is the answer for her, and probably less traumatic, as the operation of hysterectomy is simpler than myomectomy for multiple fibroids.

- For severe prolapse in an older woman who does not want more children and for whom a repair operation would be less successful than simple removal of the fallen uterus.

- For endometriosis (see page 52).

- For prolonged and severe bleeding which cannot be controlled by hormones. This condition is called 'functional bleeding' and it is in this area that there is most doubt about the value of hysterectomy.

If a woman is experiencing her bleeding because her underlying tension, anxiety and distress are having an effect on her hormone balance, removing the uterus may prevent the loss of blood — but it won't remove the underlying anxiety, tension and distress. If the woman was unhappy before her operation, she will be afterwards, and perhaps more so, because now she has no obvious symptom on which to focus her unhappiness.

It is because of this group of women, which is comparatively small but still considerable in number, that hysterectomy has collected such a bad press from so many women. There is a widespread belief that the operation makes you miserable, that it ruins your sex life for ever, that it makes women old before their time, makes them put on a lot of weight and so on and so on.

This is a pity, because in fact the operation has been of enormous value to a great many. This includes those with cancer who have had their lives saved because their cancer has been removed. Those whose fibroids were huge and drained them of blood and energy and all pleasure in their sex lives. Those who no longer had the muscles they needed to support the uterus. For them the post operative time is like a new lease of life, they feel — and look — so much better.

It is obvious, then, that every woman must talk in great detail with her surgeon if hysterectomy is mooted. Never accept the operation unless you are sure that you have been given all the facts you need to make up your mind about whether the operation is right for you. It is safe to say that in a book like this; the sort of woman who would be happier leaving all decisions to the surgeons (and there are a great many who are, and theirs is a valid choice) is not the sort of woman who would be reading these pages anyway. The fact that you are suggests that you are the sort of person who wants facts, can handle them and can use them to make her own decisions.

The scope of the operation depends on why it is being performed. For removal of cancer, the operation is likely to be larger — removing more tissue. There is a form of the operation called Wertheim's hysterectomy which is done for severe cancer of the cervix. In this, the uterus, the tubes, the ovaries and the upper part of the vagina are removed, leaving a shorter vagina. This is an heroic — that is, very large — operation and is therefore only done when it is regarded as lifesaving.

For other women, the uterus only may be removed, the ovaries and tubes being left but the cervix being taken. This is called a total hysterectomy.

In a few cases (not often these days, though the operation was common thirty years ago) the cervix is left in place, in what is called a subtotal hysterectomy. It is less

Types of hysterectomy operations

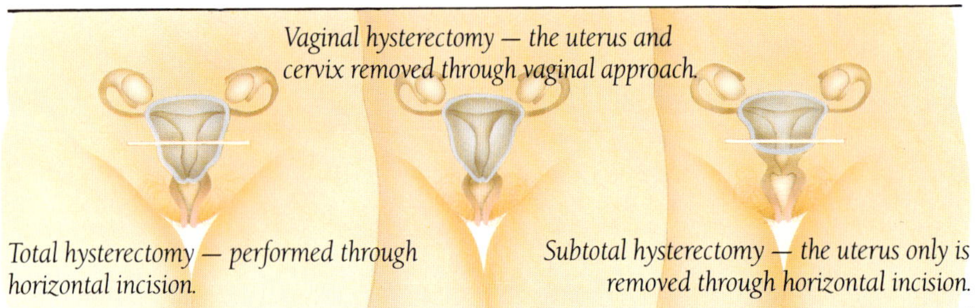

popular now because there remains the risk of cancer starting in the stump of cervix left behind.

Sometimes a surgeon removes the uterus and also the tubes and ovaries. This is called a total hysterectomy with bilateral salpingectomy and öophrectomy or panhysterectomy. This may be done for cancer, or because the surgeon fears that there is a risk of cancer in the ovaries later if they are left in place. Also a woman's age will be taken into account. Older, post-menopausal women will part with their ovaries more comfortably usually.

In practice most surgeons today do all they can to conserve the ovaries because they can and will still go on functioning by producing hormones and eggs even if the eggs can no longer be fertilized to lead to a pregnancy. The hormones will continue to provide the woman with other benefits. But some surgeons prefer to remove them and give the woman hormone replacement therapy afterwards.

And even if the ovaries are left, there seems to be a likelihood of an earlier failure of them — menopause — than there might have been. It is as though loss of the target organ — the uterus — stops the ovaries operating. So, even if the ovaries, or one of them, remains, there can be symptoms which seem to need a course of hormone replacement therapy.

It is not possible in these pages to discuss the pros and cons of ovary removal or conservation, and the balance of any risks from long term HRT. Each woman has to be regarded as an individual with individual needs. Which makes it imperative, yet again, for each woman to discuss in detail with her surgeon what he is going to do to her, and why, and what effect his work may have on her in future years. (See also Section nine.)

What is done

Patients for this operation are admitted to hospital at least a day in advance and sometimes two, so that they are well rested before surgery. It is a major operation and it is necessary to do checks of blood (to prepare for possible blood transfusion to replace that lost in operation) and to ensure that the rectum is well cleared. Also, many hospitals arrange for patients to be taught in advance useful exercises they will need to do after the operation to improve their rate of recovery. Shaving of the pubic hair is usual, especially if there is to be an abdominal approach to the operation.

In some cases a surgeon will use the vaginal approach — as he does for a repair — and this one is in fact most used for hysterectomy performed because of prolapse. (It is not a popular route in general with British surgeons). Usually the abdominal route is preferred and the incision is made low in the belly, within the pubic hair line. Then, as long as the hair regrows after the operation, the scar will be invisible.

(Some older women need to be warned that the pubic hair may not regrow. Those who have found that theirs is thinning rapidly are the ones most likely to find they are left comparatively bald afterwards. But for most the hair does grow again, if not quite so luxuriantly.)

The operation tends to be a long one (it can take up to a couple of hours, depending on what needs to be done) and that means a prolonged anaesthetic. It is this that makes the patient feel as low as she inevitably does afterwards; the operation itself is of course an insult to the body, but the anaesthetic, however skilfully given (as they are today) is even more debilitating.

So is the pain. Where there is a surface wound, there tends to be more discomfort, and painkilling drugs are given to combat this. These also make people feel less than well, though they do control the pain, so the first few days after the operation are not very agreeable.

But having said that, it must be added that some women feel fine within twenty-four hours, and get out of bed for the first time and begin to enjoy their food. Each woman varies, as does each surgeon in his techniques and in what he allows his patients to do post-operatively.

Possible complications

These are the same as for any major surgery — bleeding (which will be spotted quickly in hospital and will be dealt with even faster if it occurs — which is rare), infection, and sometimes difficulties with peeing. The bladder is so close to the uterus that it is inevitable sometimes that it will be disturbed and create problems in the early post-operative days. Catheters may be needed in some cases.

Many of the surgical complications of the past have vanished — the thromboses due to prolonged bed rest, the pressure sores due to lack of movement in bed, and so on. But in a few cases, if the patient is old and frail and otherwise in poor condition, they remain a possibility. But since most people remain in hospital for ten days to two weeks after the operation, such problems are dealt with there, and don't have to be faced at home.

After-care

Long convalescence is usually advised, two weeks at home doing nothing after the first couple of weeks in hospital, then only very light activity for a couple of weeks after that. No car driving for a month, no full time job for six to eight weeks.

When it comes to sex, opinions vary. Some surgeons put on a firm embargo for six weeks, others say that the sooner intercourse is restored the sooner the vaginal tissues return to normal, and suggest three to four weeks, as long as the man is gentle and the couple use a good lubricant. It is a matter that has to be discussed by patient, spouse and surgeons.

If a woman has her ovaries removed she may experience symptoms of sudden menopause – notably hot flushes and vaginal discomfort. To prevent this, most surgeons give HRT, unless this is inadvisable because there was cancer. In some cases, where the operation is done for this reason, the use of HRT is not possible, and the flushes have to be controlled by other means (see page 127).

It is not necessarily true that a post-hysterectomy woman will get fat, be miserable, will grow hair on her face, become deeply wrinkled and elderly and lose all interest in sex. Yes, some women do get some of these reactions – but not because of the operation. Some women feel so much better that they eat more and that is why they get fat. Some have been getting more lined and tending to grow unwanted hair before the operation, as most women do as they get older, but never really noticed. Now the operation is over they focus more on their appearance and see blemishes they never saw before. The loss of sex drive and the unhappiness and tearfulness some suffer – and it is true that some talk of it – is due more to the conditions of their lives, generally speaking, than to the operation itself. The experience of surgery may trigger a sharper awareness of what is wrong for a woman – but that doesn't mean it caused it. In later pages (see Section nine) there is an account of what can go wrong with a woman's sexual responses in later life and what she can do to improve them. But the first step is not to blame an operation that, if entered into for the right reasons, confers benefit rather than trouble.

To have or not to have

As with all other gynaecological operations, this has to be a matter for discussion with the surgeon – but there needs to be special awareness of the state of your own life and your own feelings and attitudes before you start the discussion. There are some women who almost seem to beg their surgeons to remove the uterus, seeming to feel that it is the seat of all their distress. If a woman has that idea before surgery then the likelihood is she will feel rotten afterwards, because no operation can cure unhappiness.

Breast surgery

The removal of doubtful lumps in the breasts is of obvious value; no one wants to harbour a possibly cancerous growth. The whole purpose of BSE (see page 109) is to spot such lumps early and get rid of them.

In the past women feared reporting lumps not only because they feared cancer but because they feared the loss of a breast. And breasts are very valuable to most of us and to our view of ourselves as women. There are people who could more easily face the fear of cancer than the possibility of losing a breast. (I have to be honest and say this is not an opinion I can ever share. I think life is what matters, not the bits and pieces of my body. I'll part with any of them if that's the price I have to pay for continuing health.)

Happily for many women, the options available today for breast surgery are widely increased. No longer do all surgeons opt for total removal of the breast if there is a doubtful lump. Careful removal of the lump, together with removal of any adjacent glands which might contain cancer cells which have spread there, followed by radiotherapy and/or chemotherapy – the use of cancer-killing drugs – can provide successful treatment and leave the main structure of the breasts intact.

In some cases, the removal of the breasts in such a way that reconstruction afterwards can be carried out so that the woman is left with a reasonable facsimile of her original appearance, can be offered. This operation is called a subcutaneous mastectomy and ensures that the skin and nipple are conserved so that future plastic surgery can be performed.

This is an area of surgery where it is not really possible to offer on these pages general information about what will be done and what will happen. The treatment of breast cancer is now so very flexible that each woman has her care virtually tailor made for her. As always, individual discussion with your surgeon is the best way to get the information you might need.

There are other forms of surgery women may need, for many different parts of their bodies; here it has only been possible to give an account of some of the more common ones. But the key for all of them, whether they be gynaecological or of any other kind, is to ask questions. The days are long since gone when a patient touched her forelock politely and said, 'Yes, sir,' when a surgeon handed down his opinion. He is there for her to consult, not to exert control. Her life and her body are her own – and so are the decisions made about operations on it. But better than having to ask questions about operations is to avoid them altogether. Not all illness can be avoided, of course, but a great deal can be done, by means of controlling lifestyle and diet and exercise to keep your body in such excellent condition that it needs little in the way of outside remedies.

Post-mastectomy exercises

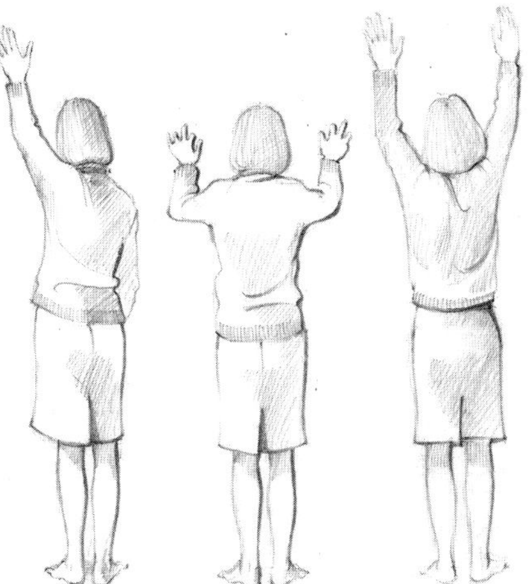

Stand close to a wall. Make a mark as high as you can with your 'good' arm. *Bend your elbows and place your arms against the wall at shoulder level.* *Work hands up wall parallel to each other, until painful; work down slowly.*

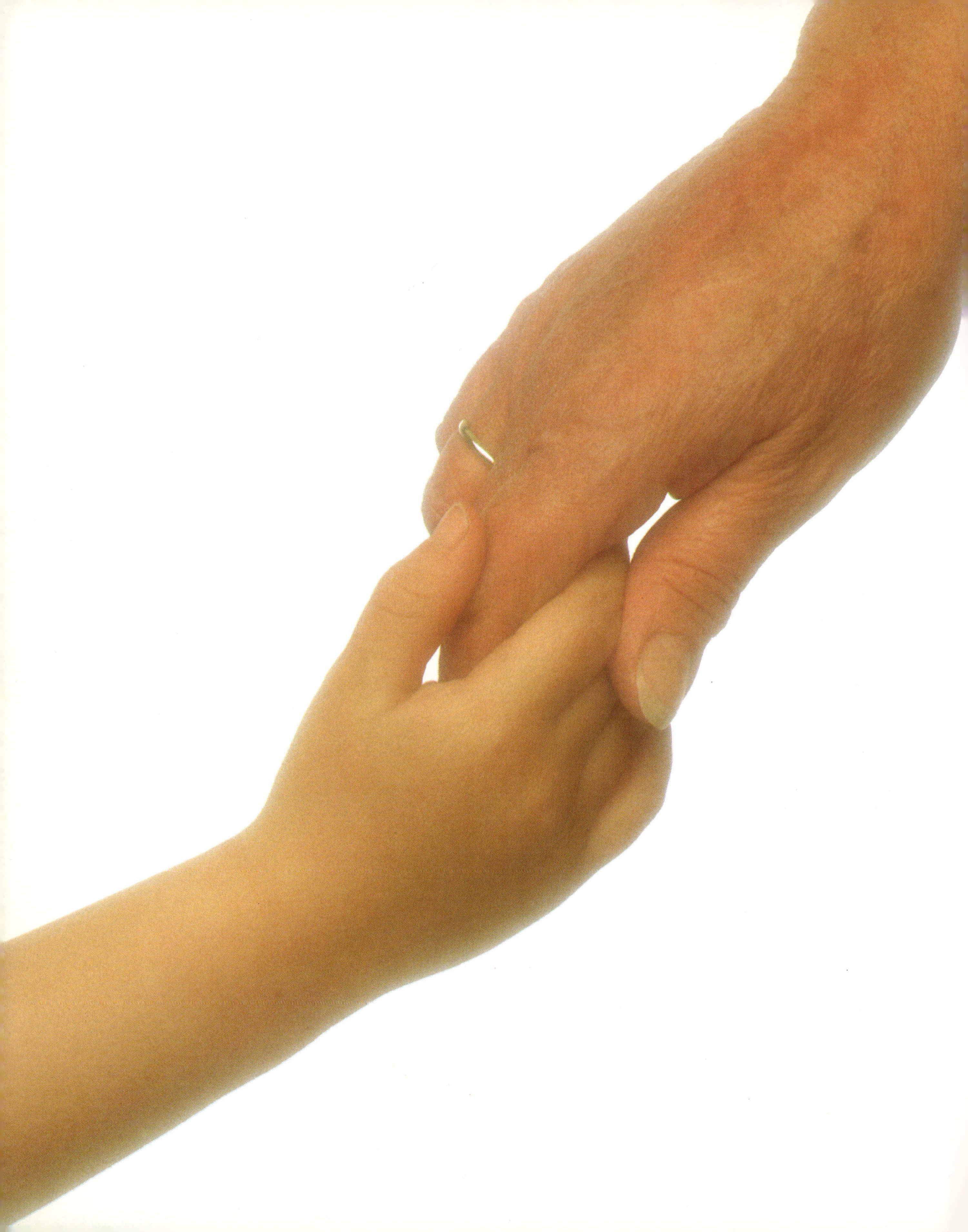

9

WOMAN IN MATURITY

This will be the shortest section of this book; not because older women are uninteresting or unimportant — far from it — but because they are not really all that different from younger ones. It really is absurd how often the apparently intelligent assume that age changes people so totally that they cease to be individuals, but need to be lumped together under one label as 'the old folk'. (And have you noticed how that pseudo-cosy word 'folk' is always used to diminish people? 'Little folk', 'old folk', call them that and you needn't take them seriously, or pay them any attention.)

It is also absurd how coy people can be about the age of women. 'I'm twenty-nine', flutters a particular sort of silly one when someone asks her on her forty-fifth birthday how old she is. Indeed, there are people who think it the height of ill manners to comment on a woman's age at all once she passes her twenties, although when she reaches her late forties or so, people who want to insult her or show how much they despise ber ability and judgement will say disparagingly, she's 'of a certain age', as though that were the worst thing that could be said about anyone and that it actually explained anything. It's all so stupid. As if getting older were some sort of sin, a crime against femininity.

The facts are that women, like men, change physically as they grow older, but not necessarily for the worse. The smoothness of the very young may look superficially appealing but beneath it inevitably lies a smoothness of mind due to inexperience and lack of training in thinking, in talking, in just being interesting. Older people of both sexes are, by and large, rather more fun to be with and have more to contribute to their relationships with others because they have rubbed off their boring bits and sharpened their interesting ones. They have learned to leave behind them the deep selfishness of the young (it's natural to be self-absorbed when you're still not sure who or what you are) and can give a great deal of pleasure to themselves and to other people because of the way they relish their own maturity.

Having said that the smoothness of the young can be appealing, in many ways the lining and sagging and shaping of the older face and body can be even more attractive. Without for one moment wanting to dismiss young beauty, it has to be said that it can be very satisfying to look at the mature face, although it's important to remember that we all get the mature faces we deserve. If you're bad tempered and sulky all through your youth and growing years you'll reach your middle and later years with the lines of your moods etched for all to see at all times.

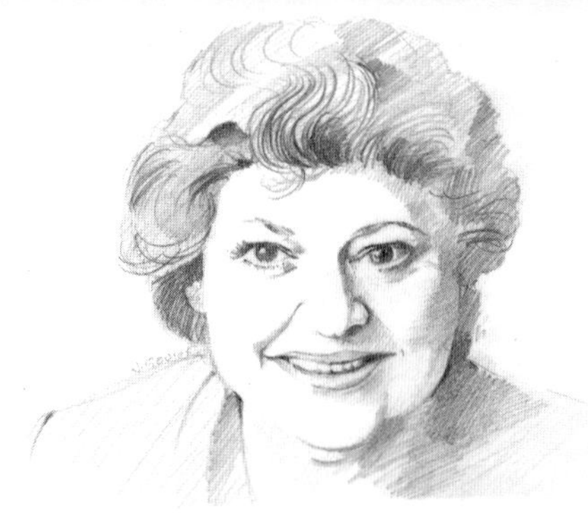

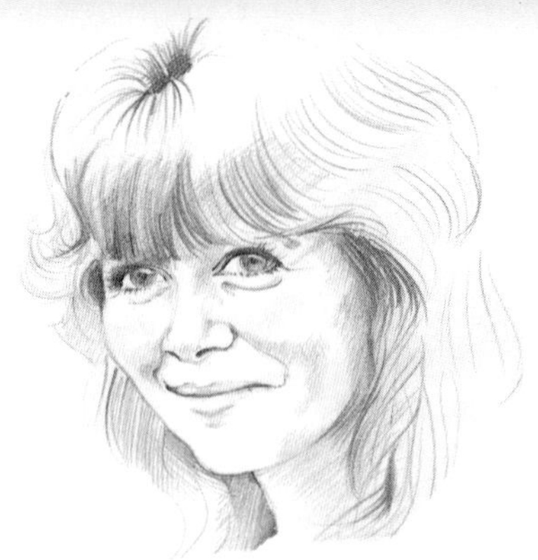

The physical changes of ageing that affect men and women alike are shown on page 129. There is one change in the middle years, however, that affects only women — the alteration in the reproductive system known as the menopause.

Menopausal changes

The word menopause means literally 'end of periods' and no more than that. It is not a description of an illness, nor a description of what happens over a period of time. It is not accurate to say that a women is 'going through the menopause' because the word can only be used accurately to define what has happened after the last loss of blood from the vagina has occurred. However, it is so common a phrase it might as well be accepted by all of us, though a more correct label would be climacteric; this is a Latin word which means 'a critical point in human life' which, though it can be used for other times of life, such as when a child enters puberty, tends to be used for this middle stage. It can be applied to men, too, in this context. They don't have periods, so have no menopause, but they often have the 'mid-life crisis' experience.

The process of climacteric change commences in women sometime in the late forties. It is not possible to foretell when any one woman will start hers (there is no proof of the old belief that the younger a girl is when she starts her periods, the older she will be when they end) but the average age in the UK seems to be about forty-nine though this may be altered by the effects of cigarette smoking. (There is evidence that the menopause occurs on average two or three years earlier in smokers.) But since this is an average it means that some will start as young as forty or so, and some will not start till they are fifty-five. In a few cases, it may happen under the age of forty or after the age of fifty-five, but this is rare.

Equally variable is the sort of experience a woman will have and the sort of signs and symptoms she will recognize. For some women — these are only a few — there is a sudden cessation of periods and that is that. They have no problems of any kind.

For some there is a pattern of changing periods — sometimes short, sometimes long, but with the flow diminishing as the years go on until, after three or four years, they cease altogether.

For others there is a great storm of symptoms, some of which can be directly related to what is actually happening in the body, others which it seems are more likely to be due to the woman's emotional profile, her life experience and psychological stresses.

Hormonal changes

What is happening inside the body is that the hormone control which has been steadily ebbing and flowing for the past thirty-five years or so begins to falter. The ovary, by now an ageing scarred organ which shows by its pitted surface that a great many of the eggs it carried have been ripened and shed, ceases to respond as it once did to the surges of stimulating hormone from the pituitary. It doesn't shed an egg, and doesn't send out its own estrogen, so a period is missed.

The pituitary, failing to get the message (from estrogen levels, in the blood) that its stimulation has worked, redoubles its efforts and sends out another surge of stimulating hormone. This may trigger the tiring ovary so that it does go into action — and it may go into uneven action, producing enough estrogen to make the uterus respond with a heavy period at an unexpected time.

As time goes on, the pituitary will continue to try to stimulate the ovaries, but will eventually stop. This is why the periods are so erratic in these last years, and why there can be heavy, flooding periods, which can be very debilitating (see menorrhagia, page 52, Section four).

There may still be an occasional ovulation — egg shedding — and it is possible for a woman to become pregnant because her erratic periods make planning her contraception difficult. There is a higher risk of producing a damaged infant in older women (a two per cent risk of a Down's Syndrome baby which increases with age) and as very few women approaching fifty want more children, often an abortion has to be decided upon. To avoid such distressing experiences, women are usually advised to use contraception till they have had two period free years under the age of fifty, and one period free year after the age of fifty. Then it is felt that the ovaries no longer function and fertility has gone.

Hot flushes/sweats

Because estrogen affects other parts of the body as well as the uterus, the effects of its changing balance are experienced elsewhere, and one of the most tiresome for the woman it happens to (and that is about eighty per cent of menopausal women) is the effect on heat control mechanisms; the blood vessels, which can expand and contract to carry blood to the surface to be cooled when necessary, are so confused by the changes in estrogen and related hormone levels that they suddenly send a good deal of blood to the body's surface to be cooled. The result is the hot flush; in the USA it's called the hot flash — a slightly alarming term to some British ears, seeming to suggest a bolt of lightning rather than the somewhat slower surging up of heat which is what actually happens.

Whatever the label, it can be an uncomfortable experience. A feeling of being extremely hot washes over the woman, while her upper chest, arms, neck and face redden. The reddening can be widespread, reaching down to the belly, and she feels so fiery that she is sure everyone can see what is happening. There is also often a marked sweating response which can be embarrassing for some. In fact it never looks as obvious as the women thinks it does; many say that if they can be near a mirror when a flush happens and watch the effect they are surprised how little it actually shows, considering how intense the sensation can be.

Anxiety reactions

In some women the flush makes them feel giddy and sick and it may be accompanied by a surge of adrenalin (remember all the hormones work together) so that there is also a sense of fear, trembling and belly fluttering — all the familiar sensations of panic.

If a woman knows what is happening and understands there is nothing dangerous going on inside her, however uncomfortable she may feel, she should be able to let the flush roll over her and away. It usually will within thirty seconds or so, though in some unfortunate women it can persist for a minute or two. It is much more likely to last a long time in the woman who becomes agitated about what is happening. Her agitation will increase the adrenalin response and with it the flushing and unpleasant sensations.

Sadly, some women become so unnerved by their early experiences of flushing that they become over anxious and hyperventilate; they breathe deeply and rapidly as a reaction to their fear (a useful thing to do if you need extra oxygen to run away or to fight; not useful if you don't) and this leads to other symptoms including pins and needles affecting hands and arms; giddiness, dazzling of vision ('spots before the eyes') and sometimes painful cramps of the hands so that they go into a claw-like spasm. All very frightening. But only remotely due to the effects of the pituitary trying to whip the tired ovaries into action; most of the response is due to the woman's exaggerated reaction to that.

Once women know what is happening and are reassured there is no dire illness at work, many of them learn very rapidly how to relax when a flush occurs, and how to sit or stand quietly till it fades away. Sometimes a flush can be short-circuited by using cooling techniques — running cold water over the pulse points at the wrist, sipping cold drinks and sitting in a direct breeze, and so on. If it happens at night, and causes night sweats, which are not uncommon (the actual hormonal action which causes night sweats is slightly different from that which causes daytime flushes, but the basic mechanism is the same) then throwing off the bedcovers so that sweat can dry on the skin and so cool it is all that is needed. It's better not to dry yourself laboriously (unless you are very uncomfortable and get too cool) because that can sometimes send you off into another sweat. The simplest way to short circuit an overbreathing attack is to breath in and out of a paper bag. That reduces the amount of oxygen you get, increases the amount of carbon dioxide, and so regulates the breathing and banishes the hyperventilation symptoms.

Skin reactions

Other body effects due to alterations in estrogen levels are noticed in the skin; the loss of elasticity that is inevitable in the fifth and sixth decades of life is accelerated, and an underlying thinning which had been happening anyway becomes more apparent and a woman may say she has 'gone wrinkled overnight'. This isn't in fact true; it's just that the deepening of the lines that were already there make her actually see them for the first time (it's amazing how you can look in the mirror regularly to do your hair and makeup and yet not actually see what is going on on your own face).

Something else which may suddenly become more apparent is hair in the moustache and beard areas. All women have some, but often it is so soft and light it is not apparent (though some women may inherit hairiness; it's a marked feature of Mediterranean women, for example, and is often much admired in them). As the estrogen is withdrawn from the circulation, this hair may thicken and increase, and become noticeable for the first time.

It happens because the male-type hormone all women naturally have — it's called androgen — and which in the reproductive years is damped down by high blood levels of estrogen, becomes more powerful. This creates the new hairiness. For some women it does something else — it increases their sexual desire. The ribald music-hall style jokes about sexually insatiable old women are based on this observation.

Even more significant however, than what happens on the facial skin, is what is happening to the sexual skin — the mucous membrane that lines the vulva and vagina.

This becomes thinner and less able to produce quantities of lubricating liquid. This can alter the normal acid balance of the vagina and allow infection to get in and establish itself. The result can be a particularly uncomfortable form of thrush, or other types of infection, which can be hard to eradicate.

Sexual reactions

The thinning of the vaginal lining also means that the mucous membrane is tighter   it loses some of its elasticity just as skin does. This can make the vagina tighter and drier — an effect which may increase the tenderness and fragility of the vulva, and lead to attacks of cystitis (see Section seven) and also, obviously, can affect a woman's sexual responses. She may find she takes longer to lubricate when she is sexually aroused and, not realising how dry she is, allows the penis to penetrate too soon and finds it painful. There can be 'burning' sensations (there is no actual burning of course) generalized soreness, possibly some bleeding and, naturally, an inability to reach orgasm (it's hard to relax and enjoy yourself when you hurt).

Since hormone levels do play a part in sexual arousal (though by no means the only or even the most important part) there may side by side with all this be some loss of sexual desire. The tendency to get a little more tired after a day's work, the effects of the worries and anxieties there may be in the woman's life can also make her less willing to embark on sex. It all becomes lumped together with the changes in the vagina to make the woman more and more unwilling to try. And there is great truth in the old adage that 'if you don't use it, you lose it'. The less a woman engages in sexual arousal, the less she wants to, so it all becomes a downwards spiral.

If she also has the totally unnecessary notion that 'people of my age shouldn't have sex anyway' that can be enough to turn her into a complete celibate, much to her partner's distress. He too is likely to be at a stage of his life when he is noticing some loss of his sexual powers and this can make him very uneasy. If his partner spurns him he is, sadly, unlikely to see this as a problem she is trying to cope with; he will see himself as 'unsexy' and may either lose his own potency, or more distressing still, try to prove to himself and to his partner that he is still the sexy creature he always was, by rushing off to have an affair with a younger woman. There are far too many marriage breakdowns of this sort in this age group that could be avoided if only both partners knew what middle age and the menopause actually does and how some of its less agreeable effects can be circumvented.

The important thing to know is that the hormonal action of the body can be stimulated; it is all controlled via a series of feedback loops; the pituitary sends out gushes of stimulating hormone whenever there is too little ovarian hormone in the blood. It also does so when it is triggered by the thinking part of the brain — the cortex — which responds to the sexual stimuli of words, pictures or emotional reactions.

What all this means is that a woman who makes a deliberate attempt to be sexy, turning herself on by whatever means she chooses, can lift her own hormone levels and make herself enjoy her sexual encounter. She needs, of course, to overcome any local discomfort that might have led to the first unwillingness to engage in sex — the dryness. She can use a simple water-based lubricant (KY Jelly is probably the best) which is very effective at smoothing the vaginal mucous membrane and making sex pleasurable. The tightness won't be affected by the KY Jelly but since that can actually increase the couple's pleasure (the woman can feel the penis more strongly and the man can feel the vagina more closely) most people don't mind that.

The more often a woman engages in sex at this stage of her life, the more she will improve her own hormone levels by perfectly natural means.

Eventually, of course, the pituitary gland will give up trying to thump the ovaries into action and the hormone surges will stop. The flushes will cease, and the thin, dry vagina won't get any thinner or drier. The woman can then go on enjoying her sex for a long time, because although she has lost the hormonal fragment of her drive, she will still have the emotional and intellectual elements. And they remain unchanged, or can even be enhanced with the years.

A note to those women who find that because of the increase in their androgen levels, as estrogen fades, they become more amorous; this is nothing to be ashamed of or to fear. It's something to be glad of, and will be envied by those women who find their drive fades as their estrogen does. The best advice the high-androgen woman can be given is to enjoy, enjoy!

Structural alterations

The body of the woman at the menopause does alter in shape. The breasts lose a good deal of their now no longer needed milk-making tissues, and the inner lips of the vulva become smaller and thinner. The uterus starts to diminish in size too, and this shrinking will go on until, in old age, the woman's reproductive organs are much the same size as they were before she started puberty. She comes, as it were, full circle. But this is a later stage, and for many women doesn't happen until the late seventies or even after.

Ageing effects include loss of skin elasticity, muscle power, bone tissue, cartilage density, hair colour and thickness, speed in nerve impulses and alteration of fat distribution.

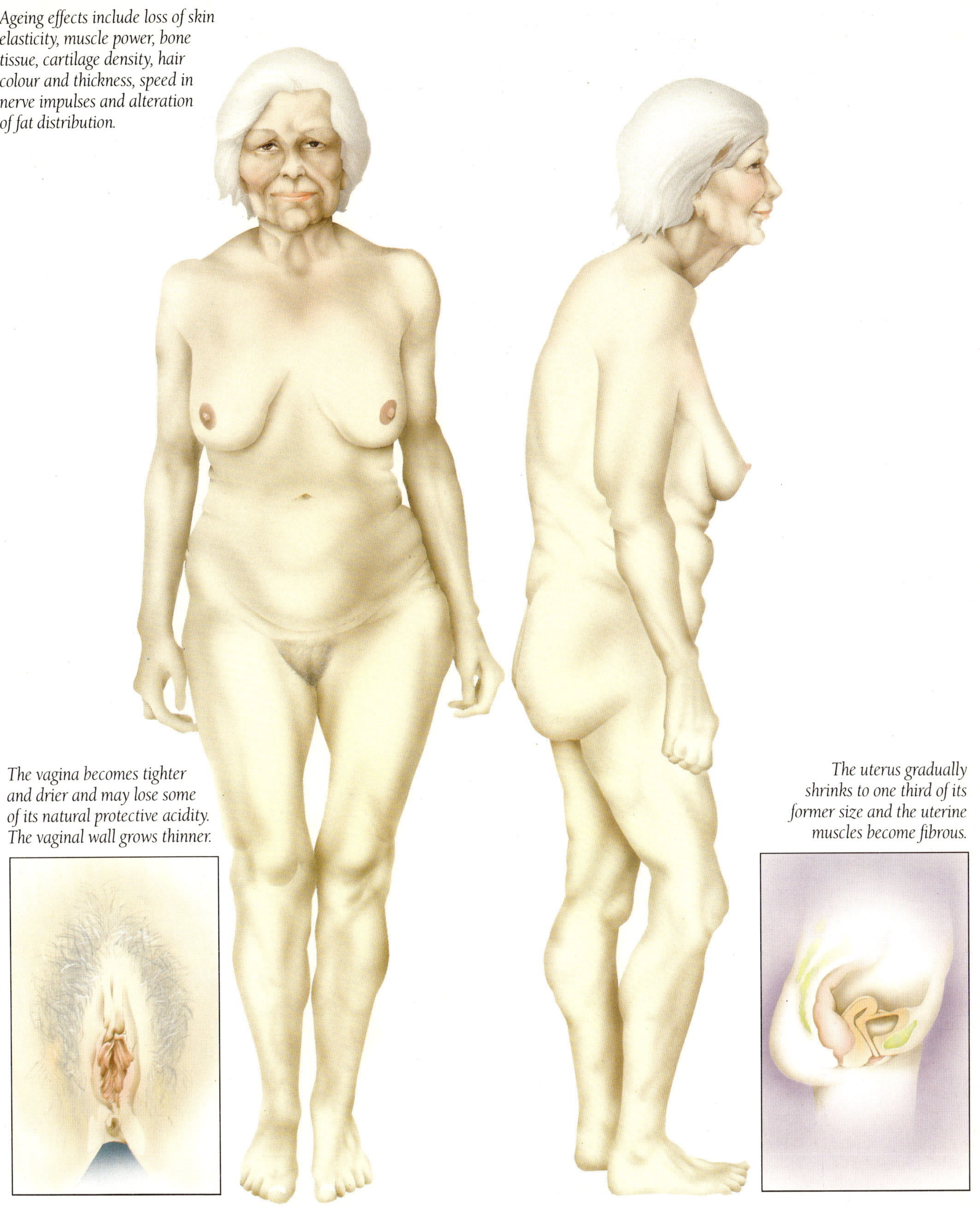

The vagina becomes tighter and drier and may lose some of its natural protective acidity. The vaginal wall grows thinner.

The uterus gradually shrinks to one third of its former size and the uterine muscles become fibrous.

This is one time of life when being rather plump is a blessing. Women get their estrogen not only from their ovaries but from their fat stores (estrogen is a steroid hormone — that is, it has a fat-like molecule). Women who are fat therefore are likely to have added estrogen in their blood long after the ovaries are no longer functioning. Thin women on the other hand will not, and in their later years become very much thinner and more frail, particularly in regard to their bones.

Osteoporosis is the name given to the condition in which the bones become diminished in mass, and sometimes so weak that they break easily, or in the case of the spine, collapse. This accounts for the high incidence of broken wrists and legs among the elderly in icy weather and also for their occasional humped backs.

It happens to men as well as women but more commonly to women because estrogen plays so important a role in the way bone is made and maintained. Once again, fatter women are better off than thin ones when it comes to this problem. Not only do they have more estrogen; the heavier a person is the more dense and strong do their bones become. Weightlessness can lead very rapidly to bony loss, as the NASA people found when they checked on the health of the astronauts who had spent long periods in space.

Smoking too contributes to bony loss; the mechanism by which this happens isn't quite clear, though it may possibly be linked with the way nicotine causes blood vessels to constrict, and so reduces the blood supply to the bones as well as other body parts.

It is possible to avoid some of the effects of osteoporosis (see page 131) and this is important because prevention is the only answer. Once bony mass has been lost it can't be replaced.

Muscular changes

In addition to the ordinary loss of muscle strength that comes with age, women after the menopause have a greater problem because of the loss of hormone which is closely involved with muscle tone. This can have a particularly marked effect on the strength of the pelvic floor muscles. Some women experience a sudden prolapse of the uterus and bulging of the vaginal walls, and need treatment — possibly surgery — to correct the weakness. (See Section eight.)

Aches and pains

Often women experiencing their mid-life changes complain of a whole range of symptoms that appear not to be linked with any changes of estrogen levels. Pains in joints and muscles and belly; headaches; nausea; depression; sleeplessness; changes in appetite; changes in thinking patterns; nightmares and many more are reported. It is these symptoms, which seem not to be due directly to the hormonal changes of the menopause, that cause most of the misery women talk about, rather than the two symptoms which can be proven to be directly attributable to it, which are hot flushes and vaginitis (the thinning and drying of the vagina).

Hormone replacement therapy

For many years women seeking help with problems like this felt their doctors shrugged them away with a dismissive 'It's your age, my dear. You'll just have to grin and bear it,' and felt very angry as well as miserable in consequence. But to be fair to the doctors, it wasn't necessarily just a masculine refusal to take women seriously that created this response. Women doctors who have themselves reached menopausal age have been known to say the same thing to their patients.

The point is that though it may be possible that some of these symptoms are linked with the experience of fluctuating estrogen levels, it is hard to prove they are. And if it is not proven, the answer that some women seek — the replacement of their lost natural hormones with supplements — may be dangerous for them. It sounds so simple; if a woman has symptoms during the years of the menopause, it must be because she is short of hormone. Give her back the hormone and all will be well. And, after all, if women who have their ovaries removed at hysterectomy operations have this treatment, why not give it to women whose ovaries have failed because of the menopause? But it isn't so simple. Hormones are powerful and when used as a drug — to treat symptoms — they can behave like any other drug and cause side effects. The more power a treatment has to do good, remember, the more it has to do harm.

And over the years, there has been much anxiety about the possibility that hormone replacement therapy — HRT — can do harm as well as good. High estrogen in the blood can contribute to thrombo-embolic disease in which blood clots within blood vessels, and can lead to a heart attack or stroke, and it has also been suspected of contributing to cancer of the uterine lining. Research in the USA suggested that a marked increase in the incidence of this sort of cancer was linked with an increase in the use of HRT. Also it has been suggested that it might be involved in heart disease, though some research results have appeared which suggest that maybe estrogen protects against breast lumps and so against cancer too.

Altogether the findings have been confusing. Some of the doubts about the safety of estrogen have been soothed by the use of a special form called conjugated estrogen which is said to be safe, but even so, many doctors — and their patients — are still very cautious. There are still questions unanswered about the effects of HRT in otherwise healthy women which British doctors worry about. And surely while the questions remain unanswered it is right and proper that we should all be cautious about prescribing and using HRT unless we can be certain a patient is suffering from deficiency.

And the only proven deficiency symptoms are flushes and vaginitis. Not depression or migraine headaches or aches and pains. These can be due to other causes, the more cautious doctors point out, and it's wiser to treat them with other remedies. Anti-depressants and/or psychotherapy for depression and anxiety; painkillers for headaches; and even for those with proven estrogen deficiency, if there is a history in an individual woman which makes her an extra doubtful candidate for treatment with it (say she has had a cancer in her reproductive system or breasts, or has had episodes of thrombosis) the use of a drug called clonidine which is not a steroid, but which acts on the central nervous system and so on blood vessel activity, can be very effective for hot flushes and for migraines.

There is only one other condition for which HRT is the only remedy and that is osteoporosis. The evidence that it is possible to prevent bony loss in middle aged women by improving the level of calcium in the diet — calcium being the stuff of which bones are made — is not impressive. Calcium can only be taken up and used by the bones via a complex biochemical process, and estrogen has an important role to play in that process. So, a woman who is thin and who smokes may need estrogen in the menopausal years to protect her from the effects of osteoporosis (though she'd be better off giving up smoking).

Apart from these three problems — flushes, vaginitis, and osteoporosis — medical caution about the giving of HRT is to be respected and appreciated rather than damned. It has become an article of faith with some women to complain most bitterly that doctors who refuse to give HRT to all women who ask for it are anti-feminine — but aren't such women actually being more anti-feminine than the doctors they complain about? To suggest that all older women are suffering from some sort of deficiency disease, simply because they no longer fizz with estrogen, is to insult them much more than to behave with caution about prescribing a potentially risky therapy. There were doctors, notably in America, who espoused the cause of HRT with enormous enthusiasm, announcing that with its use women could be 'feminine for ever' — thus implying that without it we are neutered. That has to be the most insulting nonsense ever; we *are* feminine for ever, whether we're being pumped full of steroid drugs or not.

The fact is that by no means all women have a bad time at the menopause. Some, those who are busy and happy and fulfilled in their work and their relationships, may not notice or can brush aside the occasional irritating effects of changes in their hormone balance due to the menopause. These are the older bolder women who know that their greater experience of living, their learned wisdom and their applied intelligence make them as exciting and attractive and interesting as personalities as ever they were in their youth.

Some women have a stormier time, but still manage to cope without taking hormones, preferring not to and using other remedies as they require them — notably the self-help systems of relaxation and exercise and sensible diet (see Section ten). But finally there are those women who, despite their commonsense approach and sensible self-care, have a very difficut time with waves of hot flushes — and some do — or really uncomfortable vaginitis that causes constant cystitis and thrush attacks. They may indeed need HRT. And for them, if their general health is good and their lifestyle healthy, it will work well.

HRT administration

Because of the risk of endometrial cancer when estrogen is given unopposed, it is usual today to give it in tandem with progestogen for part of each four week cycle of pills, so that the uterus builds up and sheds a lining regularly. This mimics a period and can be a drawback for those women who find it tiresome to have to deal with a monthly (or three monthly) bleed when they are well into their fifties, but it is the price that has to be paid for safety. (Added safety measures may include regular examinations of the lining of the uterus, necessitating D and C operations from time to time.)

A common pattern is for estrogen alone to be given for sixteen days and then progestogen is added for twelve days, though there are different systems. It can also be given as an implant which means a pellet of the hormone is inserted under the skin to release its contents over a period of around thirty-six weeks.

If the main symptom is vaginitis it may be simpler to use a local cream containing estrogen. This has the benefit of putting the hormone where it is most needed, while reducing its general effects on the body, though some is absorbed into the circulation from the walls of the vagina and the vulva. (Never use it just before intercourse, by the way; a man can absorb it through his penis with alarming effects — he may get a little 'breasty'.)

A woman having HRT should be checked regularly by her doctor. Her blood pressure should be at normal levels; if it rises, this can be dangerous because of the possible effects of thrombo-embolism. Regular cervical smears and breast checks are also needed during the use of HRT. It is rare that it can be continued much after the age of sixty, and there may in some women be some rebound symptoms for a while once the treatment is stopped. After hysterectomy the use of HRT is much safer — no uterus in which cancer might arise — and it can be given continuously.

One extra word of warning; it is possible to become dependent on estrogen, just as on any other drug (and used as HRT estrogen is a drug). For these women, coming off after prolonged use can create problems.

Lifestyle problems

No good doctor will give HRT to a woman who does not show that she has actual estrogen deficiency symptoms. Those who complain only of depression and headaches and loss of sex drive and so on will need other help. It has been suggested that one reason for the distress menopausal women suffer is the contrast with their own daughters who are going through puberty just as they reach their difficult years. This has to be poppycock, spouted by people who can't do arithmetic. For a woman to reach her menopause at the same time as a daughter reaches puberty she would have to have given birth to the girl when she was around forty, since puberty happens around twelve or so. The average woman has her babies in her twenties and thirties. Most of them are still ten or fifteen years ahead of their menopause when their daughters are pubertal.

Similarly it is silly to suggest that women suffer symptoms of the menopause just because they are 'getting old'. Forty-nine or fifty isn't old at all; it's still a peak time in any healthy person's life. Many are the people appointed to high political office who are described as 'young' because they are only fifty-five or so.

But it is true that some women suffer what can be labelled as menopausal symptoms because of their life experience. Women still, in many areas of life, get a bad deal. We have to work harder, push more, shout louder and generally shove a great deal longer to get equality of opportunity with the men in our lives. We tend too often to be lumbered with all aspects of domesticity, and not just the care of babies. We often hold ourselves back by our own poor opinion of our capabilities and our low aspirations for ourselves. That this can lead to depression, anxiety and assorted aches and pains in mid life is perfectly understandable. There are men who feel that they have been passed over, have failed in some way, are losing their drive and their energy who display exactly the same symptoms. They are not menopausal. They are experiencing a mid-life crisis. Women need to be sure that when they have problems in their forties and fifties they are correctly identifying the causes. It isn't reasonable to blame your hormones when it's your home or your husband or your housework or your hatred of your job that is to blame. And it's surely foolish to think that taking a potentially risky drug like estrogen is going to relieve such feelings.

Generic Name	Trade Name UK	Trade Name USA	Trade Name Australia	Trade name Canada
conjugated estrogens	Premarin	Premarin	Premarin	Premarin; Oestrilin
conjugated estrogens + norgestrel	Prempak-C	not available	not available	Enovid-E
danazol	Danol	Danocrine	Danocrine	Cyclomen
Dienoestrol	Ortho-cilag	Ortho-cilag	Ortho-cilag	Orthocilag
dydrogesterone	Duphaston	not available	Duphaston	not available
ethinyl estradiol	no trade name	Estinyl	Estigyn	Estinyl
ethinyl estradiol + methyltestosterone	Mixogen	Estratest	Mixogen; Primodian	Climacteron (injection)
medroxyprogestrone	Provera	Provera; Amen	Provera	Provera
mestranol + norethisterone	Menophase	not available	not available	Program
norethisterone	Primolut N; Utovlan	Aygestin; Norlutate	Primolut N	Norlutate
estradiol	Progynova; Hormonin*	Estrace	Progynova	Estrace
estradion + levonorgestrel	Cyclo-Progynova	not available	Ovestin	Ovulen 0.5
estriol	Ovestin	not available	Ovestin	not available
estrogen-progestogen	Ovran; Eugynon 50	Ovral; Nordette	Ovral; Eugynon	Ovral
piperazine-estrone	Harmogen	Ogen	Ogen	Ogen
quinestradol	Pentovis	not available	not available	not available

*The product contains active ingredients other than that in the generic name column

Avoiding problems

According to research in South Africa some women can be identified as particularly likely to suffer disagreeable menopausal symptoms. Others are particularly resilient and will have few symptoms and will cope well. The value of this research is that it shows women some aspects of their personalities that they can modify to make themselves less vulnerable. The research shows that there are three areas which indicate how a woman is likely to react.

The first is her psychosomatic responsiveness. Some people tend to develop physical reactions to emotional states more easily than others — a response that is, to an extent, self-taught. These women condition themselves to be aware of every bodily sensation, instead of blocking out many of them, as non-physical reactors do.

The second is a woman's personal life satisfaction. The amount of pleasure and reward she gets seems to have a direct effect on how she will cope with new physical changes.

And the third is sex stereotype attitudes. A woman's view of what is 'womanly' and what is 'manly' and her own opinion of how she fits into the stereotype can again have a direct action on her physical health.

The following 'quiz' is based on this research. Answering the questions could help you to identify your own potential to react in less than happy ways to your mid-life years and your menopause.

Tick **a**, **b** or **c** answers and then add up your score.

Quiz

1 When you are worried, under stress or depressed, do you get physical symptoms, such as headaches, nausea, diarrhoea, breathlessness, dizziness, palpitations?
a. Yes
b. No
c. Occasionally.

2 When you have a period do you suffer from cramps, nausea, diarrhoea, headache, bloatedness?
a. Yes
b. No
c. Occasionally.

3 When pregnant, did you experience sickness, fainting, aches, constant anxiety? (If you have never been pregnant, mark **b**.)
a. Yes
b. No
c. Occasionally.

4 If you are married or live with a partner, does the relationship in all aspects — sexual, financial, companionable, intellectual — give you
a. More strain than satisfaction
b. More satisfaction than strain
c. About equal strain and satisfaction?
(If you are alone, mark **c.**)

5 If you have children, does your relationship with them give you
a. More strain than satisfaction
b. More satisfaction than strain
c. About equal strain and satisfaction?
(If you are childless, mark **c.**)

6 Do you enjoy looking after other people — especially children — listening, sympathizing, feeding, cuddling?
a. No
b. Yes
c. Sometimes.

7 Do you feel that when crises arise in your life you have ample support from family and friends?
a. No
b. Yes
c. Sometimes.

8 Whatever your work, be it shop, office, factory, or housewife, do you find it

a. Unsatisfying
b. Satisfying
c. Neither one nor the other?

9 When you look at yourself — appearance, personality — do you
a. Like nothing you see
b. Like all you see
c. Like and dislike yourself equally?

10 Are you
a. More interested in your home and relationships than in outside activities like work and social life
b. Equally interested in both
c. More interested in your work and social life than your home and relationships?

11 If your ordinary routine collapses — the washing machine breaks down, a child gets ill, extra work is loaded on to you in your job, unexpected guests arrive for dinner — do you
a. Find you can't cope at all and panic
b. Rise to the challenge, cope well, pleased with your own resourcefulness
c. Plod on regardless, neither panicking nor coping?

12 Would you describe yourself as
a. Timid
b. Self-assertive
c. Sometimes assertive, sometimes timid?

To score, give yourself 0 for every **a** you ticked, 2 for every **b** and 1 for every **c**.

If you scored zero, then you are very rare; a totally vulnerable person who has frequent aches and distressing symptoms, almost an invalid in fact — and have been so all your life. You'll almost certainly have as stormy a menopause as your life has been already.

If you scored twelve or less then you are on the vulnerable side. It could be that you are a psychosomatic reactor (look at questions 1 to 3 — you probably answered 'Yes' to all of them). Or you could be unsatisfied with your relationships (see questions 4 to 8 — your answers were probably 'Yes' again).

If you scored between fourteen and twenty-four, you're resilient. You have your vulnerable spots which you can strengthen, but you're not doing badly. You'll probably have a tolerable menopause with symptoms you'll cope with well.

If you scored twenty-four then you are rare indeed — a totally resilient woman who never gets psychosomatic disorders, loves her job, her lifestyle, her partner, her children. You will have a very comfortable menopause even though you may have a few minor problems such as occasional hot flushes, but you won't allow even these to perturb you unduly.

Whichever it is, you will now know which areas of your life need to be changed. If you're a psychosomatic reactor you can teach yourself to relax, and not to respond to stress with physical symptoms and to refuse to listen to the inner workings of your own body. Even something as simple as taking up yoga can teach you to do this. Or, learning the art of relaxation (see Section ten) can give you more resilience and remove some of that vulnerability.

If the problems are in your relationships and your workload, be it as housewife or as earner, then again the road to the remedy is clearly signposted. You may need counselling to put the satisfaction back in your marriage, or in your relationship with your children. You may need a radical rethink of your job, and a more determined effort (even in these hard times) to get better and more satisfying employment.

If you have a negative view of your role as a woman, then you need other women to shore you up and give you back some self-esteem, and with it some resilience. Joining a lively women's group can offer just that. Women working at anything together help each other to feel more positive, more able to cope with life and less liable to unpleasant menopause symptoms, because the research does show that the way a woman experiences and copes with her life is powerfully affected by psychological and lifestyle factors which are, to a large extent, in her own hands.

Nowhere in this section is there any information on how to 'look your best', what makeup or clothes to use to 'disguise your faults' or any similar suggestions. No woman who has reached her middle years really needs someone else to tell her how to do that. She is perfectly capable of searching out her own style of makeup and clothes to make the best of herself, so that she likes the way she looks and is content with the effect she has on others. To suggest that any woman needs a makeover, or lots of earnest advice on How To Be A Successful Woman just because she is in her forties or fifties is to be insulting. This is, as I know very well on my own account a marvellous age to be. I can say with total honesty that I have never felt better than I do now, never thought I looked much better, never cared less about other's disapproval, never felt better able to listen to and act on constructive criticism. The best thing about maturity is the marvellous freedom it has brought me to be myself, and to run my own life in my own way. Children grown and responsibility for them lessened means I — and my partner — can be cheerfully selfish again; any loss of physical power due to age is more than made up for by my gathered knowledge and trained mental agility.

10

WOMAN'S WELLBEING

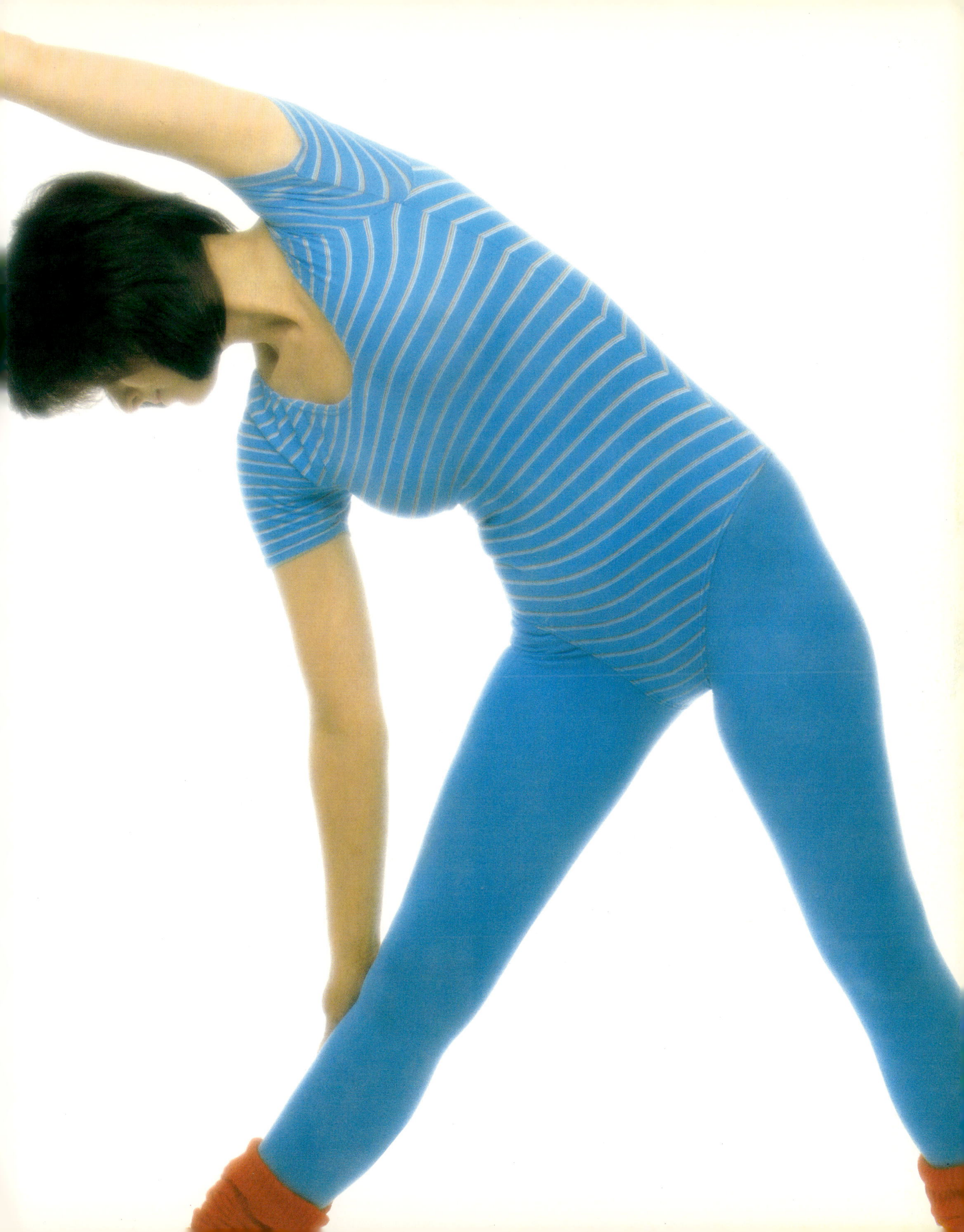

Some of the prophets of our times preach so loudly of the vital importance of what we eat and what exercise we do and how due attention to such matters is all that is needed to ensure perfect health, you would be forgiven for getting the idea that feeling ill or indeed being in anything less than absolutely top condition at all times is a personal failure. If you just put your mind to it, watching every mouthful you eat, counting the calories, checking the additives and training each and every muscle till it is as finely tuned as a Rolls Royce about to enter a Grand Prix race, then, the gurus seem to assure us, you can be Superwoman. Poppycock.

To become so perfectly 'in health' would demand a degree of concentration that would border on the obsessional. There would be no time for anything else, like reading or thinking or making love or sitting staring at the sky. It's like the rules we are offered for being beautiful. It is clear we could all look like polyurethane sprayed angels of light if we were prepared to invest fifteen hours of every day, seven days a week, fifty weeks a year — and a great deal of money — in beauty regimes. But that wouldn't make us really beautiful. We'd just look like expensive polyurethane sprayed angels of light on the surface, while inside we'd be deeply, jaw-crackingly boring. In the same way, being obsessive about physical health would not make us healthy inside. In fact it would make us psychologically somewhat sick.

So this section is not designed to bring you perfect health in a handful of easy-to-read pages. It offers only an overview of the present accepted wisdom as regards healthy regimes, with special reference to food and exercise and relaxation. By the time this book is published it may well be that some of this wisdom will have been superseded by new information about how the human frame should be fed and worked.

And in a hundred years or so, people may well laugh themselves sick at what we, in our benighted late twentieth century foolishness, thought was good for us, just as we tend to laugh now at the quaintness of Victorian books on women's health and welfare. (Actually, not all of them; there are some that are very wise indeed.)

Since people are made largely of food (there is also water and oxygen and other items in us) nutrition is a reasonable point at which to start looking at basic health regimes.

Food

The human animal is omniverous; it can and does eat everything and anything that can provide the essential building materials it needs for its body, and to supply the fuel that drives it. In different cultures, in different parts of the world, at different times in history, humans have eaten a startlingly wide selection of materials. Every animal that ever moved, from ants via bees, grubs, worms, snakes, rats and mice and birds even to each other (human flesh was considered a special delicacy in many societies, having a mystical symbolic value to add to its calorie content) has been brought to the human dinner table. It is indeed a great asset to have so obliging a digestive and metabolic system; animals that are able to eat only very limited forms of food are far less adaptable than we are. That is one of the reasons why *homo sapiens* is the species that dominates the world, while the giant panda, which lives entirely on bamboo shoots, is dwindling into extinction any day now.

But like all assets, this one has its damaging side. Because we can eat anything and everything (well, almost everything; we're not as well adapted to living on grass as are cows, though we can do it for a while, if we have to) and are able to develop a taste for a bewildering variety of food, many of us are in danger of a particular form of malnutrition; over-nutrition. While a great many human beings lack enough of any food at all to live (famines in Ethiopia and other parts of Africa have killed literally millions) there are parts of the world where most people eat too much. It has been estimated that one person in four in the rich Western world has more fat on his or her body than they need. Furthermore, study of mortality patterns has shown that people in that twenty-five per cent have a much higher likelihood of suffering from arthritis (painful and inefficent joints) high blood pressure, which can damage heart and kidneys and contribute to sudden death from stroke or coronary thrombosis, and a few other unpleasant and potentially life-shortening disorders.

So it makes health sense for that twenty-five per cent of people to recognize their faulty diet and aim to put it right, so that they burn off the excess fat they are carrying. But only these people need to do this.

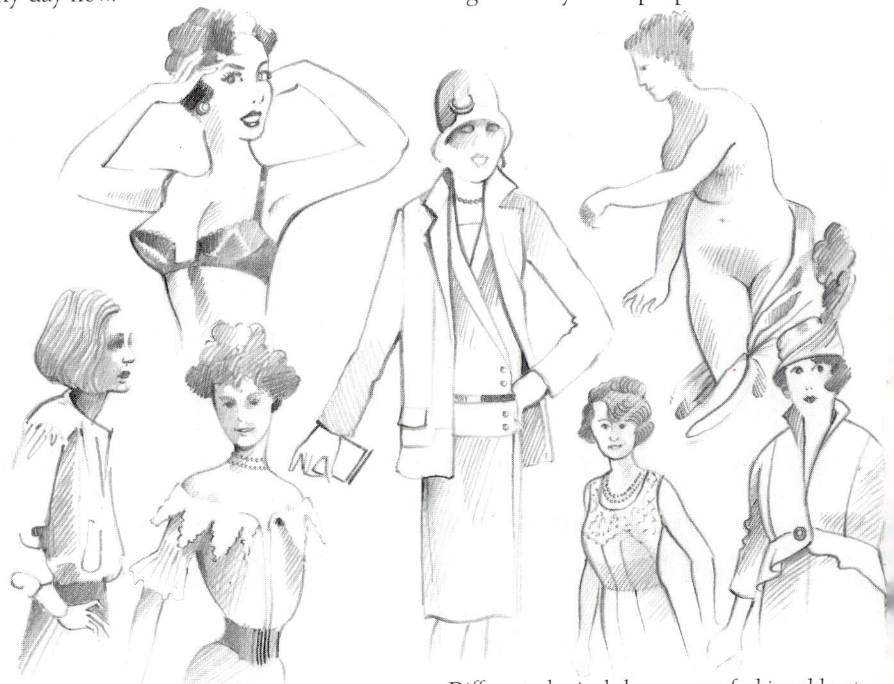

Different physical shapes were fashionable at different periods in history.

The rest of us can continue to eat as we always have, as long as we feel well and comfortable and are functioning normally on the food we swallow.

Yet, at any one time in the UK, around sixty-five per cent of women are dieting, that is, consciously altering their style of eating in order to reduce their fat stores and change their bodies. And when in surveys some of these dieting women were asked why they were so behaving the majority replied it was for cosmetic reasons, not for health ones, (unlike men who when they diet — and far fewer do — almost always do so for health reasons).

This is very unhealthy behaviour. We need our fat stores. They are necessary for continued health and normal functioning. Women who are too thin, remember, find that their periods cease, and that they have difficulties in conceiving (see Sections three and six). We need fat for cosmetic reasons, too. It is fat which gives women their rounded feminine shape that is so attractive to our sexual partners. Yet over and over again, women in the West are found to be obsessed with the need to diet away their normal body fat, and to make themselves unhealthily thin.

It really is very silly. In the past decades the fashion was for fat women; look at Rubens' models, at Edwardian ladies, at the pin-ups of the forties. Then there were periods when women were supposed to look like adolescent boys — the Regency, the twenties, the sixties. Now the aim is to 'look good on a camera' — and that tends to demand a hollowness of face and a thinness of body that resembles a victim of starvation.

We all need to accept ourselves for what we are; fat or thin, 'beautiful' or 'ugly' — none of these matter in any real way. It is self-acceptance, which goes hand-in-hand with self-esteem, that makes us interesting and attractive people, and therefore should govern us, not the opinions of people with goods to sell who use pictures of abnormally thin women to try to make us unhappy enough to buy those goods. A woman is a woman. We don't have to be starved into attractive feminity. We are attractive whatever we look like as long as we feel good about ourselves.

Effects of food deprivation

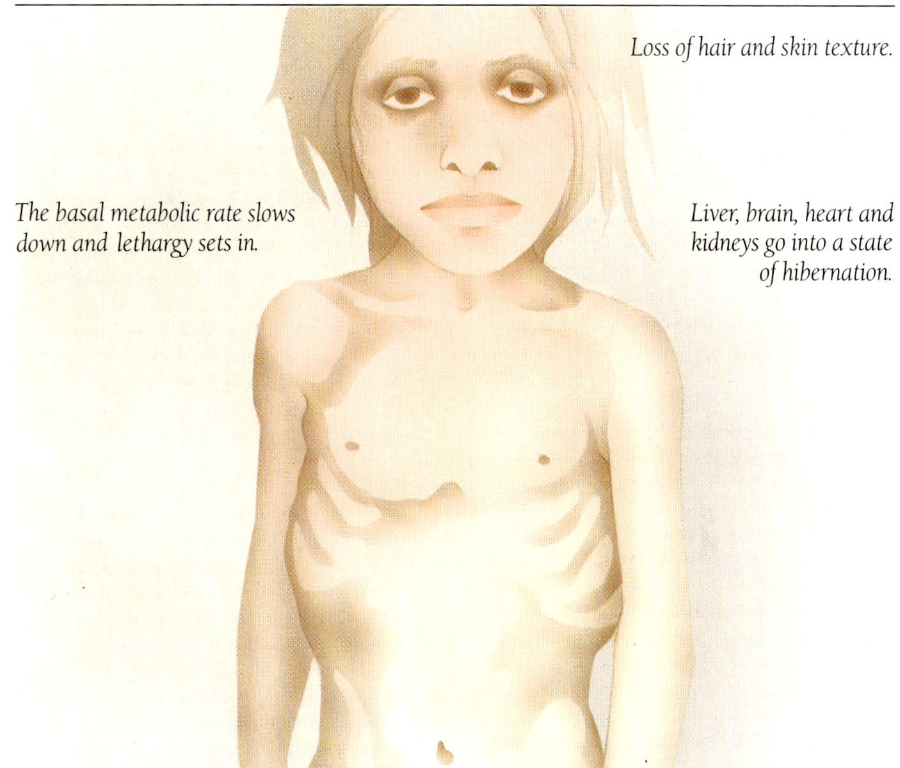

Loss of hair and skin texture.

The basal metabolic rate slows down and lethargy sets in.

Liver, brain, heart and kidneys go into a state of hibernation.

Fortunately, the idea that we do have to conform to a physical ideal in order to be successful women is slowly being eroded. Feminists are saying loud and clear that women diminish themselves as people rather than as physical bodies if they allow themselves to be brainwashed into constant dieting.

They are also pointing out a very important fact; continuous attempts at dieting can even make you fat. The human body is designed to survive at times of food failure — if you look at the people who have been starving in African famines these past years, you will see that, amazingly, they exist on incredibly low amounts of food. That is because we have physiological mechanisms that enable us to use minimal calories when few calories are available.

The basal metabolic rate — the speed at which the body burns fuel — slows down when food is withheld. The lungs use less oxygen. The level of vitamins, enzymes, hormones in body fluids — is disturbed and that means cell replacement and building ceases.

The whole body goes into a sort of hibernation state — vital organs such as liver, brain, heart and kidneys cut down to a marked degree their demands for calories. The person feels lethargic, anxious, withdrawn, often sleeps a good deal.

Then, as and when food again becomes available, the body immediately sets to work to convert as much of it as possible to fat, to store in case of yet another famine in the future.

This happens whether the lack of food is due to failure of crops and resulting famine in Africa, or a crash diet in a rich city suburb in Europe or America, and it accounts for the fact that many sad women discover too late — that the more they diet, and the more weight they lose, the more fat they put on as the years go by.

This is not to say that some people do not overeat, put on unhealthy fat and then need to get rid of it. This does happen. The reasons for overeating can be cultural (in some societies it is normal to eat vast meals — in Holland and Germany for example in

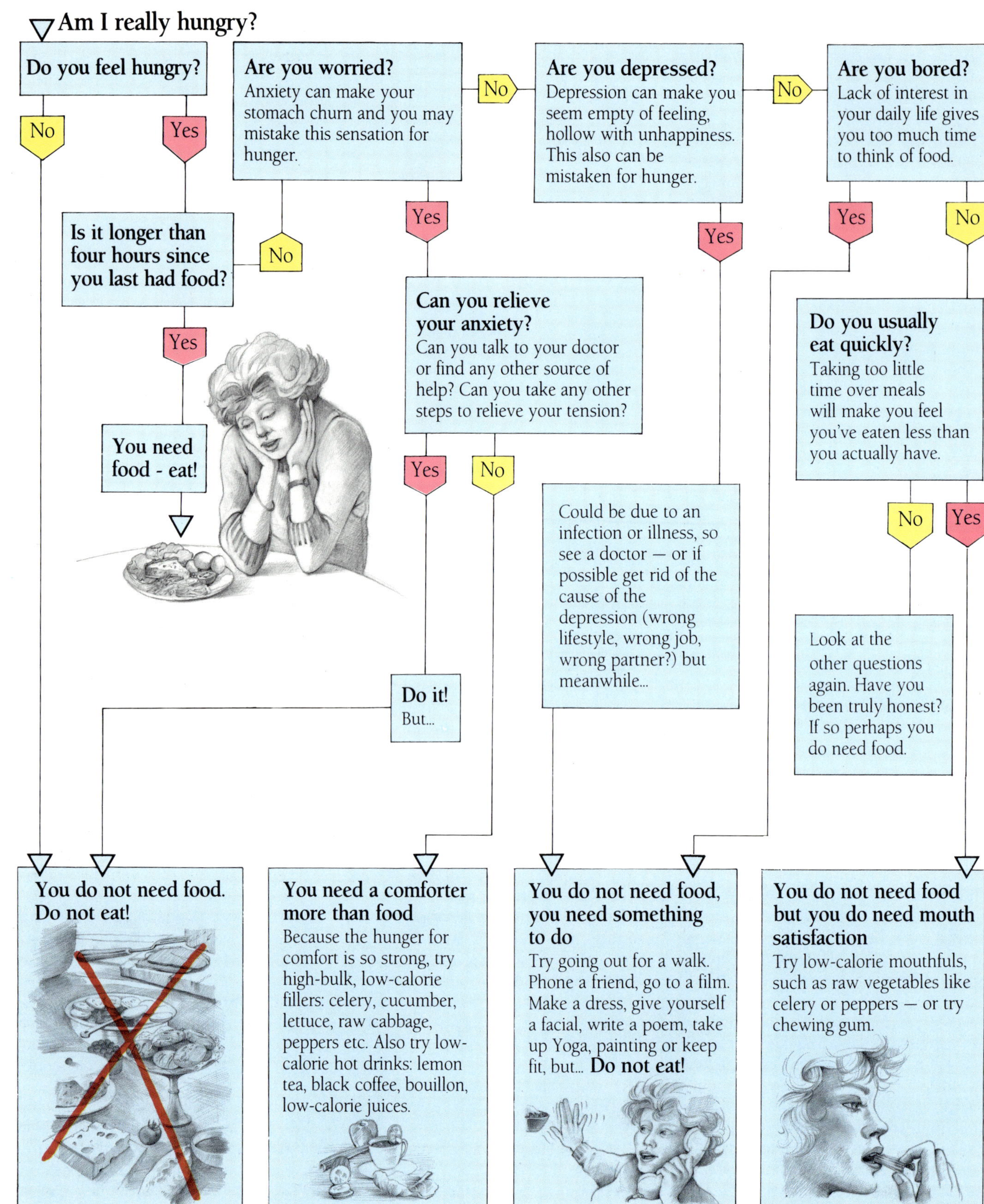
Am I really hungry?
Do you feel hungry?
No
Yes
Is it longer than four hours since you last had food?
No
Yes
You need food - eat!
Are you worried?
Anxiety can make your stomach churn and you may mistake this sensation for hunger.
No
Yes
Can you relieve your anxiety?
Can you talk to your doctor or find any other source of help? Can you take any other steps to relieve your tension?
Yes
No
Do it!
But...
Are you depressed?
Depression can make you seem empty of feeling, hollow with unhappiness. This also can be mistaken for hunger.
No
Yes
Could be due to an infection or illness, so see a doctor — or if possible get rid of the cause of the depression (wrong lifestyle, wrong job, wrong partner?) but meanwhile...
Are you bored?
Lack of interest in your daily life gives you too much time to think of food.
Yes
No
Do you usually eat quickly?
Taking too little time over meals will make you feel you've eaten less than you actually have.
No
Yes
Look at the other questions again. Have you been truly honest? If so perhaps you do need food.
You do not need food. Do not eat!
You need a comforter more than food
Because the hunger for comfort is so strong, try high-bulk, low-calorie fillers: celery, cucumber, lettuce, raw cabbage, peppers etc. Also try low-calorie hot drinks: lemon tea, black coffee, bouillon, low-calorie juices.
You do not need food, you need something to do
Try going out for a walk. Phone a friend, go to a film. Make a dress, give yourself a facial, write a poem, take up Yoga, painting or keep fit, but... Do not eat!
You do not need food but you do need mouth satisfaction
Try low-calorie mouthfuls, such as raw vegetables like celery or peppers — or try chewing gum.

the past a great many people ate hugely — and some still do). It may be due to anxiety; to misunderstood inner signals; to a sense of loneliness and sadness interpreted as physical rather than emotional hunger. The possibilities are many, and the flow chart opposite will show you how to identify them. Once you know, you can modify your behaviour. You do not need to go on a 'crash' diet. You just need to eat sensibly.

But if you are one of the twenty-five per cent of us who is overweight, how can you do that, and get rid of the fat you may have collected in the past?

The answer to this dilemma is not to diet, that is, deliberately reducing the amount of food you eat. You need to change the pattern of your eating, so that you take as much food as your hunger dictates, and so prevent your body putting up its defences against starvation, but seek out foods that provide fewer calories. (Calories incidentally are the units of heat that are produced by burning a set weight of each food, and are the measurements normally used to define the quantity and value of the food we eat.) To be able to discriminate you need information about what food is.

The food basics

There are seven constituents of food; protein; fats; carbohydrates; chemicals known as vitamins; metals and salts known as minerals; fibre; and water.

Proteins

These are the compounds forming the basic structure of living matter. We have to have a regular daily intake of protein for the repair, replacement and growth of all body cells and tissues. There are two kinds of protein; animal derived proteins (that includes meat, fish, eggs, cheese) and vegetable proteins (commonly found in peas, beans and other pulses and also in grains such as wheat and, therefore, in bread). Animal proteins can provide our essential intake in precisely the form the body needs it, but tend to be accompanied by fairly high quantities of animal fats. Even the leanest piece of steak, for example, will include fat in among the muscle fibres. Vegetable proteins are also accompanied by fat or oils in a large number of vegetables, but the amount of fat with vegetable protein tends to be less. It is also different in type (see below).

Protein is not a very bulky food but is very high in calories. It is very easy to eat more protein than you actually need at any one time, because of its lack of bulk; if you eat more protein than you require for replacement of your body tissues, the excess will be used to provide extra energy or — more likely — will be converted to fat for the body's fat store.

Fats

Fats provide energy and very small quantities are required for body repair and growth of tissues. It is also required to provide fatty tissues for insulation, and is essential to the body's use of certain vitamins (see page 140).

Fats are described as either saturated or unsaturated; generally speaking saturated fats are derived from animal foods and they tend to increase the amount of cholesterol in the blood. It has been suggested in many studies that cholesterol is the substance that must be incriminated in atheroma — the blocking up of the arteries which leads to high blood pressure and possibly to stroke and heart attack. Unsaturated fat which is found in vegetable oils and in fish and poultry is regarded as more healthy because it does not cause the increase of the amount of blood cholesterol.

Of all the vegetable fats, those derived from the sunflower, safflower, corn or soya bean are regarded as the healthiest, because they are polyunsaturated.

Fats are very high in calories; they are the most calorie rich foods of all.

Carbohydrates

These are the foods which contain carbon, hydrogen and oxygen, and this is what gives them their name. Anything that is sweet or starchy is a carbohydrate. Sugar, biscuits, bread, potatoes and other root vegetables and cereals, all are high in carbohydrates. Carbohydrates are an excellent source of energy and essential in the daily diet. They are not as high in calories as fats or proteins and are much bulkier. It is possible to eat a great deal of carbohydrate in volume to get the same number of calories that you would from a comparatively small quantity of fat or protein.

Fibre

This is the tough material that resists digestion in the human alimentary tract and is largely excreted in the stools. In the past it was regarded as an unnecessary part of food and great efforts were made to remove it from most staple items of diet. Bread was regarded as more palatable and agreeable if the bran was removed (the bran is the outer husk of the wheat and very rich in fibre). Today, fibre is regarded as an essential part of the diet, for many reasons. We suffer today from diseases that our ancestors of a couple of hundred years ago knew nothing about. For example, appendicitis. The first operation for removal of this little organ was done in 1848, and over the next fifty years or so it was still a very rare illness. Yet today, it is a common problem, and one which every schoolchild knows about. Many researchers today believe that this disease, together with many others, is a direct result of a profound change in our eating habits.

Over thousands of years, the human gut was evolved to deal with a bulky diet, largely vegetable in origin, and with a high proportion of cereals among those vegetable foods. Mankind learned to store his cereals and so for the dark months of the year this was his main food. In summer and autumn months he could eat fresh vegetables and fruits, and some meat and fish of course, but it was grain that was the most important. And he ate the whole grain. In a harsh world, not a scrap was ever wasted. He ate the lot.

But then humanity got clever — and richer. And people in the wealthiest areas began to demand a diet richer in fancy foods and lower in rough foods. So, the outer covering of the grain — called the bran — began to be

Vitamins

VITAMIN	VITAMIN A Provitamin, Carotene	VITAMIN B1 Thiamine	VITAMIN B2 Riboflavin	VITAMIN B3 Nictotinic acid, Anti-pellagra vitamin	VITAMIN B6	VITAMIN B12 Cyanoco-balamin
SOURCES	Butter, cheese, egg yolk, whole milk, fish liver oil, liver. Green leafy vegetables; all yellow vegetables, carrots. Artificial concentrates available in several forms.	Widely distributed in all plant and animal tissues but seldom occurs in high concentration. Whole grain cereals, peas, beans, peanuts, oranges, offal. Many vegetables, fruits, nuts.	Eggs, green vegetables, liver, kidney, lean meat, milk, wheat germ, dried yeast, enriched foods.	Yeast, lean meat, fish, vegetables, whole grain cereals and peanuts.	Red meat, cereal grains, wheat germ, blackstrap, molasses.	Liver, kidney, dairy products, We need only tiny quantities so no need to seek it out.
FUNCTION	Essential for maintaining membranes, especially in lungs and eyes. Helps maintain resistance to infections. Necessary for the formation of rhodopsin, needed for provision and prevention of night blindness.	Important in releasing energy from carbohydrates. Essential for maintenance of normal digestion and appetite. Essential for normal functioning of nervous tissue.	Important in utilization of food energy, formation of certain enzymes and in cellular oxidation.	As the component of two important enzymes, it is important in glycolysis — the way sugars are used — tissue respiration and the way fats are dealt with in the body.	Metabolism of amino acids. Formation of haemoglobin.	Produces remission in pernicious anaemia (a fairly rare form of anaemia.) Essential for normal development of red blood cells.
EFFECTS OF DEFICIENCY	Retarded growth; lack of resistance to infection. Abnormal function of gastro-intestinal, genito-urinary and respiratory tracts. Skin dries, shrivels, thickens. Pimples may form. Xerophthalmia, an eye disease, may occur. Other local infections are possible.	Appetite loss; impaired digestion of starches and sugars. Colitis, constipation or diarrhoea. Various nervous disorders. Loss of co-ordinating power of muscles.	Impaired growth, lassitude and weakness, atrophy of skin, anaemia, cataracts.	Pellagra (a deficiency disease). Gastro-intestinal disturbances. Mental disturbances.	Dermatitis round eyes and mouth. Neuritis, Anorexia and vomiting. Possibly pre-menstrual syndrome.	Pernicious anaemia *note:* Vegans who eat no dairy products or meat should take Vitamin B12 supplements — they risk severe anaemia otherwise.
CHARAC-TERISTICS	Fat soluble; not destroyed by ordinary cooking temperatures. Is destroyed by high temperatures when oxygen is present. Can be stored in liver. Excessive intake of carotene may produe yellow discolouration of the skin.	Water soluble; not readily destroyed by ordinary cooking temperature. Destroyed by exposure to heat. Cannot be stored in the body.	Water soluble and alcohol soluble. Not destroyed by heat in cooking. Unstable in light and in the presence of alkalies.	Soluble in hot water and alcohol. Not destroyed by heat, light, air or alkalies.	Soluble in water and alcohol.	Soluble in water or alchohol. Unstable in hot alkaline or acid solutions.

FOLIC ACID Folacin	VITAMIN C	VITAMIN D	VITAMIN E	PANTO-THENIC ACID	BIOTIN	VITAMIN K
Offal, yeast, green leafy vegetables, fruit.	Most fresh fruits and vegetables, especially citrus fruit and juices, tomato and orange. Can be factory made as ascorbic acid.	Butter, egg yolk, fish liver oils, fatty fish, liver, oysters, yeast. Formed in the skin by exposure to sunlight when tanning.	Lettuce and other green leafy vegetables, wheat germ and sunflower oil, margarine, eggs, cereals, breast milk.	Egg yolk, meat, nuts, whole grains	Liver, kidney, egg yolk, nuts, most fresh vegetables.	Made by intestinal bacteria; leafy vegetables.
Essential for formation of red blood cells. Aids the formation of some proteins. Can possibly help prevent birth defects.	Essential for formation of healthy tissues, including skin, teeth, cartilage and bone. Important in the healing of wounds and fractures of bones. Facilitates absorption of iron.	Regulates absorption of calcium and phosporus from the intestinal tract — so is involved in health of teeth and bones.	Anti-oxydant — protecting the body's polyunsaturated fats from destruction by oxygen. It also protects Vitamin A.	Needed by all cells for energy production.	Needed by skin and circulatory system.	Needed for normal blood clotting.
Anaemia. Deficiency may arise when the body's need for red blood cells increases, as in pregnancy. (Often given as a pregnancy supplement for this reason.)	Lowered resistance to infections. Joint tenderness, susceptibility to dental decay, pyorrhoea (gum disease) and bleeding gums. Haemorrhage, anaemia, scurvy, (a deficiency disease). *Note:* The infant diet is likely to be deficient in Vitamin C unless orange or tomato or blackcurrant juice is added.	Irritability, Muscle weakness. Dental decay. Rickets in young children. Osteomalacia (bone softening in adults.)	In premature babies could lead to anaemia. Deficiency unlikely in adults with a good general diet.	Lethargy, muscle weakness.	Various skin reactions.	Excessive bleeding from injuries. Bleeding gums.
Slightly soluble in water. Decreases when food is stored at room temperature. Much is lost in cooking.	Soluble in water. Easily destroyed by oxidation; heat hastens the process. Lost in cooking particularly if water in which food is cooked is discarded. Quick frozen foods lose little of their Vitamin C. Stored in the body to a limited extent.	Soluble in fats and organic solvents. Relatively stable under refrigeration. Stored in liver. Often associated with Vitamin A.	Fat soluble.	Probably fat soluble	Fat soluble.	

Vitamins are complex chemicals which are found in a wide range of foods and are essential for a variety of different bodily processes as the chart shows.

discarded to meet this new demand for a fine diet. People ate more and more refined foods such as sugar, as well as refined flour, until we reached the stage we are at today, where most food is bland and smooth, with all the roughness processed out of it.

The increase in gut diseases seems precisely to match the decline in the food intake of whole cereals. The food that is eaten now is low in residue. Instead of the gut being full of a lot of toothpaste-like material which is soft, moist, and easy to move, it is only half-full of a meagre, dryish, tarry, slow-moving material.

But the gut still tries very hard indeed to do its job in spite of this. It squeezes down rigorously trying to push the stuff along. The result is that the contraction waves are so powerful that constricting 'rings' appear along the length of the gut and the waves of force, instead of pushing the waste along the gut to the outside, 'kick back' on the actual gut walls.

If this occurs near the appendix the result is a swollen blood-starved little organ (the blood supply is pinched off by the contraction waves) which is then very susceptible to attacks of bacteria. The same process is involved in a number of other conditions affecting the gut, especially diverticulitis. A diverticulum is a little blind pouch that appears on the gut wall, rather like a 'blow-out' on a tyre; it's 'blown' out by these powerful pressured waves that are trying to act on the viscous gut content to move it along. Once these little pouches have formed in the gut wall, they, like the appendix, can become infected. The result is a lot of pain, nausea and vomiting, alternating constipation and diarrhoea and in severe cases, which are fortunately uncommon, there may be complications of intestinal obstruction, bleeding and perforation (actual breaking down of the gut wall) all of which are very serious.

A similar condition is the irritated bowel syndrome. The patient complains of attacks of abdominal pain and alternating diarrhoea and constipation. This means that spasmodic contractions are biting down hard on inadequate bowel contents again and these vigorous bowel contractions cause pain or a feeling of discomfort.

Another effect is, obviously, constipation — a slowing down of the passage of food wastes through the bowel. The rings of contraction that appear in the gut hold up the onward movement and a vicious circle is set up; the gut contents become drier and harder as water is reabsorbed into the body, the stools become more difficult to pass, there is excess pressure on the gut wall, and especially at the outlet, leading to haemorrhoids, the enlarged inefficient veins at the anus which are popularly known as piles.

The most worrying possible effect of slow movement of gut contents is cancer of the gut. No one yet knows the precise mechanism involved, but it seems likely that the chemicals that are naturally present in the gut contents are changed by the action of bacteria and other normal body chemicals until they become highly irritant substances called carcinogens: which are cancer-causing chemicals.

If the waste material moves through quickly, then the carcinogens have no time to be formed, and even if they are, they aren't in contact with the gut wall for very long, so they exert less effect. This is still theoretical but research has been carried out on bowel transit times. People were given little pellets to swallow, and then timed to see how long it took for them to reappear at the other end using different types of diet. A typically British low-residue diet took over eighty hours to pass through the gut and produced a small quantity of stool, while Africans eating a traditional rural diet, high in residue, took only thirty-five hours to produce four times the quantity of stool. And in rural Africa the incidence of diverticulitis, cancer of the colon and other gut diseases is so very low that it is practically unknown.

Minerals

Minute quantities of minerals are needed to keep the body healthy.

	CALCIUM	PHOSPHORUS	POTASSIUM	MAGNESIUM	IODINE
SOURCES	Dairy produce, green vegetables.	Meat, dairy produce, pulses and cereals.	Avocados, bananas, apricots, potatoes and many other foods.	Pulses, nuts and cereals, leafy green vegetables.	All seafood; iodized salt, liver, meat, eggs, enriched cereals.
CHIEF FUNCTION	Essential for blood clotting, and the structure of bones and teeth. Needed for working of nerves and all other electrically active body tissues.	Basic cell energy store, key element in cell reactions.	Major mineral within body cells. Essential to fluid balance and for many cell reactions.	Needed by all cells. Important in electrical activity of nerves and muscles.	Needed by thyroid gland.

For the researchers in this field, the link seems unquestionable. They believe very strongly indeed that these diseases are largely preventable, and can also be treated to an extent by the use of a different sort of diet. They don't pretend that altering what you eat will cure you of appendicitis or gut cancer if you've already got it — but it can certainly reduce the symptoms of diverticulosis, constipation, haemorrhoids, and anal fissure (a crack occurring in the soft anal tissue). And you can certainly protect yourself against getting these disagreeable conditions.

Minerals

The derivations of metals and salts such as iron and calcium, sodium chloride and phosphorus are needed in minute quantities and very few people suffer from mineral deficiency. The chart shows from whence the most important ones in the diet can be derived and you will see it is very rarely that you need concern yourself about them.

The only one that is particularly important is sodium. An excess of sodium in the diet can lead to high blood pressure, with resulting strain on kidneys, heart and brain. Many researchers in the Western world feel our diet is much too richly provided with sodium in the form of sodium chloride (common table salt). Foods that are highly salted and very popular, such as potato crisps, salted peanuts and biscuits (often taken in surprisingly large quantities by people having a drink in a bar) really have no place in a healthy diet.

Water

About half your body is made of water. Every single cell needs its complement of water to keep it at its normal level of 'plumpness' and function. In any one day, you dispose of around two litres — up to four pints — in urine, in faeces, in sweat and in droplets breathed out with expired air. About seventy per cent of the amount of fluid you need to replace this loss is obtained from your food. Most people find that drinking up to half a litre (one pint) of fluid a day is quite enough. However, in hot climates where people sweat more a larger fluid intake may be needed. Many people drink more fluid than they need in the form of stimulant drinks, such as tea, coffee, cola drinks, cocoa.

There is some evidence that the caffeine in these drinks causes disorder in some people. There can be rapidly increased heartbeat, anxiety, excess sweating and other symptoms of stress in people who have a high caffeine intake. If an individual who has been drinking a great deal of these fluids cuts them drastically to reduce the caffeine intake, there is rarely any need to increase fluid intake to replace that loss. However, there are some people so much in need of their regular drinks, that they prefer to drink decaffeinated fluids so that they can pretend to themselves that they are still drinking their coffee, tea or whatever. There's no harm in this.

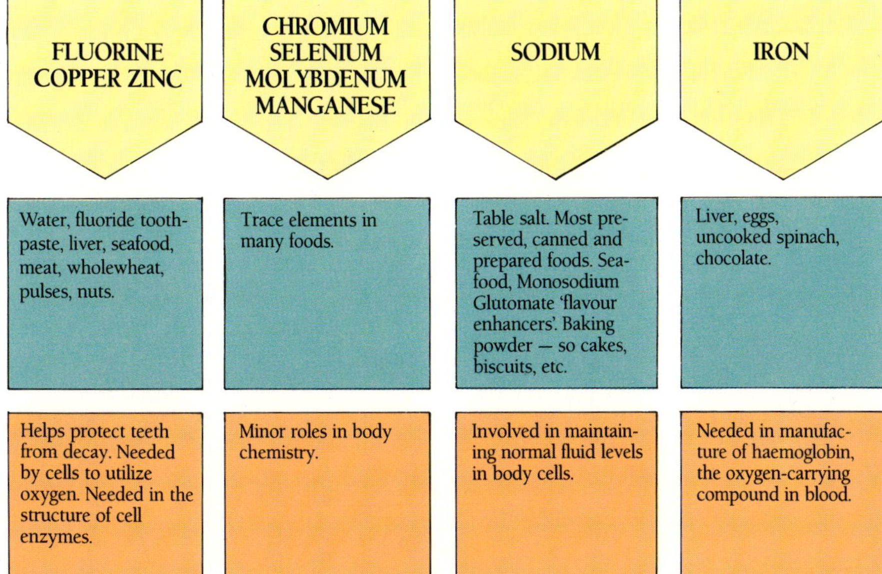

Planning a healthy diet

The current thinking about food is that in the West we are overfed. We have such a variety of foods it is difficult not to be tempted to eat too much by their sight, taste and smell.

Many of the foods which we find so tempting and which have been prepared by the food industry contain substances known as additives — colourants, preservatives, flavourings — some of which are derived from 'natural' sources, and some of which are synthesized in a factory to mimic those derived from natural sources.

There's been a great deal of anxiety in recent years about the effect of additives. Some people have believed that they are sensitive to them and suffer physical and psychological reactions. Some experts in the food industry maintain that the additives used actually protect us from a range of unpleasant disorders by preserving food and preventing bacterial pollution that can damage us, and also maintain that food made more palatable with flavourings is more beneficial to us.

The arguments will, no doubt, go on raging for a very long time, with one lobby furiously maintaining that 'all additives are bad' while the other maintains that 'additives are good for you'. The truth probably lies, as the truth generally does, somewhere between the two. But in the meanwhile, many people who would like to live as healthily as possible feel that a diet that is based on fresh foods, eaten raw when possible or freshly cooked when that is not unrealistic, is healthier than the classic 'supermarket' diet. However, disaster will not overtake somebody who has some convenient supermarket food; for a busy woman running a job and her home and

Group one

Skinned poultry, other than duck or goose
Tongue
Liver
Kidney
Sweetbreads
Potatoes
Turnips
Swedes
Parsnips
Corn
All sorts of green and leaf vegetables, eaten raw or, if possible, only lightly cooked
Skimmed milk
Low fat yoghurt
Low fat cottage cheese
Non-oily fish including cod, haddock, plaice, whiting, hake
Shellfish including prawns, cockles, winkles, oysters, crab, etc.
Bran
All fresh fruits and juices (unsweetened)

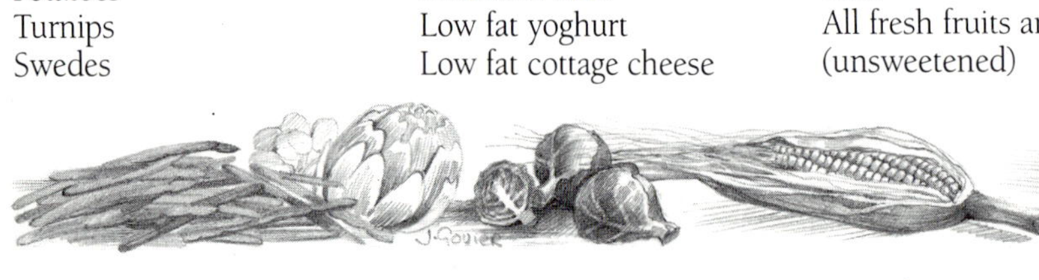

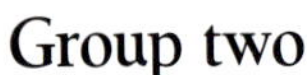

Group two

Lean beef, lamb and pork
Beans
Peas
Lentils
Eggs
Hard cheeses
Full cream milk
Full cream milk products (yoghurt, etc.)
Oily fish including herrings, mackerel, sardines, tuna, salmon
Pasta (made out of whole wheat)
Rice (brown)
Whole grain breads
Whole grain cereals (unsweetened)
Polyunsaturated margarine and vegetable oils

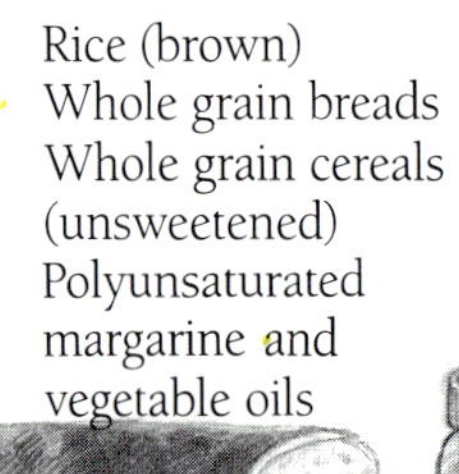

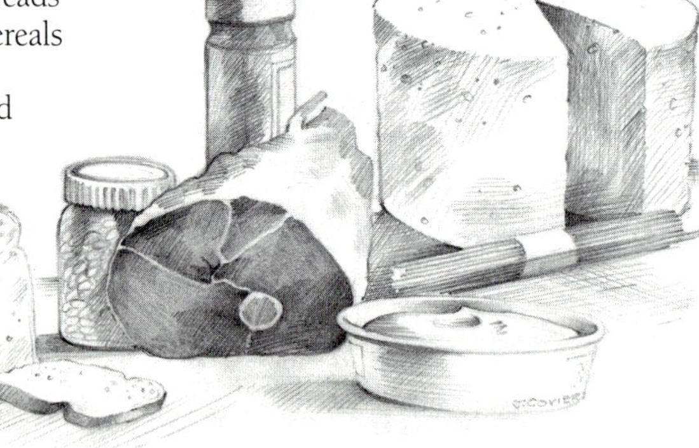

Group three

Visible fat on any meat
Bacon
Ham
Pork products of all kinds
Duck
Goose
Sausages
Salami
Pates
Most delicatessen meats
Butter
Lard
Ordinary margarine
Ice cream (including water ices if they are commercial; home made water ices based on unsweetened fruit juice are fine — they belong in Group One)
Refined sugar
Unrefined sugar — in other words, all sugars
Sweets
Chocolates
Cakes
Pies
Pastries
Biscuits
Puddings
Custards
Jellies (except home made fruit jellies made without sugar — those belong in Group One)
Canned foods which include sugar on the list of ingredients (remember to look at savoury foods as well as sweet ones — canned soups are often very high in sugar)
Dried fruits
Nuts
Jams
Honeys
Marmalades
Syrups of all kinds

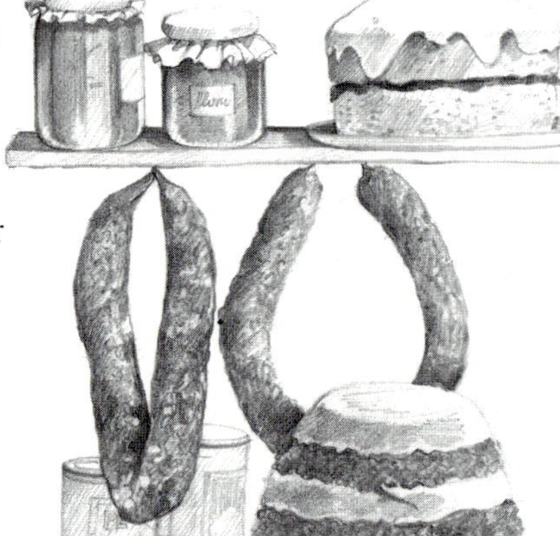

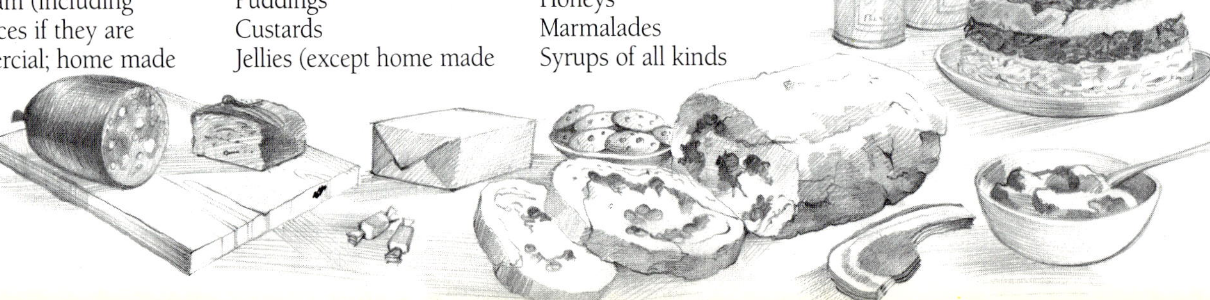

feeding other people as well as herself the saving of time and labour provided by the use of such foods is a benefit not lightly to be discarded.

A daily diet that is made up of foods from the three groups listed opposite, in the right proportions, will be a healthy one. From Group One foods, you may eat as much as you like as often as you like.

From Group Two foods you should eat at least one good portion per day.

From Group Three foods you should eat as little as possible, knowing them to be rich in sugars which provide no other nutrients apart from carbohydrate, and saturated fats, which you will remember are regarded askance by many experts on heart and arterial disease, but which are enjoyable.

Counting calories

Estimates have been made in various studies of the numbers of calories a person needs, depending on their activities. It has been estimated, for example, that a woman with a desk job needs 2,000 calories a day, whereas a woman with a fairly active job — say she's a doctor or a dentist or a full-time housewife — needs 2,500 calories. A man with a fairly active job — say he's a carpenter, a teacher, or a shopkeeper — needs 2,800 calories. Men who work as bricklayers, as road menders or coal miners need 3,300 calories a day, and professional athletes, whatever their sex, need up to and sometimes in excess of 4,000 calories a day.

But having said that, it really is of small help, because individuals vary greatly. A woman of 1.78 metres (5 feet 10 inches), for example, will have a larger frame and will need more calories than a woman of just 1.52 metres (5 feet). A short man will not require as many calories as a tall man. And it would be obsessive to be constantly counting calories to come up with some ideal total that may not suit you anyway.

More to the point is to understand how your daily diet should be balanced to give you adequate quantities of protein, carbohydrate and fats. If a diet is properly balanced according to the figures below, then the likelihood is that you will get enough calories, and also the vitamins and minerals you need.

In Britain and the USA committees have suggested that the ideal daily diet for all people should consist of about:

11 per cent protein
52 per cent carbohydrate
32 per cent fats.

It may help you to know that to provide 2,500 calories, you should take 55 grams (1.9 ounces) protein 260 grams (9.2 ounces) carbohydrate, 72 grams (2.5 ounces) fat.

But generally speaking most healthy people can allow their appetites to be their guide. People who become too anxious about the number of calories they are eating, and the quality of the food they are eating, lose the normal ability to control their diet merely by appetite. The appetite is really like the bowel; you don't need vast quantities of laxative to ensure that your bowels empty themselves. They do that perfectly well on their own without any interference from you. Similarly you do not need to exert manful control over your appetite if you are a reasonably healthy person. Of course there are some people who have been so badly trained as regards food that they have virtually been forced to become obsessed about their diet. At its most severe this sort of obsession leads to the illness of anorexia nervosa or bulimia nervosa in which periods of quite appalling self-starvation are punctuated by periods of violent over-eating and sometimes self-induced vomiting. People to whom this has happened need psychiatric help, very often for prolonged periods of time.

But for the rest of us, it cannot be said too often that eating good food as you want to, at reasonable intervals as your appetite dictates, will ensure that you are well fed and have the necessary vitamins and minerals.

Food reactions

A phrase a great many people use when they develop unpleasant symptoms is, 'It must be something I ate.' It seems logical to assume that aches and pains, especially in the belly, and disturbances of stomach or gut could be due to the swallowing of some noxious substance, and indeed it often is the case. Food badly prepared or stored may be contaminated with organisms to which the body objects violently, and of which it rids itself as fast as possible. Salmonella, which causes severe vomiting and diarrhoea, is a case in point, and there are many times people have illnesses which are labelled rather vaguely as 'food poisoning' which are indeed due to 'something I ate'.

Some people can't eat the fraction of wheat called gluten (children unable to digest it suffer from an illness called coeliac disease) and others can't cope with caffeine in coffee, tea, cocoa and cola drinks.

It is also known that some people develop a severe migraine if they eat foods rich in a chemical called tyramine. This is found in cheese, in chocolate, and to an extent in red wine, in pickled fish, and yeast extracts.

In recent years there has been an upsurge of interest in the question of food allergies. There are some substances to which an individual body objects, and which cause that body to react, via its inbuilt defensive immune system, with such symptoms as wheeziness or running nose and eyes, or skin rashes, or gut disturbances or headaches. A person who is sensitive to, say, grass pollens, finds that at the time of the year when such pollens fly far and free she suffers attacks of wheezing, running nose, red eyes and headaches — the classic 'hay fever'. A person who is sensitive to such plants as the primula may develop a rash if she touches the leaves.

It has been well known for a long time that there are people who show a violent response to certain common food stuffs. Shellfish, fruits such as strawberries, or eggs and milk can bring unfortunate sensitives out in rashes or cause debilitating sickness. The food can be scrupulously clean and perfectly fresh; there is no suggestion that the symptoms are due to bacterial pollution. It is simply that this particular individual has a body that is triggered into an exaggerated defence posture when the food enters her system.

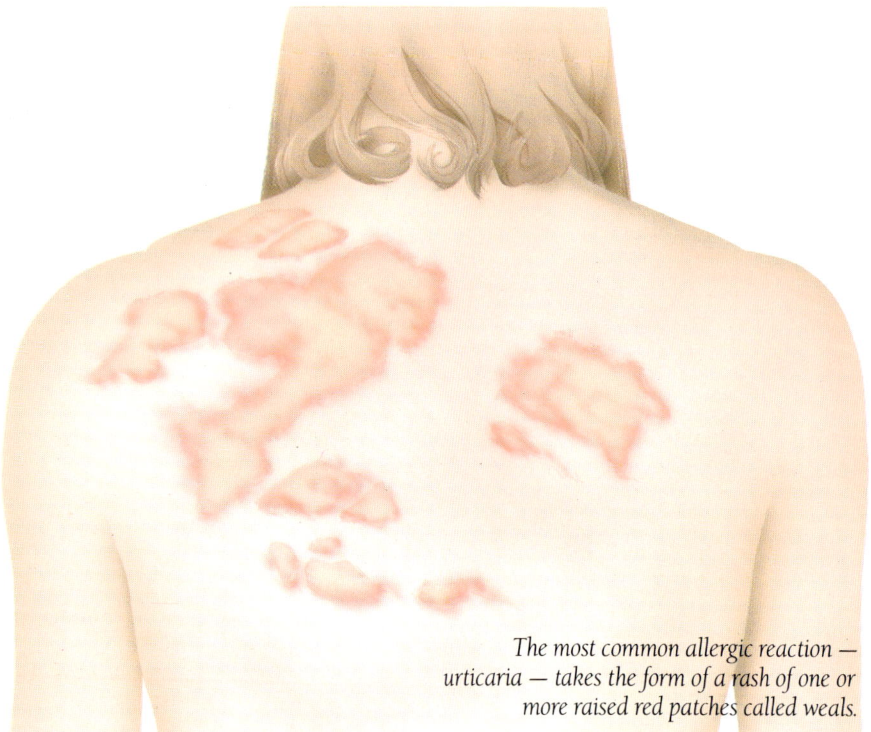

The most common allergic reaction — urticaria — takes the form of a rash of one or more raised red patches called weals.

Some people have come to the conclusion that there are far more food allergies around than have so far been identified. They claim that a wide range of sometimes bizarre symptoms, including dizziness, breathlessness, panic attacks, rapid heart beat, sweatiness, headaches, pain in the eyes, bad dreams and many many more are due entirely to food allergy. Some people have had their diets steadily reduced till they are subsisting almost wholly on lamb and green peas (why these foods are rarely accused of causing food allergy is uncertain) by doctors who are convinced that this is the only way to treat their distress.

There are other practitioners who are very dubious about the claims made by their colleagues. They point out that if it were true that there were people who were genetically unable to eat such wide ranges of foods, the likelihood is that their parents, grandparents and remoter ancestors would have been the same, and if that had been the case, they would have been unlikely to survive infancy and to have children of their own. They say there is no real scientific proof that living on severely restricted diets actually helps patients and that many of the symptoms reported resemble anxiety responses far more than allergic ones.

The food allergy controversy has been fed by increasing anxiety about the sorts of additives used in modern food technology, and especially the colourants. These have been accused of making some children over-excited — the 'hyperactive child' syndrome — and of making adults very ill indeed. Once again, it is difficult to prove these claims.

All that can be said is that while it makes sense to avoid foods you consciously dislike, (an individual's distaste may be based on the fact that her body really objects to it) it is not wise to restrict your diet severely in the search for relief from symptoms that might have other causes. Not until you have firm proof that you are suffering from food allergy should you allow yourself to become anxious about what you eat. (That proof, incidentally, can be furnished by the use of very carefully organized double blind crossover testing — in which various substances, unidentified by either patient or tester, are given and the reactions measured.) It would be wiser to consider dealing with your symptoms by other means — and relaxation can be very effective. (See page 154.)

Incidentally, it is worth remembering that doctors used to say, on the basis of no firm evidence, that acne was caused by eating chocolate or fried food. It is now known that this is quite untrue; however healthy the diet, many peope still suffer from attacks of acne. The spots are never due to 'something I ate'. They are far more likely to be linked with hormone production and its effect on the skin than with foods.

Drugs

We take more than food into our bodies. Ever since mankind found that eating fruits that had fallen to the ground and fermented gave him an interesting experience inside his head, changing his perception of his world and himself, we have used and abused alcohol. Ever since mankind found that eating certain foods such as mushrooms and some berries and leaves and barks created similar experiences, and also reduced pain, we have used and abused a wide range of drugs, and especially opiates (drugs which derive from, and/or act like the opium poppy) and tobacco.

Why? Is it simply the agreeable experiences the substances create which make them so attractive? It might seem so at first glance, because the human drive towards pleasure is a powerful one, but often the pleasurable effect of a drug is less than the unpleasant after or side effects and people soon realise this. Yet over and over again there are some who go on using a substance in ever increasing quantities which they know makes them feel more ill than well, and which causes them considerable damage, emotional, social and financial as well as physical. It seems totally irrational for a supposedly rational species.

We are indeed, but we are governed in many of our actions by brain chemicals which affect our behaviour profoundly, making the drive to a certain set of actions so imperative that it completely overrides any intellectual rational thought. And the drive to abuse drugs of all sorts seems, almost certainly, to be linked with these brain chemicals.

They were discovered by researchers who were studying brain function. They found that the human brain contains receptors which are shaped to lock precisely onto a molecule of a certain type – in this case the molecule of the opium poppy. Since it was not logical that the human brain would have evolved naturally with a special relationship to another life form, it was obvious that somewhere in the human organism there had to be a system for producing a substance that would fit the receptor sites on the brain and to which the opiate molecule bore a close resemblance. So the researchers started to look for such substances.

They found them, and labelled them 'endorphins' – that is, 'the morphine within' (morphine derives from the opium poppy). They discovered that under various forms of stress these endorphins (there are more than one) are released into the blood and travel to the brain, there to lock on to the waiting receptors. Once they are locked on, pain is reduced and a sense of euphoria and happiness is experienced.

The sorts of stresses that release endorphins are varied. Pain is one; if you damage yourself with a sharp object, say, the first reaction is acute pain, and then after an appreciable fraction of time, a different sort of pain that is duller, but lasts for rather longer than the initial sharp sensation. This pain slowly ebbs away and becomes more tolerable – because the natural painkillers, the endorphins, are damping it down.

Prolonged muscular activity can also release endorphins (this is probably why there is a marked sense of wellbeing after a period of exercise – see below) and so can certain forms of mental activity, including meditation and yoga techniques (see page 154). Also, the production of endorphins can be stimulated by quite mild pain – such as the prick of a needle. It is probably this that lies behind the successful use of acupuncture (again see page 154).

It is now suspected that some of the people who abuse drugs which offer molecules that fit the endorphin receptor sites in the brain are people who for unknown reasons lack the ability to make enough natural endorphins to keep themselves happy and comfortable. This applies not only to opiates, but to alcohol, and it is thought by some researchers, tobacco too. If they are right – that there are inbuilt differences between those who abuse drugs and those who are able to use them casually and without any sense of need – it would account for the fact that plenty of people are able to enjoy an occasional glass of wine or a mood-altering drug without becoming at all dependent, while others rapidly come to use the substance first as a crutch and then as a vital part of their everyday lives.

There are, of course, other factors involved; people who are unhappy may use drugs which dull their consciousness to blot out their thinking processes and memories, and so deal with psychic pain in that way; 'drowning one's sorrows' has a long history. Also, people who are deprived of adequate comfort, food and warmth may turn to drugs as a replacement. Hence the upsurge in alcohol abuse in the Britain of the late eighteenth and early nineteenth centuries when the desperately poor of London and other big cities could be 'drunk for a penny, dead drunk for tuppence' and in modern times wherever unemployment and poverty are high.

The damaging effects of alcohol and tobacco

Women smokers are five times as likely to get lung cancer as women who do not smoke.

Women who smoke while pregnant run twice the risk of miscarriage as non-smokers.

The risk of heart disease amongst smokers is twice that among those who don't smoke.

Alcohol acts on the brain to impair judgement and slow up reactions – lack of co-ordination and brain damage can be permanent.

About 60% of confirmed alcoholics suffer from fatty infiltration of the liver and about 10% die from cirrhosis of the liver.

The situation regarding the use of drugs and their effects is bedevilled by the fact that some drugs are legal and some are not, with the dangerous aspects of the drugs seeming to have little or no bearing on the question of legality.

Alcohol, for example, contributes to many thousands of deaths each year from drunken driving as well as from a number of alcohol-related diseases affecting liver, heart and other vital organs, while tobacco is killing more and more people every year. Yet these are legal drugs in the UK and elsewhere in the world, whereas cannabis, which is illegal, seems, as far as research can show, to be far less lethal in its effects. It is very difficult to convince people of the risks they are taking with their health by using some drugs when the governments of their countries continue to permit, even encourage, their use and gain considerable financial benefit from taxing them. Warning women that cigarette smoking can make them first ill and then may kill them prematurely is of small value when posters and advertisements for cigarettes are everywhere, albeit bearing Government health warnings. If these things can be bought over the counter in any number of respectable shops, how can people be convinced the things are potential killers?

The same applies to alcohol. There is increasing evidence that women are particularly vulnerable to the ill effects of alcohol and suffer them after what are regarded as moderate doses. Their livers find it more difficult to remove the poison – which is what alcohol is, of course – and may succumb to damage easily. Their babies, if they drink alcohol during a pregnancy, may show damage that can be directly attributed to the use of the drug. It is of course true that some women drink heavily all through pregnancy and produce perfectly normal and healthy babies, just as some women smoke heavily all their lives and not only produce healthy babies (though tobacco does restrict the supply of nutrients to the infant in the uterus) but die at a ripe old age when a bus runs over them – but that sort of anecdotal evidence does not cancel out the real and overwhelming evidence that both these drugs are dangerous to the human organism and to women in particular.

When it comes to illegal drugs, there is little more to be said than that they are illegal. Cocaine and heroin have a grisly history of damage, and anyone who risks not only their effects but the punishments of the law has to be very foolish and unhappy indeed.

Prescribed drugs

More insiduous in many ways even than licit tobacco and alcohol are the drugs that some doctors can prescribe for women, and to which they become habituated.

The pain of fear has been part of the human condition ever since we came down from the trees — before, probably. We shake and shiver, we weep and wail, we hide away from others, feel sick and our bowels turn to water — all because of a fear we can't describe or a threat we can't identify. There will be more about the painful effects of anxiety in the next few pages, but here it's important to look at what was regarded, some thirty or so years ago, as at last the answer to this widespread problem.

Researchers into other drugs (notably those used to treat tuberculosis) found that some compounds had the effect of bringing tranquillity to anxious people. The first compound actually marketed to be used for this purpose was named Miltown and was seized on, notably in the USA, as the great drug breakthrough of all time. People with worries were popping pills as though they were sweets and all claimed to feel great. Inevitably more and more such drugs were developed and today there is a wide range of them available.

To start with, everyone thought these tranquillizing drugs were harmless. They reduced anxiety without clouding consciousness and that had to be great. But slowly it was realised that tranquillizers were the same as many other drugs; their power for good was equalled by their power for harm. The only drugs that cause absolutely no side effects and no troubles are those that are so inert they confer no benefit at all. Even such splendid pharmaceutical weapons as antibiotics, for instance, have their drawbacks. In killing unwanted bacteria, they also kill desirable ones, and allow some bad organisms to flourish, as we saw in the treatment of thrush in Section seven.

In the case of tranquillizers it was found that people became dependent on them, and began to need larger and larger doses as they become more and more used to the effects the drugs could provide. (This happens with all drugs of dependence, not only tobacco and alcohol and illegal drugs.) Any attempts to reduce the amount used led, in some cases, to severe withdrawal symptoms which included sweating, cramps, feelings of 'depersonalization' (almost like a stranger inside your own skin), hallucinations, sickness, diarrhoea, fainting, rapid and erratic heartbeat — a wide range of very disagreeable feelings.

Nowadays few enlightened doctors prescribe tranquillizers except for firmly controlled short periods, and then only for specific situations. A person having to make a vital journey by air, and feeling very frightened of aeroplanes, might need tranquillizers for a day. The newly bereaved may feel they want a crutch to get them through the first hours of their pain. A person suffering from a severe attack of anxiety neurosis may need a week of tranquillizers to get her relaxed enough to accept long term treatment (which is more likely to be psychotherapy than drugs).

These doctors who have in the past overprescribed these drugs and who have patients who are dependent on them should know by now that it is totally wrong to make a person come off the drugs 'cold'. That increases the strength of withdrawal symptoms. the drug has to be slowly tailed off, under careful medical support and supervision, so that the body can become accustomed to the changes taking place in its internal chemistry.

Though tranquillizers have been a form of psychotropic (mood altering) drugs that have been ill used and led to problems, another type of psychotropic drug has been and continues to be very useful.

These are the anti-depressants. They act on the brain chemicals (not endorphins, as far as is known) which are out of balance in people suffering from clinical depression, and they can be very effective indeed. They do not have an immediate effect, like tranquillizers; they need to be taken for some time — up to a few weeks — before their beneficial effect is noticed, and can usually be tailed off after about three to six months.

Most depressive illnesses will get better by themselves, let alone, but they cause so much distress it seems cruel to leave a sufferer unaided when aid is available. The anti-depressants help the patient to feel well while she gets better on her own. They are not habituating as tranquillizers are, and there is no evidence that they do any harm. However, remembering that all drugs may have a power for ill to match their power for good, we have to wait and see what drawbacks might show in the future. Meanwhile many women have cause to be grateful to anti-depressants, which, wisely and carefully prescribed, have carried them over and through a very distressing illness.

Another form of prescribed drug which, in the past, did a good deal of harm — and which may in some areas still be available — is the stimulant. One particularly well-known one, amphetamine, also known as speed, used to be widely prescribed for women as an appetite suppressant, in an attempt to make them thin (which shows you just how far the neurosis that favours unhealthy thinness has spread and been nurtured by society as a whole). This drug reduces the need to sleep as well as cutting appetite and makes the user feel excited, sometimes to the point of being manic, a state of mind that may sometimes progress to aggressiveness and uncontrolled anger. Amphetamine and drugs like it are dangerous because they alter a user's behaviour and damage her ability to make sensible judgements. Any woman who is under the care of a doctor who still prescribes them as 'slimming drugs', or who offers any sort of drug supposed to promote weight loss, needs to question him closely about the drug and why he is offering it. There is no evidence at present that any drug currently in use has any real effect on safe and permanent weight loss. There may be one by the time this book is published, but it is highly unlikely. And though such a drug would no doubt make a fortune for its manufacturers, who draw on the pockets of millions of women who, no matter what they are told about the pointlessness of dieting will still want to be abnormally thin, it is to be hoped it never will be available.

Exercise

There are many people in the world today who would regard the idea of activating muscles for the sake of it, rather than for the purpose of necessary work, as sheer lunacy and we don't have to go very far back in our own history to find ancestors who would have regarded the concept with the same blank amazement.

But there it is; we in the West have progressed so far that many of the functions for which our bodies were designed by evolution are no longer required; the work has been taken over by machines. Yet the ability to perform those functions remains with us. The Stone Age physiques we inhabit are able to produce a great deal of effortful work; to run very fast indeed to escape from danger; to identify a threat in good time to deal with or evade it; to do a great many things we rarely need to do in the well-off West, like climbing trees, swinging on creepers and various other forms of Tarzan-like endeavour. Yet our bodies react all the time as though we do have to do all these things — and if we fail to respond to those demands we're in health trouble. The muscles sag, the body chemicals needed to drive the muscles to action kickback with symptoms of anxiety, tension and unresolved stress and the result is often a generalized ill health with vague but unpleasant physical symptoms, varying from headaches and stiffness of the neck and shoulders to belly aches, nausea, frequent bowel action, trembling, fleeting aches and pains and much more.

All this has led in recent years to a massive interest in exercise for its own sake. Large sums of money are being made by businessmen who have latched on to this interest. The manufacturers of running shoes, leotards, tights, leg warmers and track suits are waxing rich.

Quite where and how the craze started it is hard to be sure. There has always been a section of the population which has found physical pleasure in games that demand great expenditure of muscle energy, or in walking for miles over rough country, or in swimming or whatever, but most of their indolent neighbours (and they far outnumbered the active ones) put this interest down to some sort of mental quirk. These people liked being competitive, the sedentary ones told themselves; they enjoyed the sense of achievement they got from beating others at a game; or they liked watching birds or collecting wild flowers, and that was why they walked; or they enjoyed looking at almost naked people and swam because beaches and pools are good places to see them.

But then, a decade or so ago, the word began to creep around that there was more to it than that. People who used their muscles a lot, it seemed, got some sort of satisfaction that was far beyond the merely competitive or intellectual and slowly but steadily people who had once automatically waited for a lift to travel up one floor began to run up six flights regularly, people who normally sat in the car to drive to the corner to post a letter began to run six miles a day; and devoted TV-sleepers-in-front-of began to join gymnasia and country clubs. Books began to appear commending the joys of running, of exercising, of disco dancing six times a week and tap dancing every day and the voice of the aerobe was heard in the land.

What had happened was the discovery of endorphins. Not all the people who were now so busily filling the coffers of the track-suit and leotard merchant knew that this was what they had discovered, or course; they only knew that when they ran or disco danced or aerobically exercised they felt relaxed and happy in a way they had not done before. They found they slept better, no longer suffered the periods of gloominess that had once made life so effortful, and generally glowed with a sense of well being. Those who espoused the ideas of the more evangelical of the new prophets of the joys of perspiration also found that they could experience a 'high' of the sort that the drug users had written about in the hippy days of the sixties.

That it is the effect of endorphins that makes people who exercise a lot feel good seems undoubted. Strong muscular activity causes the body to react in just the same way that pain does; extra neuro-chemicals are released and sent to lock on to their special brain receptors in order to make the effort less painful. The longer the stress — that is, the muscular effort — continues, the more endorphins are released, the more comfortable and euphoric the person feels.

If endorphins were simply painkillers then the fashion for exercise that still grips a great many people whould have died long ago. It is the ability to lift mood and create an inner glow of contentment that has made exercise of all sorts as popular as it is. In some cases this has become too attractive to exercisers. There are some who deliberately exercise until they hurt. A muscle can work for just so long before it builds up what is called an 'exercise debt'. It cannot get rid of the by-products of the fuel-burning it is doing (lactic acid is the one that causes the most problems) and it protests loudly in order to demand rest. The over taxed muscle may go into spasm — cramp — or just hurt a great deal.

The body's normal reaction to such pain is to stop the action at once so that muscle can divest itself of waste materials, and be ready to work again after a rest. However, the brain can override this reflex response, and will do so under stress; if Stone Age Man was running away from a sabre toothed tiger, the likelihood was that he'd tolerate the screaming pain in his muscles and go on running rather than be eaten. But he wouldn't do it if he didn't have to.

Some modern 'teachers' tell their pupils in their exercise classes that they should behave like beleaguered Stone Agers and ignore the pain in their muscles and 'go for the burn'. They should deliberately work their muscles beyond the point of comfortable function.

This is a very unhealthy thing to do. It will certainly create a flood of endorphins and possibly a pyschological high — but it can also lead to permanently damaged muscles, and sometimes damaged joints too. If the joint is overstressed it can develop excess fluid in the protective capsule that surrounds it (a condition called bursitis) and may also develop permanent changes that limit its movement thereafter. There

Choosing the right exercise

If you follow this guide, you should be able to feel fit — that is, in good general health — and be able to enjoy the way you feel.

1 *Try to make your normal day more active. If you work at a sedentary job, stop using the lift inside buildings; make a point of getting up and walking somewhere in the office building every hour for a couple of minutes if you can. Where possible, use energy-intensive equipment rather than labour-saving devices — a broom, not a vacuum cleaner; hand rather than machine polishing; a manual rather than an electric typewriter.*

If you normally take a bus to work, make an effort to leave home earlier, and walk on to the further bus stop rather than the nearest. Leave the bus a couple of stops from home in the evening and walk the rest of the way. Or, if you drive a car, don't use it unless you must — walk to town to shop. If that is not possible, choose the car park furthest from the shopping centre.

This sort of activity, which may seem a nuisance and time wasting at first, will become second nature very soon if you persevere, and you will have added a considerable amount of regular exercise to your week.

2 *In addition, create a regular exercise pattern, at least two or better still three times a week. Try a keep fit class (lots are available, in workers' lunch hours in city centres as well as at evening or day-time classes). Or, swim on regular days; many local authority pools or leisure centres open for early morning swimmers before a day's work, and lunchtime sessions are also available.*

Or try a personal regime of exercises at home — though this really is the least satisfactory. Without others' company it can sometimes be difficult to motivate yourself when you're feeling less than excited at the idea of exercise. But erratic exercise sessions are better than no exercise at all.

3 *Choose an exercise system that you will enjoy. If it bores you or you do it grudgingly you won't benefit and you won't last the course. Boredom destroys the best of intentions. If competitive games are not for you, and getting to a swimming pool is difficult, invest in a stationary exercise bike. This is costly, but can be used in all weathers, all the year round. Set it in sight of a television set, so that you can watch while you work, or listen to the radio. This will make the exercise less boring.*

4 *Choose, if possible, an exercise that uses your whole body, and which promotes deep breathing, sweating and increased heartbeat (this is the sort labelled aerobic — it just means you burn up more oxygen). Walking, running, cycling and swimming are whole-body exercises; weight lifting and body-building are not — they just enlarge certain muscles. If you enjoy that sort, by all means engage in it — but also go for some aerobic exercise too.*

5 *Don't attempt to get into top condition too soon. If you choose swimming, for example, settle for doing a couple of lengths the first time you go. Work up gradually until you reach the time and distance limit at which you feel most comfortable — say half a mile in half an hour. Similarly, if you use an exercise bike, slowly increase the tension against which you cycle (all these bikes are equipped to do this) and slowly lengthen the period you spend on it.*

If you are a particularly competitive person — you'll know from the way you approach your job, and your relationships — avoid the sort of sports that are very energetic, until you are sure you are in good condition. You may be tempted to overstretch yourself and strain muscles and even your heart by struggling to win when you aren't in good enough condition.

6 *If you are very unfit (climbing two or three flights of stairs leaves you breathless, or in need of a rest on the way to breathe), if you are a heavy smoker, if you are seriously overweight, if you are over the age of sixty, if you are having treatment for a condition such as high blood pressure or kidney or heart disorder or diabetes, check first with your doctor before embarking on any exercise regime. You may need to undertake supervised exercise with a trained physiotherapist at first.*

7 *Don't ever go immediately into hard exercise from rest. A few gentle 'warm up' movements are needed to get your muscles working. And after exercise keep muscles warm till they are fully rested (those trendy leg warmers do actually have a function).*

8 *If you ever feel sick or dizzy or have dazzled vision or tightness in your chest while exercising, stop at once and check with your doctor as soon as possible that there is no underlying problem that needs checking and/or treating.*

9 *Never push yourself beyond what feels like reasonable limits. Exercise is never better if it hurts or makes you feel exhausted. After an exercise session you should feel invigorated, not devastated.*

10 *Follow exercise with a conscious relaxation session, for full benefit. Try the system shown opposite.*

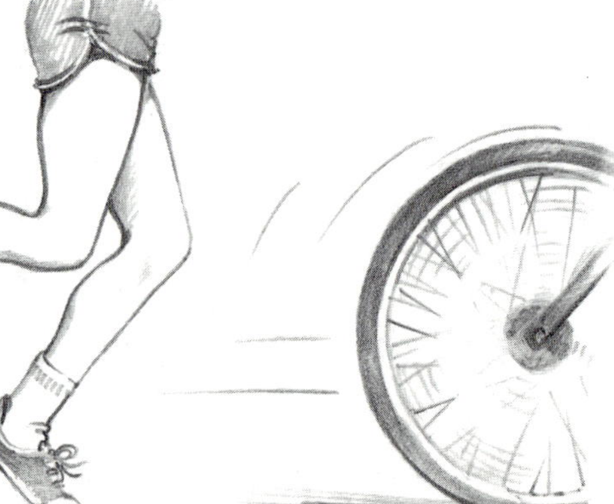

Relaxation exercises

These exercises can be used either on their own or as a follow-up to a period of formal exercises. It can be an excellent system to try in the middle of a working day, or last thing at night before you go to bed, or any time when you are feeling tense or anxious.

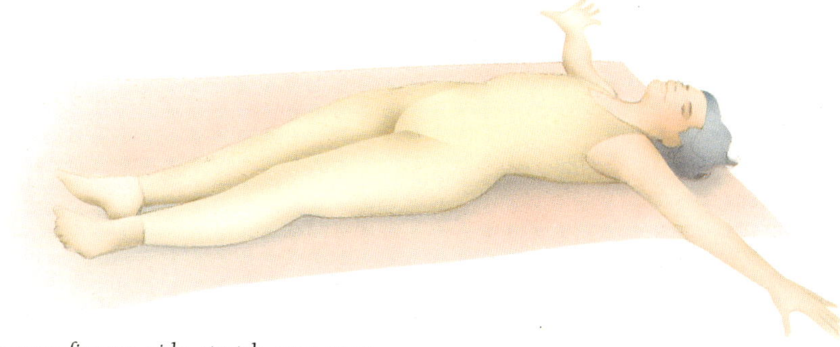

1 If possible remove or loosen tight clothing. Take off your shoes. Lie on the floor on your back with your eyes closed, in a room that is as warm as possible. Do not use a pillow. Your arms should be loosely at your side with your hands palm downwards. Your legs should be close together with your feet falling outwards.

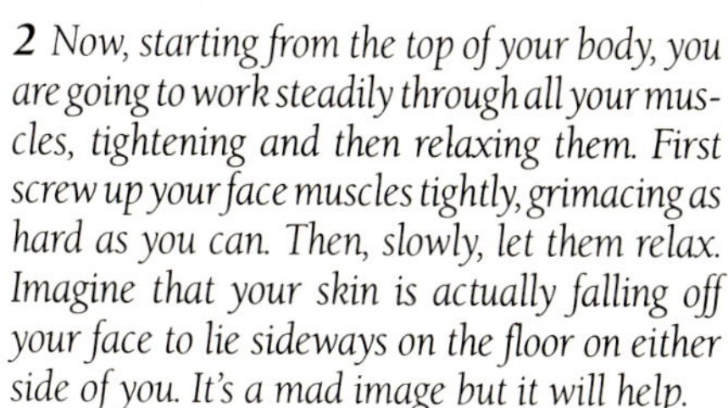

2 Now, starting from the top of your body, you are going to work steadily through all your muscles, tightening and then relaxing them. First screw up your face muscles tightly, grimacing as hard as you can. Then, slowly, let them relax. Imagine that your skin is actually falling off your face to lie sideways on the floor on either side of you. It's a mad image but it will help.

3 Next, lift up your head and pull it forwards as far as you can. Then let it fall back gently and allow your jaw and neck to relax so that you can feel your throat and your mouth opening.

4 Still continuing downwards, press your shoulders down hard onto the floor as though you were trying to push through the floor. Then, slowly relax them.

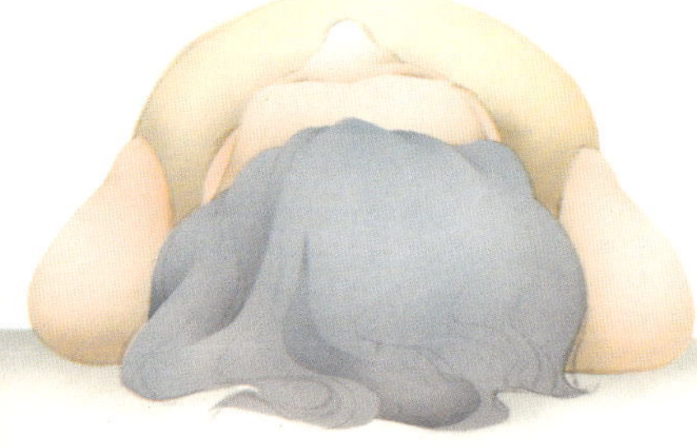

5 Open your fingers wide, stretch your arms out to your side and hold them as tight and hard as you can. Then, very slowly and steadily, let them go. Now try and imagine now that you are flying, that air is coming up under your arms and lifting you.

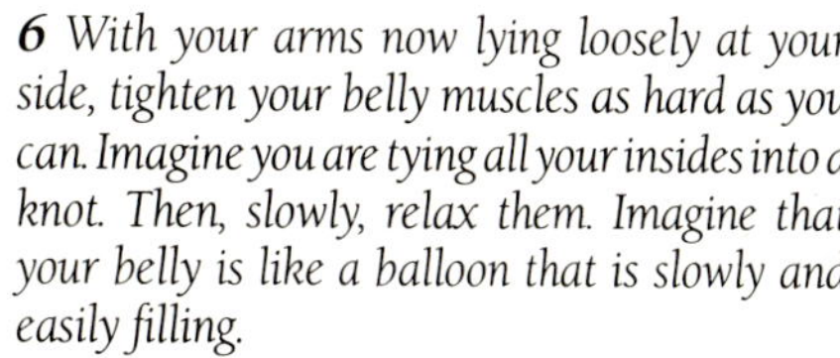

6 With your arms now lying loosely at your side, tighten your belly muscles as hard as you can. Imagine you are tying all your insides into a knot. Then, slowly, relax them. Imagine that your belly is like a balloon that is slowly and easily filling.

7 Now lift your buttocks, tightening them as they go and then gently let them fall back on the floor, stretching your spine as you do so. Relax the buttock and spine muscles, thinking consciously of the areas you are working on.

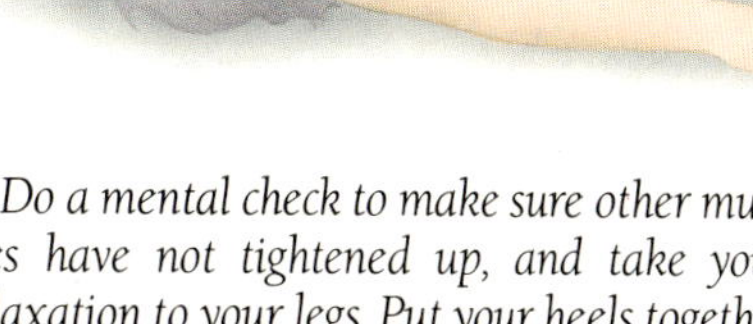

8 Do a mental check to make sure other muscles have not tightened up, and take your relaxation to your legs. Put your heels together and stretch your legs and toes as far as you can. Imagine you are trying to make your legs two inches longer. Then, slowly relax them.

9 Now, another mental check that every part of you is relaxed and floating, mouth, throat, eyelids, belly — all of you should be totally relaxed.

10 Turn on your side and lie that way for another two or three minutes with your eyes open. Sit up slowly and sit with your arms round your knees for a few seconds.

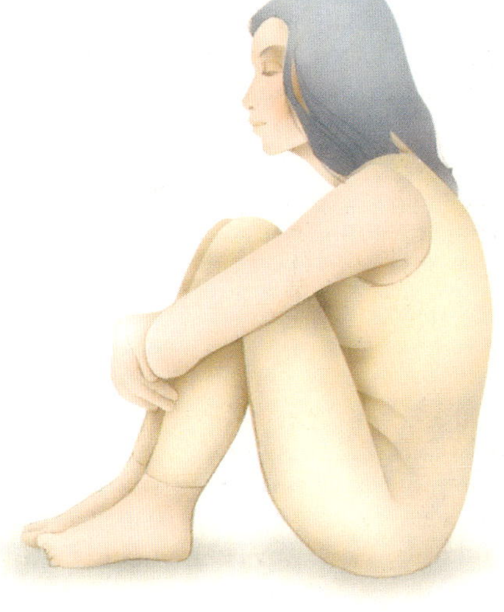

11 If you have time, repeat the whole series from the beginning. If not, lie still and fully relaxed, either imagining that your whole body is sinking through the floor because it is so heavily relaxed, or that it's so light that it's floating through the ceiling. Use whichever simile you find easiest to cope with.

will in the early twenty-first century be many doctors who will be making very comfortable livings treating the old people who did permanent damage to themselves by 'going for the burn' in the seventies and eighties of the twentieth century.

This is not to say that exercise is not good. It is. It does indeed make people feel good, and used sensibly can help the tense person to relax, because as well as releasing endorphins, exercise burns up the excess adrenalin and related stress hormones which are released when we face danger, and which create a sense of anxiety. Exercise also keeps muscles working as they should, ensures brisk circulation, heart and lung action and rids the body of excess calories that could turn into useless fat. But it must be used sensibly and steadily, not obsessively. It's a bit like the question of dieting; no one needs to spend hours pushing themselves through exercise regimes just because they thing it is expected of them, and certainly not to get an artificial 'high'. It is the sensible steady exercise that is best, just as it is the sensible steady eating patterns that are best.

Special muscle exercises

One set of muscles that are all too rarely exercised and which are particularly important for a woman are those of the pelvic floor. These are the muscles that maintain the reproductive organs — the uterus, tubes and ovaries — in precisely the position they should be, and also ensure that the rectum and bladder are supported and functioning as they should be.

Unlike other muscles in the body, these cannot be exercised by means of the general regimes already dealt with here — not even by swimming which exercises most of the body's muscles. These need direct exercise designed specifically for that purpose.

The one that needs the most exercise and attention is the *pubococcygeus* which is a sort of hammock attached to the sides and back of the pelvis and has a great many important functions. If the muscle is weak or sagging there can be stress incontinence (see Section eight), prolapse, sometimes bedwetting, occasionally menstrual distress and also difficulties during childbirth. There may also be some difficulty in sexual function since it is this muscle which grasps the penis (see Section five).

There are ways of checking whether your puboccocygeal muscle is in good tone. When you go to pee, try standing astride the loo and start to pee, and then try to stop the flow completely. This will be difficult to do if you are urgently needing to empty your bladder or if it's first thing in the morning, but if your muscle is in reasonable health it shouldn't be too difficult at other times of the day. If you can stop the flow several times, then the muscle is in excellent condition. If you can't stop it even once, then you do need exercises.

You can use this technique to check on the progress of your fitness as you do the exercises. To check on the strength of your pelvic floor muscles, sit on the floor, legs outstretched and consciously contract the muscles of the pelvic floor. Imagine you are trying to hold back when you are peeing, or that you are trying to prevent your bowels from emptying. Only contract the pelvic floor; try not to contract your back or your belly muscles. Tighten the muscles as hard as you can and hold on while you count to ten slowly. Then relax and immediately tighten again as strongly as you can while you once again hold.

If you can maintain the tightness of the hold to the end of the count of ten on both occasions, then your pelvic floor muscles are reasonably strong. If you feel the tightness ebbing away and you can't control it, then you need the exercises.

Another way to check the power of your pelvic floor muscles is to sit in the same position, regularly contract the muscle and let it go, holding each contraction for about one second. See how many of these contractions you can do before you become too tired to continue, or the muscle simply doesn't respond to your attempts to tighten it. If you can do one hundred your pelvic floor muscles are in excellent condition. If you can only do fifty or less, then you need the exercises.

Pelvic floor exercises

1 *This exercise can be performed in any position — whether you are lying, standing or sitting. It is one that you can do at any time of the day and wherever you are. It's quite useful at bus-stops, while waiting to pay your bill at the supermarket check-out, and while standing talking to people at the office.*

Contract your pelvic floor muscles tightly, as though you need to pee and you've got to stop it. Very, very slowly let it go and again tighten up tightly. Repeat this as frequently as you can, counting at the back of your mind, 'One, tight and (let go) two, tight and (let go)' and so on. It can be quite fun to time yourself. See how many times you can do this in a minute. To start with you may find that you can't do many, but with practice you should be able to do up to two hundred or more during the day. You should do a minimum of twenty contractions each time you do this exercise, but better still, try to do fifty.

2 *This is exactly the same as the previous exercise except that it is done very, very slowly. You contract the pelvic floor muscles as tightly as you can but as slowly as you can, and then hold the contraction while you count to ten slowly (one-and-two-and-three-and-) and relax at the same slow rate.*

Once again, compete with yourself, not to see how quickly you can do it of course, but to see how many you can do in the course of a day. Remember always to concentrate solely and wholly on your pelvic floor muscles; it is all too easy to tighten your belly muscles at the same time and this is not the right way to do it.

3 *Kneel on the floor, sitting on your heels with your toes stretched out behind you, and your hands on your knees. Slowly bend your back and droop your head so that your chin is as close to your chest as you can get it.*

Breathe in deeply and breathe out deeply while you pull your entire belly inwards and upwards. Try and imagine the pull of the muscles starting at the inner side of your thighs, so that you are lifting everything that you can move between your knees and your rib cage.

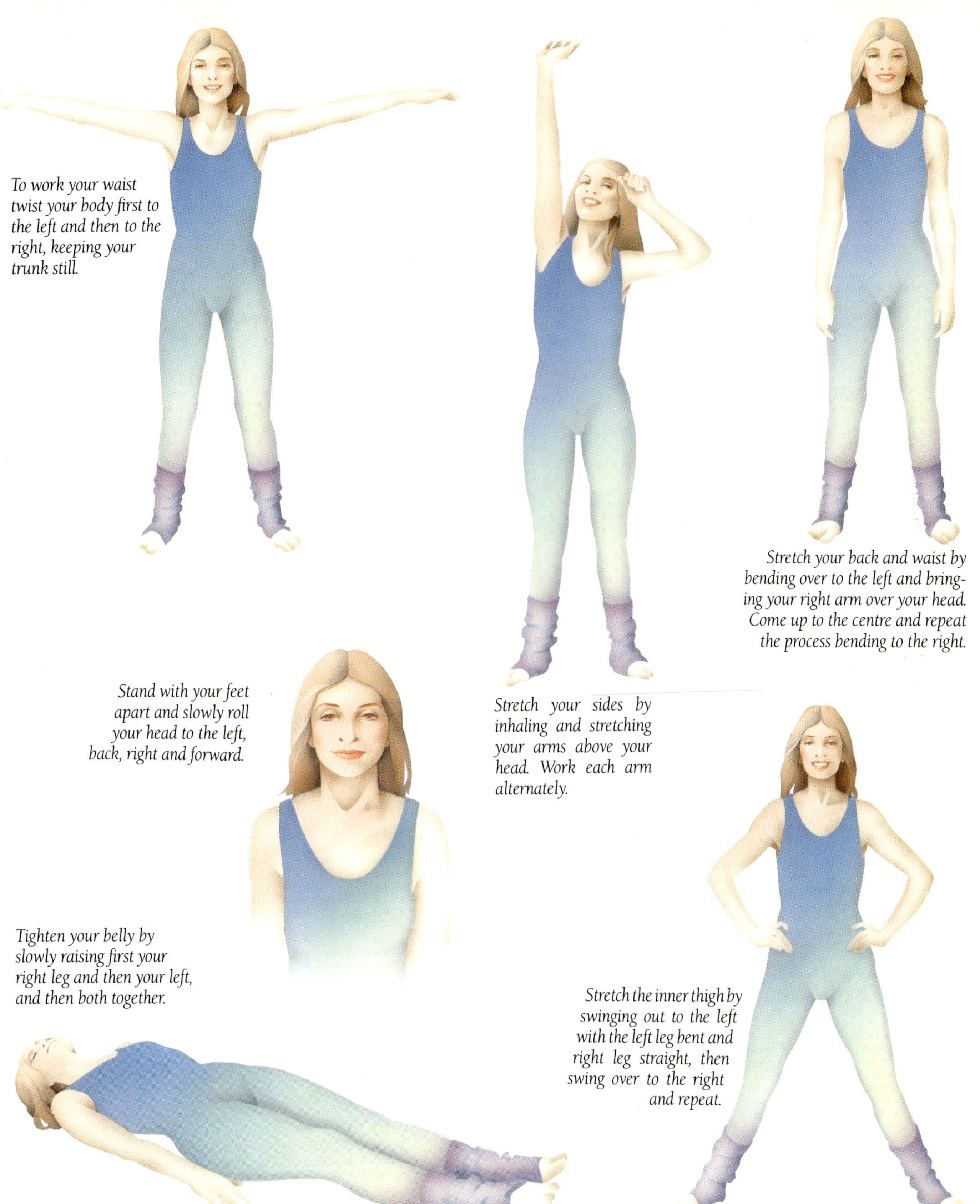

To work your waist twist your body first to the left and then to the right, keeping your trunk still.

Stretch your back and waist by bending over to the left and bringing your right arm over your head. Come up to the centre and repeat the process bending to the right.

Stand with your feet apart and slowly roll your head to the left, back, right and forward.

Stretch your sides by inhaling and stretching your arms above your head. Work each arm alternately.

Tighten your belly by slowly raising first your right leg and then your left, and then both together.

Stretch the inner thigh by swinging out to the left with the left leg bent and right leg straight, then swing over to the right and repeat.

Simultaneously with the contraction of your belly muscles, tilt your pelvis. That is, tuck your buttock muscles inwards and downwards. Try imagining that your pelvis is filled with liquid and what you are trying to do is empty some out behind you.

4 This is a much more difficult exercise which demands a good deal of concentration and imagination.

Try to think of your vagina as having distinct areas. The opening on the surface of the body; the lower section of the vagina itself; then the middle part of the vagina and finally, the upper part. It's as though you've divided your vaginal canal into four separate areas.

Next, keep your mind on the surface, that is the opening of the vagina, and try to imagine yourself tightening that bit and only that bit. Contract the muscle while you count two, and hold on.

Now, still holding that contraction, imagine you are spreading the tightening to the next segment of the vagina — the lower third. Once again tighten that area while still holding the surface tightness and count to two.

Now do exactly the same for the next two segments of the vagina so that you slowly and steadily have tightened all the muscles from the surface to the top.

Now try relaxing those contractions in reverse order from top to bottom.

Do not hold your breath at any point but just breathe normally throughout.

This is not an easy one to do; it takes a great deal of imagination (and it might be easier if you close your eyes while you are doing it) but if you persist with it, doing it up to three to five times a day, you will find that gradually you do gain more and more control over this set of muscles.

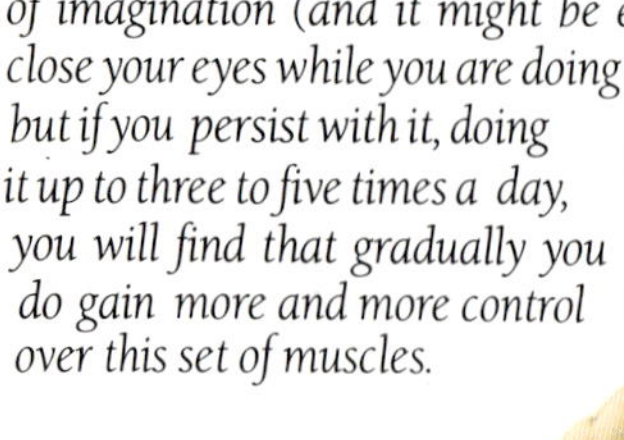

5 Sit on the floor with your knees bent. Put a soft ball or small cushion between your knees and tighten your muscles just enough to hold it there. With your hands on the top of your knees, lean back as far as you can as though you are rowing in a boat. If you find it difficult to hold your balance then put your hands on the floor instead of on your knees, though it would be better if you can practise holding on to your knees.

Now, bend your back so that your chin goes towards your chest while you hold the ball tightly between your knees, while at the same time you bring your inner thighs as close together as you possibly can. Now, while you are squeezing as tightly as you can with your knees and inner thighs, tighten the pelvic floor muscles in the way you did for the previous exercise.

Still holding on to this position and holding on to the tightness of all the pelvic floor muscles, tighten your belly muscles from the bottom upwards. You will feel very, very tight indeed, but hold on while you slowly count to ten and then very slowly release each set of muscles in the reverse order.

Once again this is an extremely difficult exercise to do, but if you practise it you will become very effective and you will improve the tone not only of your pelvic floor, but also of your belly muscles.

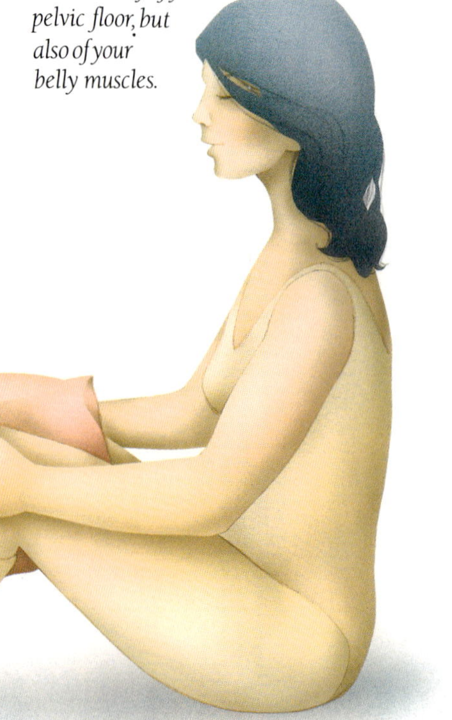

Relaxation

This ought to be the easiest thing in the world to do — just being inactive, and letting your muscles flop. In fact it is an extremely difficult thing for some people to manage and they spend most of their time in a state of high tension. Even when they lie down in bed to sleep, their faces are tight in a grimace, their shoulders are hunched and their fingers clenched.

The exercises shown earlier are designed to help you learn how a tight muscle feels, and how a really relaxed one feels, so that you can be aware of tension and deal with it before it builds up. But for many people, a much deeper form of relaxation is needed. It may be that they are over-tired; extreme fatigue can make muscles even tighter and therefore more weary. Or, it could be that some people are dealing all the time with low level anxiety, and it is this that makes relaxation seem impossible.

In many ways anxiety is the most disagreeable illness to plague modern people. Yes, you can die of cancer or AIDS or heart disease — but you can feel unutterably awful all the time if you're constantly anxious, and for many people this is the way they always are.

They spend all their lives in a state of heightened awareness, constantly fearing some nameless evil is about to befall them, constantly worrying to no purpose, (worry is useful when it leads to action that gets rid of the cause of the worry; when it can't it's pointless worry and falls into the category of Very Bad Habit;) constantly battling with all the unpleasant physical symptoms of trembling, nausea and diarrhoea, assorted vague aches and pains, breathlessness, and all the rest of the dreary litany.

Relaxation techniques

The answer to this problem seems to be in some very ancient techniques, and certainly not in the use of tranquillizing drugs (see page 148). There are however ways of teaching yourself to damp down the overproduction of adrenalin that causes the anxiety symptoms, and some of them have been used for hundreds of years in the East.

Yoga and meditation and hypnosis are methods an individual can use to change the way the conscious mind works, and with it the way the body behaves. We still know remarkably little about the way the mind operates, how consciousness is created and what is going on below the conscious level. All sorts of studies have been made yet the brain remains a largely uncharted country. But we do know that it is possible to reduce tension considerably by delving beneath what could be termed the upper level of awareness.

This does not mean to say that people practising these techniques lose consciousness or self control; they certainly do not. They remain always fully aware of themselves and it is totally untrue that any person can be made to act in a way that is foreign to their natures by means of a suggestion put in their minds under meditation or hypnosis. They can be encouraged to perform actions, but they must always be able to find a logic in the action.

For example, stage hypnotists in the past (nowadays they are banned in most sensible countries, because they can do harm due to their lack of real understanding of what they are doing) would suggest to a subject who had been put into an hypnotic state that, after being brought out of it he would take off his shoes and socks. He would not remember the instructions when he 'came round', but he would suddenly cry out that his feet were burning, or that some insects had got into his socks, and tear them off. He had done as he was told, but in a way that made sense to him. But he could not be told to kill anyone, to steal, or do anything else that was repugnant to him. It is important that this be fully understood, for many people resist the idea of hypnotism as a tool they can use to help them relax because they have these fears.

Generally speaking, the methods of yoga and transcendental meditation and hypnotism have to be learned from a reliable person. Self-teaching is not really effective, though it is indeed possible, once you have learned, to maintain the technique for yourself afterwards. To find the best teachers, choose always those who belong to recognized and respected organizations, see page 160 for useful addresses.

When it comes to hypnotism, there are many trained therapists who are also medically qualified, and generally speaking, these are the safest practitioners to use. There are some who are able to induce hypnotism but lack sufficient knowledge of medicine to treat symptoms safely, though they may be reasonable for teaching relaxation, and helping with the removal of entrenched habits like smoking or overeating. For more information about medical hypnotists see the addresses listed on page 159.

Acupuncture can be an effective therapy for some people who lack the ability to relax, and who have aches and pains of various kinds as a result. This ancient system, which involves putting fine needles into various points of the body, used to be said to act by harmonizing the two forces Yin and Yang — masculine and feminine. This is a rather mystical explanation which means little to rational thinkers, who tend to think that acupuncture works by releasing endorphins. Whatever the system does, it seems a harmless technique which might be useful, and can certainly do no harm.

And that should be the key to choosing any other sort of therapy, whether it be orthodox medicine, or one of the so-called alternative or complementary ones. If you always discuss, in as much depth as possible, what a therapist does and what he plans to do with, for and to you, you should be able to make a judgement between the possible benefit you are being offered and the possible risks. There can never be a totally risk-free treatment for any of our diseases, just as there can never be risk-free living. We're aiming at death from the moment we are conceived, and that means we take risks. But we can make the risks less risky if we apply a little common sense to our self-care.

So much happens to and in a woman's body in one lifetime that it is impossible to describe all of it in one book. And I haven't tried to do so in these pages. All I've attempted to offer is a simple account of some of the marvellous things that are you — as well as some of the tiresome things that are you. No one would pretend that thrush or painful periods should be described as 'marvellous'. But I hope all of it has been interesting, and given you what every woman is entitled to have; an understanding of and a deep pride and delight in her own femininity. To be a woman is a special privilege, in addition to the basic one of being a human. Our bodies, whatever they may look like and whatever condition they happen to be in at any particular time, are superbly engineered and functional. To be able to use and enjoy them to their full potential we need all the information we can get. That is why this book was written. To give you the information you need to make all your decades as good as the ones I've experienced — and I'm now enjoying my fifties with as much, if not more, pleasure than I found in my twenties. I hope this book helps you to enjoy your womanhood as much as I am enjoying mine.

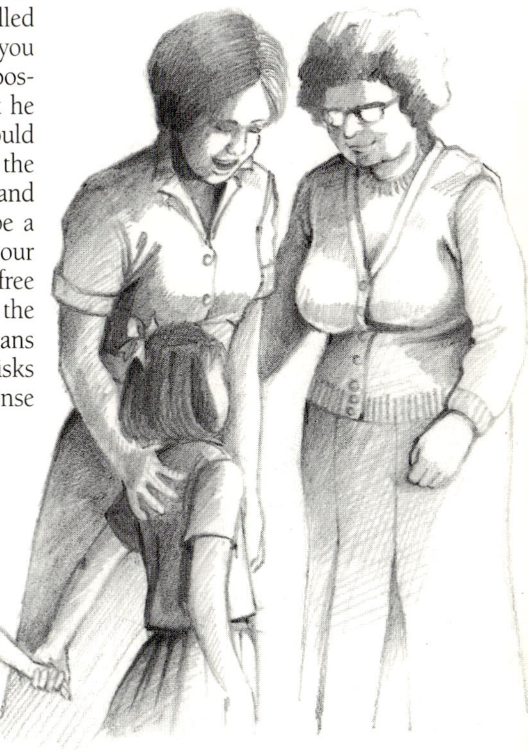

AIDS

Terrence Higgins Trust
BM AIDS Charity
London WC1N 3XX
(01 278 8745)

Department A
PO Box 100
Milton Keynes MK1 1TX
(01 981 2717)
(01 980 7222)
(0345 581151)

Alcohol addiction

Alcoholics Anonymous
PO Box 514
11 Redcliffe Gardens
London SW10

26 Essex Quay
Dublin 8

Al-Anon (for families)
Family Groups UK and Eire
61 Great Dover Street
London SE1 4YF

Accept Clinic
200 Seagrave Road
London SW6 1RG

National Council on Alcoholism
3 Grosvenor Crescent
London SW1

16 College Street
Belfast
BT1 6BX

147 Blythwood Street
Glasgow G24 EN
(041 333 9677)

Allergies

Action against Allergy
43 The Downs
Merton
London SW20 8HG

National Society for Research into Allergy
PO Box 45
Hinckley
Leicestershire

Anorexia

Anorexic Family Aid Information Centre
Sackville Place
44 Magdalene Street
Norwich NR3 1JE

The Priory Centre
11 Priory Road
High Wycombe
Bucks

Women's Therapy Centre
6 Manor Gardens
London N7

Battered wives

National Women's Aid
52-54 Featherstone Street
London EC1

143A University Street
Belfast 7

11 Colmen Street
Edinburgh

Welsh Women's Aid
Incentive House
Adam Street
Cardiff

Victims of Domestic Violence
Lifeline
℅ Mrs Turner
Glenleedle
Salen Aros
Isle of Mull
Argyll PA72 6JJ

Bereavement

London Bereavement Project
℅ The Magistrates' Association
28 Fitzroy Square
London W1

Compassionate Friends
(for parents whose children have died)
6 Denmark Street
Bristol BS1 5DQ

Cancer

Association for New Approaches to Cancer
231 Kensal Road
London W10 5DB

BACUP
(British Association of Cancer United Patients)
121-123 Charterhouse Street
London EC1

Cancer Aftercare and Rehabilitation
Lodge Cottage
Church Lane
Tinsbury
Bath BA3 1LF

Cancer Link
46A Pentonville Road
London NW1

Marie Curie Memorial Foundation
28 Belgrave Square
London SW1

National Society for Cancer Relief
Michael Sobell House
30 Dorset Square
London NW1 6QL

Women's National Cancer Control Campaign
1 South Audley Street
London W1Y 5DQ

Caring for others

Age Concern
Bernard Sunley House
60 Pitcairn Road
Mitcham
Surrey

Asian Women's Resource Centre
134 Minet Avenue
London NW10

Association of Carers
Medway Homes
Balfour Road
Rochester
Kent ME4 6QU

National Council for Carers and their Elderly Dependants
29 Chilworth Mews
City of Westminster
London W2 3RG

Chest, Heart and Stroke

Tavistock House North
Tavistock Square
London WC1

Childlessness

Child
367 Wandsworth Road
London SW8 2GJ

Artificial Insemination by Donor/Husband
Austy Manor
Wootton Wawen
Wolihull
West Midlands B95 6BX

NAC (National Association for the Childless)
318 Summer Lane
Birmingham B19 3RL

Contraception

BPAS (British Pregnancy Advisory Service)
Austy Manor
Wootton Wawen
Solihull B95 6DA

Brook Advisory Centre (full service for those under 26)
233 Tottenham Court Road
London W1P 9AE

FPA (Family Planning Association)
27-35 Mortimer Street
City of Westminster
London W1 7RJ

International Contraception, Abortion and Sterilization Campaign
374 Gray's Inn Road
London WC1X 8BB

International Planned Parenthood Federation (full information service across countries and religions)
18-20 Lower Regent Street
London SW1

Life (for those *not* wanting abortion)
7 Parade
Leamington Spa
Warwickshire

Lifeline UK (Pregnancy care service for those *not* wanting abortion)
15 Kensington High Street
London W8

Marie Stopes House
108 Whitfield Street
London W1

Dublin Well Woman Centre
63 Lower Leeson Street
Dublin

Irish FPA
5 Cathal Brugher Street
Dublin 1

FPA
47 Botanic Avenue
Belfast BT7 1JL

FPA
4 Clifton Street
Glasgow GF3 7LA

FPA 6 Windsor Place
Cardiff

Diabetes

British Diabetic Association
10 Queen Anne Street
London W1M 0BD

Drug addiction

Adfam (for addicts and family)
Box 219
Harrow
Middlesex HA1 3HA

Families Anonymous (UK)
88 Caledonian Road
London N1 9DN

Narcotics Anonymous
PO Box 246
London SW10

Release
1 Elgin Avenue
London W9 (Has leaflet Trouble with Tranquillisers (40p) and list of self-help groups)

Standing Conference of Drug Abuse
1-4 Hatton Place
Hatton Gardens
London EC1N 8ND

Turning Point
9-12 Long Lane
London EC1A 9HA

Endometriosis

Endometriosis Association
℅ 65 Holmdene Avenue
Herne Hill
London SE24 9LD

Herpes

Herpes Association
41 North Road
London N7

Homosexuality

Albany Trust
24 Chester Square
London SW1 (Counselling organization)

Campaign for Homosexual Equality
274 Upper Street
London N1 2UA

Friend
BM National Friend
London WC1N 3XX (List of local groups)

Lesbian & Gay Youth Movement
LGYM BM/GYM
London WC1N 3XX

Parents Enquiry
16 Honley Road
Catford
London SE6 2HZ

Hypnosis

British Society of Medical and Dental Hypnotists
42 Links Road
Ashstead
Surrey

Hysterectomy

Hysterectomy Support Groups
11 Henryson Road
Brockley
Lewisham
London SE4 1HL

Incest *see also* Rape

Incest Crisis Line
Shirley Edwards
66 Marriott Close
Bedfont
Feltham
Middlesex TW14 9PZ
(01 890 4732)

Richard Johnson
33 Newbury Close
Northolt
Middlesex
(01 422 5100)

Marriage Guidance

Catholic Marriage Advisory Council
15 Lansdowne Road
London W11 3AJ

Jewish Marriage Education Council
23 Ravenshurst Avenue
London NW4 4EL

National Marriage Guidance Council
Little Church Street
Rugby
Warwickshire

Association of Sexual and Marital Therapists
Box 62
Sheffield S10 3TS (will send details of counsellers in any area — send sae)

Catholic Marriage Advisory Council
35 Harcourt Street
Dublin 2

Marriage Counselling Service
24 Grafton Street
Dublin 2

Northern Ireland Catholic Marriage Advisory Council
Cana House
Corry Square
Newry
Co. Down BT35 6AW

Northern Ireland Marriage Guidance Council
76 Dublin Road
Belfast BT2 7HP

Scotland Catholic Marriage Advisory Council
18 Park Circus
Glasgow G3 6BE

Scottish Marriage Guidance Council
26 Frederick Street
Edinburgh EH2 2LR

Mastectomy

Mastectomy Association
26 Harrison Street
Kings Cross
London WC1H 8JG

Menstruation

National Association for Pre-Menstrual Syndrome
33 Pilgrim's Way West
Otford
Sevenoaks
Kent

Migraine

British Migraine Association
178A High Road
Byfleet
Weybridge
Surrey

Migraine Trust
45 Great Ormond Street
London WC1N 3AY

Multiple Sclerosis

ARMS
11 Dartmouth Street
London SW1 9BL

Multiple Sclerosis Society
25 Effie Road
London SW6 1EE

Mental Health *see also* Phobias

MENCAP
123 Golden Lane
London EC17 0RT

MIND (National Association for Mental Health)
22 Harley Street
London W1N 2ED

Nutrition

British Nutrition Foundation
15 Belgrave Square
London SW1X 8PS

Silhouette Slimming Clubs Ltd
103 Harlestone Road
Northampton

Slimnastics
11 East Sheen Avenue
London SW14

Vegan Society
47 Highlands Road
Leatherhead
Surrey

Vegetarian Society of UK Ltd
53 Marloes Road
London W8 6LA

Weight Watchers
635-637 Ajax Avenue
Slough
Berkshire

One-Parent Families

National Council for One-Parent Families
255 Kentish Town Road
London NW5 2LX

Scottish Council for Single Parents
13 Gayfield Square
Edinburgh EH1 3NX

Pelvic Inflammatory Disease (PID)

61 Jenner Road
London N16

Phobias

Action on Phobias
17 Burlington Place
Eastbourne
Sussex (send large sae)

Phobics Society
4 Cheltenham Road
Chorlton-cum-Hardy
Manchester M21 1QN

Relaxation for Living
29 Burwood Park Road
Walton on Thames
Surrey KT12 5LH

The Open Door Association
(agoraphobia)
447 Pensby Road
Heswall
Merseyside L61 9PQ

Pregnancy and Childcare

Aims (Association for
Improvements in Maternity
Services)
163 Liverpool Road
London N1 0RF

Association for Post-Natal Illness
7 Gowan Avenue
Fulham
London SW6

Association of Radical Midwives
℅ 8A The Drive
Wimbledon
London SW20

Caesarian Support Link
Sue Johnson
11 Duke Street
Astley
Manchester M29 7BG

Compassionate Friends
6 Denmark Street
Bristol BS1 5DQ

Cry-sis (for parents of crying
babies)
52 Haig Road
Stretford
Manchester
(061 865 4273)

Foresight (Association for the
promotion of pre-conceptual care)
The Old Vicarage
Church Lane
Witley
Godalming
Surrey

Foundation for Study of
Infant Deaths
5th Floor
4 Grosvenor Place
London SW1X 7HD

Gingerbread
(for one-parent families)
35 Wellington Street
London WC2

291 Ormeau Road
Belfast BT7

4a Rawiston Gardens
Edinburgh EH3 3HH

La Leche League of Great Britain
(for breast-feeding mothers)
BM 3424
London WC1V 6XX

Maternity Alliance (Campaign for
Rights of Mothers, Fathers and
Babies)
59-61 Camden High Street
London NW1 7JL

Meet-a-Mum Associations
26A Cumnor Hill
Oxford
OX2 9HA

Miscarriage Association
18 Stoneybrook Close
West Bretton
Wakefield WF4 4TP

NSPCC (National Society for
Prevention of Cruelty to Children)
67 Saffron Hill
London EC1N 8RS

16-20 Rosemary Street
Belfast BT1 1QD

Melville House
41 Polworth Terrace
Edinburgh EH11 1NG

National Association of Ovulation
Method Teachers (for those
interested
in Billings Method)
45 Heathhurst Road
Sanderstead
South Croydon
Surrey

National Childbirth Trust
9 Queensborough Terrace
London W2 3TB

National Childminding Association
204-206 High Street
Bromley
Kent BR1 1PP

OPUS (Organization for Parents
Under Stress)
223 Westgate
Guisborough
Cleveland TS14 6NJ

PETS (Pre-Eclamptic
Toxaemia Society)
33 Keswick Avenue
Hullbridge
Essex SS5 6JL

SANDS (Stillbirth and Neonatal
Death Society)
Argyle House
29-31 Euston Road
London NW1 1SD

Society to Support Home
Confinements
17 Laburnham Avenue
Durham

Rape

Box No 69
London WC1X 9NK
(01 837 1600 — 24 hour service)

PO Box 1027
Dublin 6
Dublin 601470

105 Royal Avenue
Belfast
Belfast BT1 1FF

PO Box 220
Belfast BT7 1RL
Belfast 22 68 03

Restricted growth

Association for Research for
Restricted Growth
8 Herbert Road
Clevedon
Avon BA21 7ND

Rheumatism and Arthritis

Arthritis and Rheumatism Council
41 Eagle Street
London WC1R 4AR

Arthritis Care
6 Grosvenor Crescent
London SW1X 7ER

Smoking

ASH
5-11 Mortimer Street
London W1N 7RH

National Society of Non Smokers
Latimer House
40-48 Hanson Street
London W1P 7DE

Irish Association of Non Smokers
PO Box 1024
Sheriff Street
Dublin 1
Eire

Joint Committee on Smoking
and Health
4 Clyde Road
Dublin 4

Step-parents

National Stepfamily Association
Maris House
Maris Lane
Trumpington
Cambridge CB2 2LB

Transcendental Meditation

Transcendental Meditation Centre
Mentmore Towers
Mentmore
Leighton Buzzard
Bucks

Widows

CRUSE
126 Sheen Road
Richmond
Surrey

National Council for Divorced and
Separated
13 High Street
Little Shelford
Cambridge CB2 5ES

Yoga

British Wheel of Yoga
Grafton Grange
York YO5 9OP

This information was correct at the time of going to press.